Guidebook for Pediatric Hypertension

By

Arno R. Hohn, M.D.

Professor of Pediatrics
University of Southern California
Head, Division of Cardiology
Childrens Hospital Los Angeles
Los Angeles, California
Former Professor of Pediatrics
Medical University of South Carolina
Director, Division of Pediatric Cardiology
Charleston, South Carolina

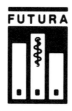

FUTURA

**Futura Publishing
Company, Inc.**
Mount Kisco, NY

Library of Congress Cataloging-in-Publication Data

Hohn, Arno R., 1931-
    Guidebook for pediatric hypertension / Arno R. hohn.
        p.   cm.
    Includes bibliographical references and index.
    1. Hypertension in children.   2. Hypertension in adolescence.
    I. Title.
        [DNLM: 1. Hypertension—in infancy & childhood. 2. Hypertension-
    -in adolescence.   WG 340 H719 1994]
    RJ426.H9H66   1994
618.92'132—dc20
DNLM/DLC
for Library of Congress   93-33059
                                                                           CIP

Copyright © 1994
Futura Publishing Company, Inc.

Published by
Futura Publishing Company, Inc.
2 Bedford Ridge Road
P.O. Box 330
Mount Kisco, New York 10549

L.C. No.: 93-33059
ISBN No.: 0-87993-573-1

Every effort has been made to ensure that the information in this book is as up to date and accurate as possible at the time of publication. However, due to the constant developments in medicine, neither the author, nor the editor, nor the publisher can accept any legal or any other responsibility for any errors or omissions that may occur.

Printed in the United States of America on acid-free paper.

To Mary Elizabeth Hohn, R.N.,
my wife of over 30 years,
whose love, support and encouragement
during all this time led to
the inception and completion of this work.

and

In memory of Mitchell I. Rubin, M.D.
former Professor and Chairman,
Department of Pediatrics,
University of New York at Buffalo and
Professor of Pediatrics,
Medical University of South Carolina
who introduced me to pediatrics,
nurtured my academic career in Buffalo,
and collaborated in my work at MUSC.

Acknowledgments

Credit for this work does not reside entirely with the author. Much of the inspiration and investigative production must be ascribed to collaboration and help from many individuals. I would like to particularly acknowledge the friendship and counsel of Ronald M. Lauer, M.D. during pursuit of a career in pediatric cardiology in general and hypertension, in particular.

For work done at the Medical University of South Carolina (MUSC) I would first like to acknowledge with gratitude my long and productive association in research and practice with Donald A. Riopel, M.D. His energetic approach and insights started the Hypertensive Progeny Study at MUSC. The assistance of the entire MUSC Pediatric Heart Center team, especially Ashby Taylor, M.D., Mr. Charles Kline, and Mrs. Debbie Bryant, allowed the study work to proceed. The critical humoral-substance analyses for the study were performed in the laboratories of Harry S. Margolius, M.D. (kallikrein), Perry V. Halushka, M.D., Ph.D. (urinary prostaglandin), Philip J. Privitera, Ph.D. (plasma renin), and Jerry G. Webb, Ph.D. (norepinephrine). Julian E. Keil, P.H. provided epidemiologic support and C. Boyd Loadholt, Ph.D. biostatistical support for the study. The counsel and guidance of these collaborating investigators is acknowledged with thanks.

Work done at the University of Southern California was largely centered in the Pasadena Study and its outgrowth: the Pasadena Prevention Project. Much of the credit for the project is due to James H. Dwyer, Ph.D. whose biostatistical and epidemiologic insights permitted planning and inception of the project and then guided the data analyses. His collaboration and that of Kathleen M. Dwyer, Ph.D., whose operational skills allowed the project to function, and Richard A. Scribner, M.D., M.P.H., as well as the entire project team developed by Lisa Nicholson, M.S., R.D. is acknowledged with thanks.

I am grateful for the support of colleagues and partners at Childrens Hospital Los Angeles (CHLA): Alan B. Lewis, M.D., Leonard Linde, M.D., Barry Marcus, M.D., Robert E. Stanton, M.D., Masato Takahashi, M.D., and Pierre Wong, M.D. The entire CHLA Heart Center team led by Mrs. Donna Fondren-Lee (administration), Gary Richie, R.T., C.R.T. (invasive laboratory), and Kathryn Sivazlian, R.D.C.S. (noninvasive laboratory), must also be credited for their assistance. Special gratitude is due Mrs. Betty Negri whose incredible patience and secretarial skills allowed the completion of the manuscript after many drafts. Finally, I am indebted to Mr. Steven Korn of the Futura Publishing Company without whom the text would not have been planned and it was his patient understanding that saw it through to completion.

Foreword

This guidebook will be of help to physicians-in-practice, house officers, nurses, and those interested in the well-child management of children whose blood pressure measurements should be part of continuing health care.

In the adult population, high blood pressure has been linked to stroke, renal disease, and coronary heart disease. These diseases are major causes of death and disability of adults throughout the world. The subject of blood pressure and its measurement in the pediatric age group has received considerable attention in the past several years because it is suspected that the origins of adult hypertension begin in childhood. Blood pressure during infancy and childhood is lower than in adults and rises throughout the pediatric age. Thus, the definition of high blood pressure must change throughout infancy, childhood, and adolescence. In this monograph, Dr. Hohn provides a review of the subject of blood pressure, its control, measurement, and a working definition of hypertension in infants, children, and adolescents. He also leads the reader through the causes of overt hypertension in childhood, the orderly workup, and the treatment of children whose blood pressures are elevated. This presentation is an important reference guide for blood pressure measurements in children.

Ronald M. Lauer, MD
Professor of Pediatrics and Preventive Medicine
Director, Division of Pediatric Cardiology
Department of Pediatrics
University of Iowa

Preface

This text, conceived over 10 years ago, has at its roots the purpose of presenting practical information on hypertension in the young. It is a work from two institutions as I first began my studies of hypertension in the Department of Pediatrics at the Medical University of South Carolina (MUSC), then relocated to Childrens Hospital of Los Angeles (CHLA) and the University of Southern California (USC). Both universities are situated in areas with significant minority populations, making them ideal for the student of a "disease" which may affect certain minorities disproportionately.

How does a pediatric cardiologist come to write about hypertension, a physical finding long considered the domain of nephrologists? The answer lies in the unique model of hypertension, coarctation of the aorta. I began studies of the impact of surgical relief of the aortic obstruction in the early '70s. Both physical parameters in terms of blood pressure response, and humoral substance change were investigated. Some of the information gained is presented in Chapter 5. Once acquainted with problems surrounding secondary hypertension, I became aware of the far greater problem of primary hypertension. I then began collaborative studies of the disorder with support from the National Heart Lung and Blood Institute.[1,2] These investigations were and are searches for etiologic clues and possible preventive measures applicable to young people who may be destined to suffer from hypertensive disorders as adults. Insights gained are presented throughout the text.

Why then a single-authored text? As an avowed student of hypertension, be it a finding, disorder, or disease, I wish to offer the reader the benefit of distillations of the problem through a single set of eyes. A practical view is put forward including my synthesized approaches to diagnosis and treatment. At the same time, it is acknowledged that the text, mainly based on my review and distillation of the work of others, is not a meta-analysis of the enormous entire hypertension literature. As much as possible, current works are cited, but it must be recognized that new information on the subject is constantly accumulating.

While secondary hypertension or that of known cause first comes to mind when a child is found hypertensive in a health-care program, it is my finding that primary hypertension or that without known cause is more common even in childhood. Despite the fact that individuals in young age groups with predisposition for or actual findings of primary hypertension are largely asymptomatic, the disorder has been labeled the "silent killer" for good reason. Hypertension affects nearly one in five of our population and is a leading cause of death in older age groups both by itself and by contributing to atherosclerotic processes. Because it is my belief that the stage for these unhappy events is set in young people, a major focus of this book is on primary or essential hypertension.

The plan of this "coast to coast" bi-institutional text is first a review of blood pressure regulation and pathophysiologic processes affecting it. Attention is then directed to blood pressure measurement which may not be so simple. Etiologic and risk considerations for hypertension are followed by review of diagnosis and treatment of hypertension of known cause in chapters on cardiovascular, renal, endocrine, and neonatal hypertension. Next, an extensive scheme for the diagnosis of hypertension is presented, including a thorough self-history form. The chapter on management, initially by preventive measures then by an individualized stepped approach with an emphasis on nonpharmacologic means, completes the text.

References:

1. Work at MUSC supported by Grants HL 19870 and HL 17705 from the National Institutes of Health.
2. Work at USC supported by Grant RO1-HL 42932-O1A1 from the National Heart, Lung and Blood Institute.

Contents

Foreword—*Ronald M. Lauer, MD* .... *vi*
Preface .... *vii*

Chapter 1. **Blood Pressure Regulation** **1**
          Hemodynamic Principles 2
          Renal Architecture 4
          Blood Pressure Control 6

Chapter 2. **Blood Pressure Measurements and**
          Normal Pressure Values **37**
          Techniques of Blood Pressure Recording 38
          Normal Blood Pressure 46

Chapter 3. **The Epidemiology of Hypertension**
          in Young People **53**
          Prevalence 54
          Age 55
          Racial Considerations 58
          Obesity 60
          Dietary Influence 61

Chapter 4. **Risk Factors in the Young for Adult**
          Onset Hypertension **75**
          Blood Pressure 76
          Heredity 77
          Obesity 79
          Race 80
          Dietary Cations 82
          Exercise, Stress, and Anxiety 85
          Smoking 87
          Alcohol, Medication, Drugs 89
          Maternal and Newborn Factors 91
          Diabetes Mellitus 93
          Uric Acid 93
          Left Ventricular Hypertrophy 94

Chapter 5. **Cardiac Hypertension** **105**
          Coarctation, Embryology, and Anatomy 106
          Pathophysiology 107
          Clinical Patterns 109
          Protocol for Diagnosis 111
          Treatment 112

Postcoarctation Repair Syndromes 116
Persistent Postoperative Hypertension......................... 119
Abdominal Coarctation.. 121

Chapter 6. **Renal Hypertension**... **127**
Investigation for Renal Forms of
Hypertension 128
Specific Renal Parenchymal Disorders
Causing Hypertension.. 132
Glomerular Diseases... 137
Renovascular Hypertension... 142

Chapter 7. **Hypertension Caused by Endocrine**
Disorders **159**
Adrenal Cortical Coditions 159
Mineralocorticoid Disorders 161
Glucocortoid Disorders 165
Pheochromocytoma 171
Hyperthyroid and Hyperparathyroid
Conditions... 177
Diabetes Mellitus 178

Chapter 8. **Hypertension in the Newborn** **185**
Blood Pressure Measurement... 185
Factors Influencing Blood Pressure in
Neonates.. 187
"Normal" Blood Pressure Values 189
Causes of Hypertension in the Newborn...................... 189
Findings-Diagnosis in Hypertensive Newborn
Infants 199
Treatment of Hypertension Found in
Newborns 201

Chapter 9. **Clinical Features and Evaluation**
for Hypertension in the Young................... **209**
Clinical Features 210
Evaluation 214

Chapter 10. **Treatment of Pediatric Hypertension** **233**
Prevention (A Hope)... 234
Making the Diagnosis 236
Workup and Need for Treatment 237
Nonpharmacologic Treatment of Hypertension 239
Specific Treatments for Curable Forms of
Hypertension 249

Appendix **279**
Index... **281**

Chapter 1

Blood Pressure Regulation

Introduction

The force generated by the arterial circulation has been recorded at least since medieval times. Indeed, medieval artists painted arterial blood spurting from victims of violence,[1] and, in 1628, the great William Harvey wrote about the force of arterial flow from a severed artery.[2] However, the first actual measurements of arterial pressure were not made until about 1730 by Stephen Hales, minister at Teddington in England. He recorded direct measurements of arterial pressure in a horse and published an account of his work in an extraordinary book: *Statical Essays: Volume 2, Containing Haemastaticks....*[3] With the development of the mercury manometer for indirect blood pressure measurements by Poiseuille and his equation summarizing the quantities concerned with the pressure measurement in 1846,[4] the basis of thinking about high and low pressure was established.

Recognition that various disease states caused hypertension began with Richard Bright's observation in 1827 relating myocardial hypertrophy with "albuminous urine."[5] Later, in 1872, William Gull extended Bright's observations to include widespread alteration in small arteries.[6] Subsequent observations led to the conclusion that two types of high blood pressure existed. The first was related to specific disease processes, such as Bright's disease, and was termed secondary. In the other, no known cause for the hypertension could be found. It was named primary hypertension. With the finding that hypertension was often synonymous with a shortened life span,

1

questions were raised concerning the mechanisms of hypertension in the secondary form and the nature of the primary type of hypertension. The search for answers has led to an enormous research and clinical effort. The results are being synthesized so that some understanding of the pathophysiology of the disorder is available. This text will begin with a review of our current knowledge of these processes. References are made available to the reader to expand the information presented and include those deemed most pertinent, as well as summary articles.

Hemodynamic Principles

At the onset, certain hemodynamic principles must be understood when hypertension is being considered. It is appropriate to begin with Poiseuille's equation.[4] This originally related fluid flow (q) directly to the pressure difference (dP) from one end of a tube to the other and to the fourth power of the radius of the tube (r^4) times a constant ($\pi / 8$) and indirectly to the length of the tube (l) and to the fluid's viscosity (v). Thus, equation 1:

$$q = \frac{\pi \, dPr^4}{8lv} \qquad\qquad 1.$$

A second and most important hemodynamic equation is derived from Ohm's law in physics: voltage (pressure) equals current (flow) times resistance (r). Transposed to fluid flow and rearranged, the equation states that resistance to blood flow equals mean blood pressure fall (drop in pressure across the circulation from aorta to right atrium) divided by blood flow (cardiac output). Thus, equation 2:

$$rS = \frac{dP}{qS} \qquad\qquad 2.$$

(where rS = total systemic resistance, qS = cardiac output, and dP = mean pressure drop from aorta to right atrium. Since right atrial pressure is low, it is generally neglected and dP is taken to indicate mean arterial pressure, therefore dP = 1/3 (systolic pressure – diastolic pressure) + diastolic pressure.)

It can be readily appreciated that the total systemic resistance can be calculated from measured blood pressure and cardiac output as determined by echocardiography or any one of a number of other means. Cardiac outputs, by age and race, determined from echocardiographic data at the Medical University of South Carolina (MUSC) are listed in Table 1. Neither age nor race differences were seen in the young people surveyed. While it can be seen that an assumed value could be used to estimate the cardiac output/meter squared, and while this would allow an estimate of resistance from the measured blood pressure, this value is not clinically useful. For, as will be noted in the discussion of primary hypertension, knowledge of cardiac output is important when assessing hypertension.

A third set of equations can be derived from the first two by substitution. Thus, equation 3:

$$rS = \frac{\dfrac{dP}{\pi\, dPr^4}}{8lv} \qquad\qquad 3.$$

(substitution of the "q" equivalent from equation 1 into equation 2) or, simplified:

$$rS = \frac{8\, l\, v}{\pi\, r^4} \qquad\qquad 3a.$$

This equation relates peripheral systemic vascular resistance directly to vessel length and demonstrates the often overlooked fact that viscosity plays a direct role in peripheral resistance.[7] It also reveals how important vessel lumen size is in resistance to blood flow. That is, with vessel narrowing or hypoplasia, systemic vascular resistance increases dramatically because the fourth power of the

Table 1.
Cardiac Output (L/min per m²)
Determined Echocardiographically by Age and Race

Age (y)	Blacks			Whites		
	(N)	Mean	SD	(N)	Mean	SD
10–12	(23)	4.36 ±	2.70	(34)	3.36 ±	0.36
12+–14	(19)	3.85 ±	0.98	(26)	4.02 ±	1.20
14+–16	(27)	4.36 ±	1.50	(21)	4.10 ±	0.93
16+–18	(19)	4.36 ±	1.70	(15)	4.36 ±	2.30
18+	(5)	4.36 ±	1.10	(6)	4.36 ±	1.30

(A.H., unpublished MUSC data, 1982).

radius makes the denominator much smaller. Hence, the value for the resistance becomes much larger.

Despite the importance of the foregoing hemodynamic considerations, homeostatic mechanisms play the decisive role in blood pressure regulation. It is generally agreed that the kidney is the major organ involved in such regulation. The remainder of this chapter will be concerned with renal and other pressure regulatory mechanisms.

Renal Architecture

A brief review of renal architecture follows. Basically, the kidney is divided into a cortical and medullary portion. (Fig. 1A). The cortical portion is composed mainly of nephrons and the medullary portion is made up of the collecting system which ultimately drains urine via the renal pelvis and ureter into the bladder. The nephron includes both the renal corpuscle and its collecting tubules (Fig. 1B).[8]

The renal corpuscle is concerned with the filtration of the blood and is composed of the glomerulus, which is a group of capillary loops leading from the afferent to the efferent arterioles, and of the surrounding Bowman's capsule, the blind end of the proximal uriniferous tubule (Fig. 1C). Of some importance is the enlargement of cells of the afferent arteriole near its entrance into the glomerulus, called the juxtaglomerular cells. These cells are thought to be the site of renin production of which will be addressed in more detail.[9] It is held that renin release may be stimulated by activity in the macula densa. Enlarged cells of the distal convoluted tubule which has wound its way back to the area of the juxtaglomerular cells comprise the macula densa. Together, the macula densa and juxtaglomerular cells are called the juxtaglomerular apparatus (Fig. 1D).[10]

The urinary tubules of a nephron are divided into the proximal convoluted tubule, loop of Henle, and distal convoluted loop. These segments play vital roles in reabsorption of water and electrolytes from the glomerular filtrate. The long-term regulation of blood pressure, as we shall see, depends upon their function.

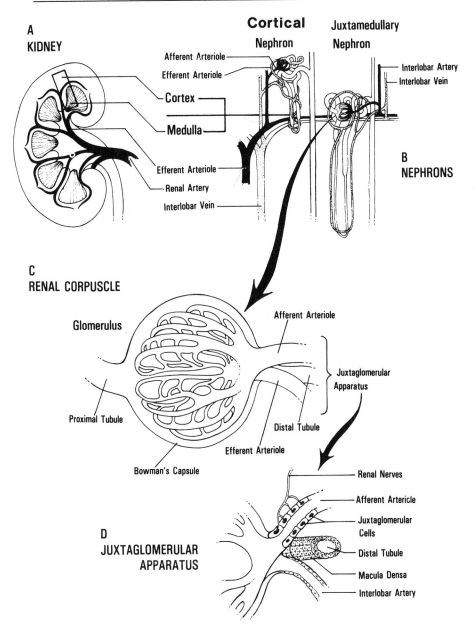

Figure 1: Renal architecture from gross anatomy (A) to microscopic depiction of juxtaglomerular apparatus (D). Illustrations by Betty Goodwin at MUSC.

Blood Pressure Control

Present concepts of hypertension are based on existing understanding of blood pressure control. Mechanisms of blood pressure homeostasis may be categorized as those which influence immediate responses and those which regulate long-term control. The *immediate mechanisms* of blood pressure control affect the changes necessary for moment-to-moment or hour-to-hour and longer control. These control systems have sensors and afferent or input loops which transmit signals of change (error) in blood pressure, and feedback (efferent) loops to effector mechanisms for responses aimed at correcting the perceived error. Superimposed on the systems are controls from higher central nervous system centers. The sum of these mechanisms is to preserve the flow of blood to the various tissues of the body in accordance with the needs of each tissue, and to preserve the required blood pressure to insure that needed flow.[11]

Immediate Blood Pressure Control Mechanisms

Nervous System Mechanisms

Initial regulatory mechanisms run the gamut from those which act within seconds to those which require minutes, hours, or even days to act. In the scheme of *immediate* responses to change or error in blood pressure, the nervous system mechanisms for pressure control result in the most rapid circulatory adjustments. Such changes are needed in daily activities as well as in emergent situations.

It has been known for some time that hypothalamic stimulation can elevate blood pressure.[12] Such responses are mediated by the sympathetic nervous system and form the basis for behavior-related hypertension,[13] perhaps through reaction with the renin-angiotensin system (see below).[14] This important etiologic consideration will be discussed further in the text.

Some basic understanding of nervous system blood pressure control through sympathetic nervous mechanisms is necessary. Although neurotransmitters are humoral substances, they are considered here because of their intimate relationship with the sympathetic nervous system.

Norepinephrine and Neurotransmitters

Anatomically, small vessels are rich in sympathetic nervous innervation.[15] This allows rapid reaction to a wide variety of activity and metabolic states. Maintenance of homeostasis by stable perfusion of vital organs and tissues is thus ensured. The principal neurotransmitter of sympathetic impulses from nerve fibers to effector cells is norepinephrine. Vasoconstriction follows attachment of norepinephrine to α-receptors on arteriolar and vein-effector cells while vasodilation results from attachment to β-receptors. β-receptor stimulation is also responsible for increased heart rate and myocardial contractility (Fig. 2).[16]

Tyrosine metabolism to DOPA, then dopamine at the nerve endings, leads to the production of norephinephrine with the aid of the enzyme dopamine β-hydroxylase. The latter is often measured as an indicator of sympathetic activity. These reactions are shown in Figure 2. Norepinephrine so produced is metabolized locally to metanephrine and vanillylmandelic acid (VMA) which is excreted in the urine. Vanillylmandelic acid urine level constitutes another measure of sympathetic activity.[16] Currently, however, plasma norepinephrine values can be measured directly, and a study from the Medical University of South Carolina lists these values by age and activity (Table 2). Sympathetic adjustments to changes in status are evidenced by the dramatic rise in levels with exercise.

Very little free norephinephrine is released into the circulation from nerve endings. However, stimulation of the adrenal medulla results in secretion of both norephinephrine and its product, epinephrine, into the circulation.[17] These catecholamines cause major alterations in the circulation in response to stress. The action pathways are diagramed in Figure 2. Whether or not this powerful mechanism has a significant role in hypertension remains debatable.

In the scheme of nervous system regulation of blood pressure, a number of reflexes have been described. Foremost among the nervous system mechanisms are the baroreflexes and the chemoreflexes.

Baroreflexes[18,19]

Baroreflexes originate in receptor nerve endings (pressor receptors) located mainly in the arch of the aorta and carotid sinus region of the internal carotid artery. The receptors in the aorta are "set" about

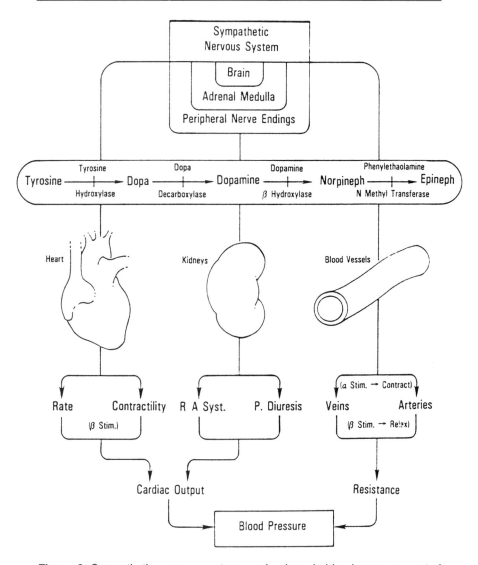

Figure 2: Sympathetic nervous system mechanisms in blood pressure control as they impact on cardiac output and resistance with resultant blood pressure (BP = cardiac output × resistance).

Table 2.
Plasma Norepinephrine Level for Blacks and Whites
by Age and Activity
(ng/mL)

Age: (y)	10–12	12+–14	14+–16	16+–18	18+
			Blacks		
(N)	(26)	(28)	(29)	(17)	(1)
Supine	0.35 ± 0.16	0.30 ± 0.20	0.29 ± 0.19	0.31 ± 0.31	0.37 ± 0
Standing	0.57 ± 0.33	0.57 ± 0.36	0.56 ± 0.27	0.57 ± 0.50	0.50 ± 0
Exercise	1.36 ± 0.66	1.40 ± 0.64	1.94 ± 0.88	1.74 ± 0.97	0.98 ± 0
Ex. Recovery	0.62 ± 0.26	0.56 ± 0.29	0.72 ± 0.38	0.73 ± 0.30	0.93 ± 0
			Whites		
(N)	(52)	(51)	(42)	(23)	(7)
Supine	0.34 ± 0.23	0.31 ± 0.32	0.25 ± 0.14	0.24 ± 0.13	0.14 ± 0.04
Standing	0.57 ± 0.26	0.55 ± 0.24	0.60 ± 0.29	0.61 ± 0.37	0.45 ± 0.23
Exercise	1.78 ± 0.84	2.51 ± 1.45	2.95 ± 1.82	2.54 ± 1.76	1.88 ± 1.85
Ex. Recovery	0.81 ± 0.38	0.86 ± 0.39	0.89 ± 0.46	0.83 ± 0.37	0.67 ± 0.58

Values given are means ± the standard deviation. (A.H. Unpublished MUSC data, from the laboratory of J.O. Webb, Ph D. 1982).

30 mm Hg higher than those in the carotid arteries. Impulses are generated by these receptors in response to stretch of the vascular walls by blood pressure in the range of 60 to 80 mm Hg. At lower pressures, there is not enough stretch to stimulate impulses, while at higher pressures the signal pathway becomes "saturated." The efferent limb of the reflex is mediated by inhibitory impulses from the vagal center. The effector mechanism consists of peripheral vasodilation and decrease in heart rate as well as contractility, all of which contribute to lowering the blood pressure. Baroreflexes mediate moment-to-moment shifts in pressure such as those that occur during changes in posture. In time, the responses become fatigued so that their effect is felt for several days at the most (Fig. 3). In hypertensive individuals, the pressure needed to stimulate the threshold level of the receptors is set at a higher level so that the reflex remains effective.

Chemoreceptors[20]

Chemoreceptors are located in the carotid and aortic bodies. They operate at the lower end of the blood pressure scale, responding

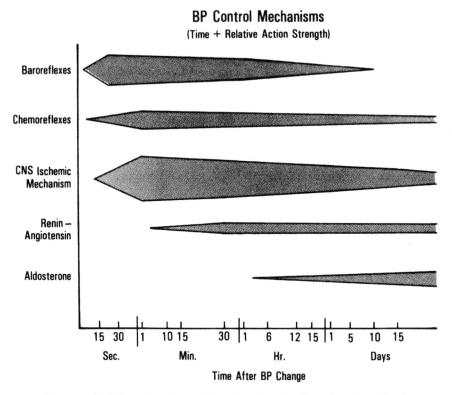

BP Control Mechanisms
(Time + Relative Action Strength)

Figure 3: Relative strength and time duration of action of various blood pressure control mechanisms.

to chemical changes (increasing CO_2 and decreasing O_2) which occur with ischemia from decreased perfusion. While primarily concerned with respiration, the chemoreceptors provide powerful impulses when arterial pressure falls toward shock levels. These effect constriction of both veins and arteries, the former leading to increased cardiac-filling pressure. As in the case of baroreceptors, these responses are relatively short-lived (Fig. 3).

Other Reflexes

A number of other nervous system blood pressure control mechanisms are concerned with correction of low pressures. The powerful *central nervous system ischemic mechanism* is a "last ditch stand" against circulatory collapse.[21] Activation of this reflex occurs with hypotension-induced medullary center ischemia. Marked sympathetic nervous system-mediated vasoconstriction ensues which may virtually stop renal and peripheral blood flow. The *low-pressure receptor "feed forward" mechanism* responds to low blood volume pressure by peripheral vasoconstriction and volume expansion through renal retention of sodium and water.[22] In this reflex, low pressure is sensed in the low pressure areas of the circulation such as the right atrium. Impulses are then "fed forward" to the arteriolar side of the circulation for the described effects. Conversely, the *Bainbridge reflex* responds to venous hypervolemic stimulation (through fluid overload) by tachycardia and concomitant elevation of blood pressure.[23] However, the tachycardia occurs only if the heart rate is suboptimal prior to the hypervolemia. As in all nervous system mechanisms for blood pressure control, these above mentioned reflexes have a rapid onset of their action and short duration of effect. A 1979 symposium reviewed other nervous system reflexes which remain to be tested by time.[24]

Humoral Mechanisms

Considerable insight has been accumulated about the influence of humoral factors on blood pressure. In 1898, Tigerstedt and Bergman showed that injection of homologous kidney extract into anesthetized rabbits resulted in a prolonged rise of blood pressure.[25] Work on their active principle, called renin, remained in question until 1928, when reproducible techniques were developed to extract the pressor substance.[26] The subsequent discovery that renin was inactive of itself, but in plasma, resulted in the formation of a new substance, variously termed hypertensin[27] and angiotonin,[28] but was later renamed angiotensin.[29] This unleashed a torrent of investigations leading to our present knowledge of the *renin-angiotensin system* as well as other humoral controls for blood pressure regulation.[30, 31] While some are classified among the immediate control mechanisms, these systems are less rapid in their onset of action than are the nervous system mechanisms (Fig. 3), beginning their effects after several moments and lasting as long as several days. Additional long-term effects have been postulated for the renin-angiotensin system through its effect on renal retention of sodium and water, which will be discussed further in the text.[32]

Renin-Angiotensin System

The *renin-angiotensin system* functions to adjust low blood pressure through vasoconstriction and extracellular fluid regulation. The system responds to physical, humoral, and neural factors. When renal blood pressure falls, receptors responding to decreased renal arterial wall tension stimulate the juxtaglomerular cells (Fig. 1D) to release renin from their intracellular granules.[33] Among humoral factors, an inverse relationship is known between the tubular sodium load and renin secretion. Sodium fluctuation is detected by the cells of the macula densa in the distal tubule which then influence renin release.[34] Although the exact neural mechanism for renin stimulation is not known, central sympathetic nervous system stimulation increases renin secretion.[14] Adrenergic nerve endings in the juxtaglomerular cells may be able to stimulate renin production as well. Both α- and β-catechol stimulation appear to be involved. The former appears to act through vasoconstriction with subsequent decreased glomerular filtration, in turn, resulting in decreased distal tubule sodium levels. The latter (β-stimulation) acts through direct stimulation of the juxtaglomerular cells. It is known that β-blockade can reduce renin secretion.[35]

Once in the blood stream, the enzyme renin acts upon the glycoprotein angiotensinogen (renin substrate), an α_2-globulin which has been produced by the liver. The result is the formation of inactive decapeptide, angiotensin I. The angiotensinogen level may be an important factor in the renin-angiotensin system. Usual levels are less than those required for maximal reaction velocity.[36] When the angiotensinogen level is increased by such medications as corticosteroids or estrogens (contraceptive pills), elevation of blood pressure may ensue.[37]

Cleavage of two amino acids from angiotensin I, by the angiotensin-converting enzyme during passage through the lungs, results in the very active octapeptide, angiotensin II (Fig. 4).[38] Angiotensin I-converting enzyme blockers not only prevent the formation of angiotensin II, but also block the degradation of the vasodilator, bradykinin.[39]

The direct initial effect of angiotensin II is very powerful arteriolar constriction which develops within a few moments of stimulation.[40] A prompt rise in blood pressure ensues, but is moderated somewhat by the baroreceptor mechanism. In working together, these mechanisms effect greater pressure control than would be the

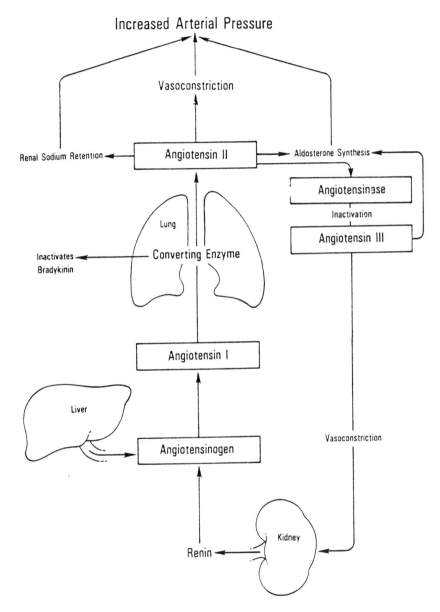

Figure 4: Renin-angiotensin system. The relationship with bradykinin as well as renal feedback are shown.

case if each operated alone.[11] Only a small amount of angiotensin II is needed to achieve its effect, for the peptide is about 50 times as potent as norepinephrine on the basis of weight for elevating pressure.[41] Stimulation of the sympathetic nervous system by angiotensin II leads to increased sympathetic tone and increase in catecholamine secretion.[42] Angiotensin II also directly stimulates the adrenal cortex and, as a consequence, is a major influence in aldosterone production.[43] Other actions of angiotensin II include stimulation of drinking and stimulation of vasopressin secretion.[44] These latter factors may contribute to a renal retention of sodium and water. The relationship of the renin- angiotensin system to various factors concerned in blood pressure regulation is presented schematically in Figure 5. It should be noted that tachyphylaxis to angiotensin develops in time but probably is not an important factor in day-to-day pressure regulation.[45]

Angiotensinases cause rapid inactivation of angiotensin II in peripheral capillary beds. It is likely that angiotensin II is only active for 1 or 2 minutes.[46] Of the metabolic products, only angiotensin III shows some activity. It acts to stimulate aldosterone formation and may result in selective renal vasoconstriction.[47]

At this point, it is important to mention the assay of renin-angiotensin system activity. While methods are now available to assay all the components of the system, generally, measurement of plasma renin activity (PRA) is equated to activity of the entire system. It is the rate-limiting substance in the renin-angiotensin system. Most commonly, a radioimmunoassay is used to measure the rate at which angiotensin I is generated when plasma is incubated in vitro under standard conditions of time, temperature, and pH.[46] In the laboratory at the Medical University of South Carolina, the results are expressed as (ng/mL per hour).[48] When determining the PRA in the clinical setting, consideration must be given to the circumstances of sampling since a large number of factors influence renin production. The more important influences of PRA level include:

1. age: young individuals have higher PRAs and levels fall with aging.
2. race: blacks have lower PRAs regardless of blood pressure levels.
3. diet: increased sodium in the diet decreases and sodium deprivation elevates PRA.

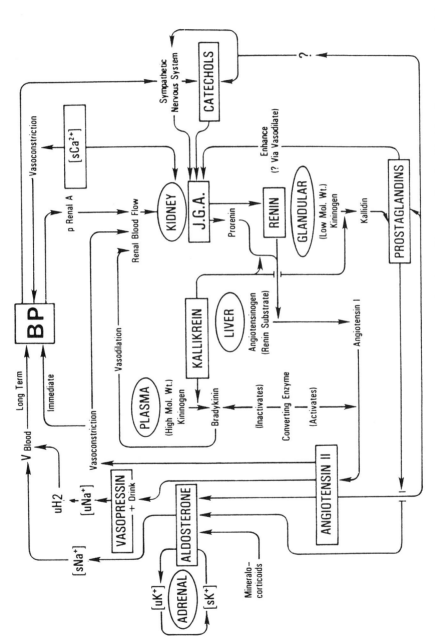

Figure 5: The formation and interaction of various humoral and cation substances involved in blood pressure control (see text).

4. position: standing evokes a sharp rise in PRA level.
5. activity: stimulates a marked increase in PRA whereas a fall is seen with sleep.
6. time of day: with supine individuals, a circadian rhythm is evident.
7. menstrual cycle: increases during luteal phase.
8. medications: diuretics, vasodilators, anesthetics, caffeine, estrogen, glucocorticoids *all* increase PRA, while β-blockers, mineralocorticoids, cardiac glycosides, phenobarbital and prostaglandin synthesis inhibitors (aspirin, indomethacin, etc.) decrease PRA.[49]

These factors are summarized in Table 3.

At the Medical University of South Carolina, a number of measurements were made in individuals of the pediatric age group in several positions and activity states. These renin values are listed in Table 4 by race and age. As anticipated, racial differences were evident in this group of young people. The mean supine PRAs of all blacks was 2.42 ng/mL per hour while the mean supine PRA value for all whites was 4.58 ng/mL per hour. These PRA values may be considered for reference but should not be considered as absolute normal data. Normal levels must be established for each laboratory. In clinical practice, use of renin determinations in pediatric patients is helpful in certain situations, which will be detailed in subsequent

Table 3.
Factors Influencing Plasma-Renin Activity (PRA) Level

Increased PRA	Decreased PRA
White race	Black race
Young age	
Sodium depletion	Sodium excess
Fluid volume loss	Increased fluid volume
Decreased renal perfusion pressure	
Catecholamine excess	Catecholamine deficiency
Hypokalemia	Hyperkalemia
Increased renin substrate	Decreased renal tissue
Acute renal damage (including J G cells)	

chapters. For each sample, factors that influence the renin level such as age, race, position, diet, and medication must be considered in interpreting the values obtained.

A number of other humoral mechanisms exist and interact with the renin-angiotensin system (Fig. 5). Production of substances such as aldosterone and prostaglandins may be directly stimulated by angiotensin II.[43,50] Other substances, such as renal kallikrein, may be produced in response to blood pressure changes in the kidneys.[51] As a rule, production of these substances follows pressure changes by several hours, peaking only days after change is discerned (Fig. 3). Thus these substances are more properly classified among the "long-term blood pressure control mechanisms," and are featured in the following section.

Long-Term Blood Pressure Control Mechanisms

The Kidney-Blood Volume

The primary site for long-term control of arterial pressure is in the kidney. In this extremely important function, the kidney acts by

Table 4.
Plasma-Renin Levels for Blacks and Whites by Age and Activity
(ng/mL per h)

Age (y):	10–12	12+–14	14+–16	16+–18	18+
			Blacks		
(N)	(25)	(26)	(32)	(15)	(2)
Supine	2.91 ± 2.4	2.03 ± 1.7	2.51 ± 2.0	2.54 ± 1.5	2.21 ± 1.6
Standing	3.80 ± 3.3	2.74 ± 2.1	3.01 ± 2.4	3.18 ± 2.2	2.00 ± 1.4
Exercise	8.62 ± 6.6	6.59 ± 4.4	6.86 ± 4.9	6.67 ± 6.4	3.77 ± 2.1
Ex.Recovery	7.85 ± 6.1	5.87 ± 3.5	7.50 ± 6.1	6.28 ± 5.2	3.62 ± 3.2
			Whites		
(N)	(50)	(52)	(42)	(23)	(8)
Supine	4.10 ± 2.4	3.72 ± 2.2	4.60 ± 3.6	3.49 ± 2.2	3.33 ± 1.4
Standing	5.84 ± 3.4	4.95 ± 2.5	4.22 ± 2.1	4.00 ± 3.4	4.00 ± 1.6
Exercise	14.11 ± 8.5	12.66 ± 7.1	11.49 ± 5.4	9.21 ± 5.1	9.90 ± 4.7
Ex.Recovery	12.20 ± 6.9	12.06 ± 6.9	11.21 ± 5.1	9.42 ± 4.8	9.11 ± 3.5

Values given are means ± standard deviation. (A.H. Unpublished MUSC data, from the laboratory of P. J. Privitar, PhD. 1982).

changing cardiac output through changes in extracellular fluid and blood volume. The renal mechanism affects the change through natriuresis and diureses, in response to changes in renal arteriolar blood pressure. Thus, a renal blood pressure increase results in an increase in sodium and water excretion. This type of response may, over time, increase the renal output of sodium and water 6 to 8 times. The "system" comprises a "feedback loop" with renal loss of sodium and water decreasing blood volume, hence, cardiac output. Then, in turn, the arterial pressure is lowered towards normal. With hypotension, a converse effect ensues.

The kidney-blood volume mechanism is perhaps the only blood pressure control mechanism that can return arterial pressure back to completely normal levels. Feedback gain can be equated to the amount of pressure correction divided by the remaining pressure abnormality according to the formula:

$$\text{Gain} = \frac{\text{Pressure Correction}}{\text{Remaining Abnormality}} \qquad 4.$$

Since there may be no remaining pressure abnormality in the kidney-blood volume system, and the denominator in this situation is zero, the gain is infinity. Hence, the system has been labeled as having "infinite gain."[52]

If, however, the daily intake of sodium or water is altered, or if a pathologic process develops in the kidney, the long-term arterial pressure level will be altered or "reset." The processes which change the set point of the kidney-blood volume mechanism include: alteration in glomerular membranes, altered plasma proteins with resultant altered glomerular filtration, angiotensin or aldosterone-induced sodium and water retention, intrinsic renovascular changes, and sympathetic nervous system-induced changes in renal blood vessels.

A schematic view of the system and site of alteration is presented in Figure 6. From these considerations, an understanding is developed that hypertension may follow decreased renal capability to form glomerular filtrate in relationship to tubular ability to reabsorb sodium and water. Conversely, hypotension may develop when the capability of tubular reabsorption is reduced below glomerular filtration capacity. In this regard, diuretics which interfere with tubular reabsorption of sodium and water reduce the "set level" for arterial pressure. Consequently, these drugs are useful for blood pressure control. However, diuretics also activate renin

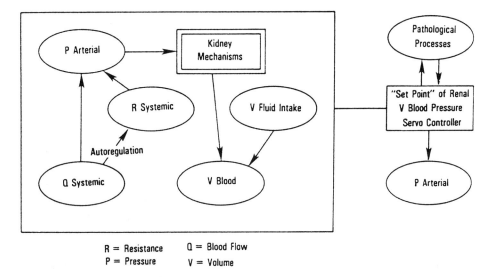

R = Resistance   Q = Blood Flow
P = Pressure   V = Volume

Figure 6: Modified Guyton arrangement of renal hemodynamic-pathophysiologic blood pressure control mechanisms. These factors dictate how the set point of arterial pressure may be changed.

production which modifies their effect and results in reduced diuretic potency.[11]

Autoregulation

The major long-term effect of the kidney-blood volume mechanism is to control tissue blood flow through changes in peripheral resistance by the "feedback loop" system described. Another means exists by which local vasoregulating changes in peripheral resistance are effected. This other system exerts its action indirectly through a mechanism called "autoregulation of blood flow." To achieve hemostasis, each tissue controls its own blood flow to meet its needs, perhaps related to endothelium or other tissue-derived factors. With excessive cardiac output, autoregulation in the various tissues will result in local vasoconstriction.[53] The effect is additive and can result in a marked increase in total peripheral resistance. Although, as indicated in the previous sections, the kidney-blood volume mechanism first controls arterial pressure by cardiac output, the long-term effect is on peripheral resistance and cardiac output returning to normal levels. Thus, chronic volume-loading hypertension is likely to have high resistance rather than high output.[54]

Humoral Mechanisms in Long-Term Blood Pressure Control

The Renin-Angiotensin System

Attention has been called to the immediate vasoconstrictor effects of the renin-angiotensin system. However, since a major effect of the system lies in its long-term affect on renal excretion of electrolytes and water, it is important to review this mode of extended actions. Angiotensin directly acts upon renal tubules to increase sodium and, to a lesser extent, potassium and water reabsorption.[55] With hypotension such stimulation may be chronic and so change the set point of arterial pressure as described for the kidney-blood volume system. The known angiotensin stimulation of the adrenal cortex to produce aldosterone contributes to this change.[56] Aldosterone-induced retention of sodium and water, however, is not the major factor, for the set point change still occurs in adrenalectomized individuals.[57] It is also doubted that the angiotensin thirst or antidiuretic hormone stimulation mechanism adds significantly to the response.

In special situations, where there is renal artery narrowing with concomitant lowering of afferent arteriolar pressure, renin production is increased. This leads to increased levels of angiotensin, some of which may be produced in the kidney. In these cases, the angiotensin maintains a near normal glomerular filtration rate through efferent arteriolar vasoconstriction. Simultaneous systemic arteriolar constriction leads to higher blood pressures. Should the renal arterial constriction be unilateral, the opposite kidney will almost cease renin production in a "feedback" type response to high plasma renin levels. Circulating angiotensin will stimulate sodium and water reabsorption in the "good" kidney leading to a higher set point of systemic arterial pressure.[58] It is important to note that blockage of this response, by the use of a converting enzyme blocker such as captopril in bilateral renal artery stenosis or in unilateral stenosis with a single kidney, may interfere with glomerular filtration and lead to renal failure.[59] In these cases, careful monitoring of urea nitrogen or creatinine is necessary. Withdrawal of the medication restores the pretreatment state.

Aldosterone

As the principal mineralocorticoid of the adrenal, aldosterone is produced in the zona glomerulosa of the cortex. Aldosterone enters into the scheme of blood pressure regulation through its renal action to cause sodium and water retention, mainly in the distal tubules. Thus stimulated, the sodium and water retention results in a gradual rise in blood pressure over a period of several days as renal function is altered to a new set point of pressure regulation (Fig. 3). The most potent effect of aldosterone is sodium retention with water reabsorption following along the osmotic gradient.[60] An almost equally potent effect is the secretion of potassium into the distal tubules of the kidney which may result in hypokalemia, a feature of hyperaldosteronism.[61]

In other circumstances, aldosterone may stimulate the hypothalamic-posterior pituitary system to increase secretion of antidiuretic hormone. With pathologic hypersecretion of aldosterone, only a mild to moderate elevation of blood pressure is seen (i.e. 10 to 20 mm Hg) unless the corticoid excess results in renal damage. These causes of pressure elevation will be discussed further in subsequent chapters on the specific types of hypertension.

Of the four major substances, angiotensin, potassium, sodium and ACTH, which stimulate aldosterone secretion, angiotensin II is generally considered to be the most powerful.[62] The peptide appears to bind to a cell-membrane receptor and facilitates the conversion of cholesterol to aldosterone.[63] Although angiotensin stimulation provides only modest elevation in circulating aldosterone level, this increase has important effects on plasma electrolytes. In turn, circulating potassium concentration provides a potent affect on aldosterone secretion. A 20% increase in potassium level results in a doubling of aldosterone production. Sodium depletion also increases aldosterone levels. This effect is not mediated through the renin-angiotensin system as it occurs in nephrectomized individuals. On the other hand, while an increase in ACTH does not affect aldosterone production, absence of ACTH will depress secretion of aldosterone. However, in usual ranges ACTH has little effect on aldosterone levels.[60] It appears that the influence of aldosterone on blood pressure is indirect, being mediated through stimulation by factors other than direct blood pressure changes. Levels of aldosterone found in childhood have been reported by Van Ackee and coworkers,[64] as well as Kowarski and colleagues.[65]

Prostaglandin

Authorities now concede that the humoral vasodilators, prostaglandin and kallikrein, are factors in blood pressure control.[66,67] They may achieve their effect, at least partially, through other hormonal systems. While these substances interact, their mechanisms of action remain controversial. Prostaglandins, present in many tissues, are formed by the metabolism of arachidonic acid. The metabolism proceeds through the formation of cyclic endoperoxides into the production of 1) prostacyclin which prevents platelet aggregation and also has vasodilator actions; 2) prostaglandin E_2, the major renal prostaglandin vasodilator which may be further metabolized to prostaglandin F_{2a}, a vasoconstrictor substance; and 3) thromboxane, which promotes platelet aggregation and constricts smooth muscle.[68] The latter is found in the urine, with renal outflow obstruction perhaps explaining the elevation in blood pressure shown in such cases. Renal prostaglandins are formed in the cortex as well as in the medulla. They are released into both blood and urine. Together with the kallikrein system, prostaglandins affect renin release and renovascular resistance.[69] The latter may result through a direct local effect on vascular smooth muscle. Infusions of prostaglandins initially result in vasodilation and a tendency to lower blood pressure. However, prostaglandin stimulation of renin and aldosterone production, with accompanying changes in salt and water excretion, may influence this effect.

In the kidney, prostaglandins appear to have a primary defensive role. With stress-induced activation of the renin-angiotensin system, production of angiotensin II causes generalized vasoconstriction. At the same time, angiotensin II activation of prostaglandin synthesis ensues and may attenuate the renal vasoconstrictor action of angiotensin, thereby helping to maintain renal blood flow.[70] Inhibition of prostaglandin synthesis by substances like indomethacin or aspirin (prostaglandin-synthetase inhibitors) may modulate the stress responses in the kidney. Indomethacin does not lead to the development of hypertension in normal individuals, although the drug may depress renal function and cause increased severity in those with an existing hypertensive disorder.[71] Some evidence exists that the antihypertensive effect of certain medications, for example, hydralazine, is mediated by prostaglandins.[72] Intrarenal prostaglandins affect aldosterone production as well as antagonize antidiuretic hormone. These effects are schematically shown in Fig. 5, along with other known vasoactive substances. Prostaglandin levels appear to vary with age. The Medical University of South Carolina data on levels of urinary prostaglandin E-like substance are presented in Table 5 and are similar to those presented by Godard, Vallotton, and Favre.[73]

Kallikrein-Kinin System

In the 80 years since it was found that injection of an individual's urine into the circulatory system causes a fall in blood pressure, much has been learned about vasodilators so injected.[74] Yet details of the mechanism of action of the kallikrein-kinin system have remained an enigma. Two forms of the endoprotease, kallikrein, are known: plasma and tissue (glandular) kallikrein. Both catalyze the cleavage of vasodepressor peptides or kinins from protein substrates or kininogens. The plasma kallikrein-kinin system relates to the coagulation cascade through the Hageman factor, and shares enzymes with the renin-angiotensin system.[75] Plasma kallikrein catalyzes the formation of bradykinin from high-molecular-weight kininogen and can activate the formation of renin from prorenin (Fig. 7), as well the Hageman factor.[76] Bradykinin degradation is mediated by the peptide hydrolase, kininase II, or angiotensin-converting enzyme (Fig. 4). Thus, the action of the angiotensin-vasoconstrictor system is aided by the simultaneous inactivation of the vasodilator bradykinin. Conversely, the antihypertensive effect of captopril blockage of converting enzyme is enhanced by reduced

Table 5.

Urinary Prostaglandin Levels in Young People
(ng/dL)

Age	(N)	Prostaglandin Level Mean ± SD
10–12	(71)	685.0 ± 57.0
12+–14	(46)	848.8 ± 82.1
14+–16	(29)	1112.8 ± 91.1
16+–18	(16)	1335.1 ± 112.1
18+	(5)	1800.0 ± 154.4

(A.H. Unpublished MUSC data, from the laboratory of
P. V. Halushka, MD PhD.1982).

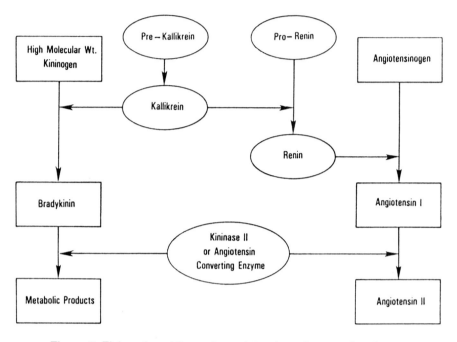

Figure 7: Elaboration of the renin-angiotensin and system interfaces.

degradation of bradykinin resulting in persistent vasodilator activity.[77]

Bradykinin and angiotensin systems usually act in reciprocal fashion as noted. They can, however, respond with changes in the same direction. Thus, assumption of upright posture causes a rise in level of plasma renin activity, angiotensin II, and bradykinin.[78] Sodium balance changes also produce parallel changes in these substances.[79] The reasons for this correlation of vasoactive substance activity and the mechanism that regulates the plasma concentration of bradykinin are unknown. The effects of bradykinin may be mediated in part through prostaglandins which vary from tissue to tissue. For example, the bradykinin-mediated arteriolar response is vasodilatation from PGE_2 production. In venules, vasoconstriction results from PGF_{2a} production.[80] Renal kallikrein is produced in the distal tubules and acts locally, being released into the urine only.[81] It catalyzes the formation of the vasodilator, kallidin (lys-bradykinin), from low-molecular-weight kininogen. Kallikrein level in the urine generally has an inverse relationship with sodium intake, but a direct relationship with plasma aldosterone concentration.[82] While urinary kallikrein is not the major determinant of the entire kinin system, low urinary kallikrein levels suggest decreased amount of the renal vasodilator kallidin. Most, but not all hypertensive individuals, especially those who have kidney disease, have lower urinary kallikrein levels than those who are normotensive.[83] Blacks, who as a group have a high incidence of hypertension, are reported to have lower kallikrein levels than whites, both in adults[84] and children.[85] In children, urinary kallikrein varies with age, and those with highest blood pressures have the lowest urinary kallikrein levels.[86] Many children of hypertensive parents also have low urinary kallikrein levels. Our laboratory findings in these groups were equivocal, but black children of hypertensive parents did have the lowest urinary kallikrein levels.[87] An age tabulation of our South Carolina values is in Table 6. These data represent a tenfold increase in levels when compared with the findings of Godad, et al,[73] perhaps representing methodologic and/or geographic variation.

Other Humoral Mechanisms

Other vasoactive substances deserve consideration when discussing vasoregulatory mechanisms. They are vasopressin or antidiuretic hormone, calcium, natriuretic hormones, and endothelium factors. Each of these substances can affect blood pressure, yet their roles are under debate. Brief mention will be made of current

Table 6.
Urinary Kallikrein Values Grouped by Age and Activity
(EU/24 h per m²)

Age	Blacks (N)	Mean ± SD	Whites (N)	Mean ± SD
10–12	(31)	3.64 ± 2.7	(54)	6.21 ± 4.8
12+–14	(30)	5.00 ± 5.5	(52)	5.28 ± 3.3
14+–16	(33)	5.94 ± 5.4	(42)	6.44 ± 4.4
16+–18	(23)	3.88 ± 2.6	(26)	5.27 ± 3.9
18+	(5)	4.15 ± 3.3	(9)	6.34 ± 3.4

(A.H. Unpublished MUSC data, from the laboratory of H. S. Margolis, MD, PhD. 1982).

thinking of their pressure regulatory function or contribution to blood pressure.

Vasopressin: Vasopressin release from the posterior pituitary may be stimulated by angiotensin II.[88] By promotion of the reabsorption of water from the distal tubules and collecting ducts of the kidney, vasopressin can cause an elevation in blood pressure through volume expansion.[89] With prolonged stimulation, however, this effect abates. In higher amounts, vasopressin secreted at times of stress can act as a vasoconstrictor.[90] Since such levels are seldom achieved, some investigators have perceived a regulatory role for vasopressin in concert with the sympathetic nervous system through both central and peripheral influences.[91] However, it is felt that vasopressin does not significantly contribute to hypertensive disorders.[92] Godard, Vollotton, and Favre recently reported vasopressin levels in healthy children.[73]

Calcium: Contraction of arteriolar smooth muscle, like all muscle, is dependent on calcium-mediated coupling of actin and myosin filaments. Thus, the availability of free "activator" calcium, whether from cellular influx or intracellular stores, influences the contractile state of the arterioles.[93] Vasoconstrictor hormones appear to mediate their effect through intracellular release of calcium for excitation-contact ion-coupling.[94] It is postulated that sodium retention in hypertension leads to increased intracellular sodium. In turn, this leads to increased intracellular calcium. Peripheral vascular smooth muscle contractility is thus increased, leading to raised peripheral resistance.[95] Animal studies have shown raised levels of cellular calcium with hypertension.[94] It is also known that patients with elevated calcium levels often have higher blood pressures than normotensive individuals.[96] Thus, it is likely that the vascular tone and reactivity increased by calcium contribute to the increased vascular resistance of sustained hypertension. These considerations furnish the rationale behind the reduction of blood pressure in hypertensive patients by calcium channel blockers such as nifedipine or verapamil.[97] On the other hand, increased calcium intake has been advocated to relieve or prevent hypertension in certain individuals (see Chapters 3, 4, and 10).

Natriuretic Hormones: Favor has been found with the hypothesis that an inherited defect in sodium excretion may be a causative factor for hypertension. It is known that hypertensive individuals respond to sodium challenge with excessive excretion of salt. At least two natriuretic substances have been identified in the urine of such individuals.[98] One of these substances is believed to be a nonpeptide hormone generated in the hypothalamus. The natriuretic hormone so produced apparently acts as a sodium transport inhibitor by a ouabain-like inhibition of Na+–K+–ATPase. In the renal tubules, this leads to decreased sodium reabsorption and natriuresis. Other effects of natriuretic hormone inhibition include sodium retention and vasoconstriction with elevation of blood pressure. This substance has been found in newborn infants causing false-positive digoxin measurements.[99]

The second substance is a peptide hormone produced in the walls of the cardiac atria. It is now known as atrial natriuretic factor (ANF). The hormone is stored in granules and released when the atrial walls are stretched by hypervolemic states or by expansion of extracellular fluid volume.[100] Release of ANF is also stimulated by epinephrine as well as by vasopressin. Atrial natriuretic factor values are highest at birth and are elevated in heart or renal failure.[101,102] Atrial natriuretic factor results in natriuresis and vasodilation. It may lower blood pressure. However, while ANF may serve to vary blood pressure in the short term, the role of ANF in overall blood pressure regulation is unclear. Much remains to be learned about these natriuretic hormones.

Endothelium-Derived Factors: The contribution of endothelium to blood pressure regulation will be unraveled in the nineties. Investigations have already uncovered defective endothelium-mediated vasodilation in hypertensives.[103] A major portion of the effect of endothelium-derived relaxing factor (EDRF) has been found to be related to the synthesis of nitric oxide (NO). Evidence holds that EDRF is nitric oxide.[104] Defective NO synthesis leads to hypertension in animals.[105] On the other hand, endothelin-1 has been found to be a potent vasoconstrictor.[106] Levels of endothelin-1 were found elevated in two hypertensive patients with malignant scalp hemangioendothelioma.[107] Both the level of endothelin-1 and blood pressure were reduced with tumor removal. When the tumor recurred in one patient, the levels again became elevated. A recent symposium presented current thinking about these factors.[108]

Summary

In this chapter, the central role of the kidney in blood pressure regulation has been emphasized and its architecture reviewed. Renal mechanisms maintain blood volume, but their set point may be altered by changes in fluid intake or pathologic processes. Superimposed on renal blood volume control mechanisms are various neural, humoral, and autoregulatory systems. The sympathetic nervous system, through intricate reflexes and mediation by norepinephrine, initiates the fine circulatory adjustments needed in moment-to-moment living. The renin-angiotensin system not only provides immediate vasoconstrictive influences when required, but also, with aldosterone, influences electrolytes and fluid balance over longer periods. The kallikrein system may provide opposite vasodilator reactions where necessary. Tissue circulatory autoregulation may account for a significant fraction of peripheral resistance. These and other factors such as prostaglandins, vasopressin, calcium, natriuretic hormones, and endothelium-derived substances interact to maintain blood pressure and tissue-perfusion hemostasis, both on a short- and long-term basis. Their interaction can be understood in terms of the hemodynamic principles outlined in the chapter and summarized in Figure 8. While not known, the etiology(s) of primary hypertension may reside among these factors.

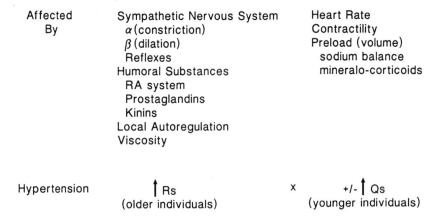

Blood Pressure = Peripheral Resistance(Rs) X Cardiac Output(Qs)

Affected By	Sympathetic Nervous System
	α (constriction)
	β (dilation)
	Reflexes
	Humoral Substances
	RA system
	Prostaglandins
	Kinins
	Local Autoregulation
	Viscosity
		Heart Rate
		Contractility
		Preload (volume)
		  sodium balance
		  mineralo-corticoids

Hypertension	↑ Rs (older individuals)	x +/- ↑ Qs (younger individuals)

Figure 8: Summary of major factors affecting blood pressure arranged according to the formula: blood pressure (hypertension) = resistance (elevated Rs) × systemic blood flow (Qs) which may be elevated or normal (+/− Qs) in younger individuals.

References

1. Pickering GW. Systemic arterial hypertension. In: Fishman AP, Richards DW, eds. *Circulation of the Blood: Men and Ideas*. New York: Oxford University Press; 1964.
2. Harvey W; Leake CD, trans. *Exercitatio Anatomica de Motu Cordis et Sanguinis in Animalibus*. Springfield: Charles C Thomas; 1946.
3. Hale S. Statical Essays: Vol 2: Containing Haemastaticks; or an Account of Some Hydraulick and Hydrostatical Experiments made on the Blood and Blood Vessels of Animals. London: Innys and Manly; 1733.
4. Poiseuille JLM. Recherches experimentales sur la mouvement des liquides dans les tubes des tres petits diametres. *Mem Acad Sci* (Paris) 9:433, 1846.
5. Bright R. *Reports of Medical Cases Selected with a View of Illustrating the Symptoms and Cure of Diseases by a Reference to Morbid Anatomy, 2 vols*. London: Longman; 1827.
6. Gull WW. Chronic Bright's disease with contracted kidney (arterio-capillary fibrosis). *Brit Med J* II:673, 1872.
7. Letcher RL, Chien S, Pickering TG, Sealey JE, Laragh JH. Direct relationships between blood pressure and blood viscosity in normal and hypertensive subjects: role of fibrinogen and concentration. *Am J Med* 70:1195, 1981.
8. Pitts RF. *Physiology of the Kidney and Body Fluids*. Chicago: Year Book Med Pub; 1963.
9. Tobian L. Physiology of the juxtaglomerular cells. *Ann Intern Med* 52:395, 1960.
10. David JO. The control of renin release. *Am J Med* 55:333, 1973.
11. Guyton AC, Hall JE, Norman RA, Smith MJ, Balfe JW, Kastner PR. Physiology of blood pressure regulation. In: Lauer RM, Shekelle RB, eds. *Childhood Prevention of Atherosclerosis and Hypertension*. New York: Raven Press; 251:1980.
12. Karplus JP, Kreidl A. Gehirm und sympathicus VII: uber beziehungen der hypothalamus zentren zu blutdruck undinnerer skretion. *Pflugers Arch* 215:667, 1927.
13. Zanchetti A, Bartorelli C. Central nervous mechanisms in arterial hypertension: experimental and clinical evidence. In: Genest J, Koiw E, Kuchel O, eds. *Hypertension Pathophysiology and Treatment*. New York: McGraw-Hill; 59:1977.
14. Zanchetti A, Stella A. Neural control of renin release. *Clin Sci Med* 48:215, 1975.
15. Mellander S, Johansson B. Control of resistance, exchange capacitance functions in the peripheral circulation. *Pharmacol Rev* 20:117, 1968.
16. Kuchel O. Autonomic nervous system in hypertension: clinical aspects. In: Genest J, Koiw E, Kuchel O, eds. *Hypertension Pathophysiology and Treatment*. New York: McGraw-Hill; 93:1977.

17. Axelrod J, Weinshilboum R. Catecholamines. *N Engl J Med* 287:273, 1972.
18. Burton AC. *Physiology and Biophysics of the Circulation*. Chicago: Year Book Med Pub; 173:1965.
19. Guyton AC. *Arterial Pressure and Hypertension*. Philadelphia: WB Saunders Co; 13:1980.
20. Comroe JH Jr. *Physiology of Respiration*. Chicago: Year Book Med Pub; 1965.
21. Sagowa K, Taylor AE, Guyton AC. Dynamic performance and stability of cerebral ischemic response. *Am J Physiol* 201:1164, 1961.
22. Mancia G, Lorenz RR, Shepherd JT. Reflex control ofcirculation by heart and lungs. In: Guyton AC, Cowley AW Jr, eds. *International Review of Physiology Vol 9, Cardiovascular Physiology II*. Baltimore: University Park Press; 111:1976.
23. Burton AC. *Physiology and Biophysics of the Circulation*. Chicago: Year Book Med Pub; 184:1965.
24. Tarazi RC. Symposium on the heart in hypertension. *Am J Cardiol* 44:845, 1979.
25. Tigerstedt R, Bergman PG. Niere und kreislauf. *Skand Arch Physiol* 8:223, 1898.
26. Pickering GW, Prinzmetal M. Some observations on renin: a pressor substance contained in normal kidney, together with a method for its biological assay. *Clin Sci* 3:211, 1938.
27. Braun-Menendez, Fasciolo EJC, Leloir LF, Munoz JM. La sustancia hypertensora de la sangre del rinon isquemiado. *Rev Soc Argent Biol* 15:420, 1939.
28. Page IH, Helmer OM. A crystalline pressor substance (angiotonin) resulting from the reaction between renin andrenin-activator. *J Exp Med* 71:29, 1940.
29. Fasciolo JC. Historical background on the renin-angiotensinsystem. In: Genest J, Koiw E, Kuchel O, eds. *Hypertension Pathophysiology and Treatment*. New York: McGraw-Hill; 134:1977.
30. Laragh JH. The renin system and four lines of hypertension research: nephron heterogenecity, the calcium connection, the prorenin vasodilator limb, and plasma renin and heart attack. *Hypertension* 20:267, 1992.
31. Guallery EN, Robillard JE. The renin-angiotensin system and blood pressure regulation during infancy and childhood. *Pediatr Clin North Am* 40:61-79, 1993.
32. Cowley AH Jr, Coleman TG, McCaa RE, Young DB. The renin-angiotensin system: its vasoconstrictor function. In: Guyton AC. *Arterial Pressure and Hypertension*. Philadelphia: WB Saunders Co; 166:1980.
33. Davis JO. The control of renin release. *Am J Med* 55:333, 1973.
34. Vander AJ. Control of renin release. *Physiol Rev* 47:359, 1967.
35. Buhler RF, Larach JH, Baer L. Propranolol inhibition of renin secretion: a specific approach to diagnosis and treatment of renin-dependent hypertensive disease. *N Engl J Med* 287:1209, 1972.

36. Reid IA, Morris BJ, Ganong WF. The renin-angiotensin system. *Ann Rev Physiol* 40:377, 1978.
37. Newton MA, Sealey JE, Ledingham JGG, Laragh JH. High blood pressure and oral contraceptives. *Am J Obstet Gynecol* 101:1037, 1968.
38. Soffer RL. Angiotensin-converting enzyme and the regulation of vasoactive peptides. *Ann Rev Biochem* 45:73, 1976.
39. Ondetti MA, Cushman DW. Inhibitors of angiotensin-converting enzyme. In: Soffer RL, ed. *Biochemical Regulation of Blood Pressure.* New York: John Wiley and Sons; 165:1981.
40. Oparil S, Haber E. The renin angiotensin system. *N Engl J Med* 29:389, 1974.
41. Cowley AW, Guyton AC. Quantification of intermediate steps in the renin-angiotensin-vasoconstrictor feedback loop in the dog. *Circ Res* 30:557, 1972.
42. Cline WJ Jr. Role of released catecholamines in the vascular response to injected angiotensin II in the dog. *J Pharmacol Exp Ther* 216:104, 1981.
43. Laragh JR, Sealey JE, Brunner HR. The control of aldosterone secretion in normal and hypertensive man: abnormal renin-aldosterone patterns in low renin hypertension. In: Laragh JH, ed. *Hypertension Manual.* New York: Yorke Med Book Dun-Donnelley; 197:1973.
44. Brooks VL, Malvin RL. An intracerebral, physiological role for angiotensin-effects of central blockade. *Fed Proc* 38:2272, 1979.
45. Steward JM. Anaphylaxis to angiotensin. In: Page IH, Bumpus FM, eds. *Angiotensin.* New York: Springer-Verlag; 170:1974.
46. Reid IA. The renin-angiotensin system. In: Radzialowski FM, ed. *Hypertension Research.* New York: Marcel Dekker; 101:1982.
47. Goodfriend TL, Peack MJ. Angiotensin III (des-aspartic acid)-angiotensin II: evidence and speculation for its role as an important agonist in the renin-angiotensin system. *Circ Res* suppl II:38, 1975.
48. Halushka PV, Kaiser HR. Acute effects of α-methyldopa on mean blood pressure and plasma renin activity. *Circ Res* 35:458, 1974.
49. Kaplan NM. Clinical Hypertension, 4th ed. Baltimore: Williams and Wilkins Co, 1990.
50. Zusman RM, Kaiser HR. Prostaglandin E_2 biosynthesis by rabbit renomedullary interstitial cells in tissue culture. *J Biol Chem* 252:2069, 1977.
51. Carretero OA, Scicli AG. The renal kallikrein system. *Am J Physiol* 238:F247, 1980.
52. Coleman TG. Infinite gain feature of the kidney-blood volume-pressure regulator: the three laws of long-term arterial pressure regulations; renal servocontrol of arterial pressure. In: Guyton AC. *Arterial Pressure and Hypertension.* Philadelphia: WB Saunders Co; 117:1980.
53. Stainsby WN. Local control or regional blood flow. *Ann Rev Physiol* 35:151, 1973.
54. Guyton AC. Personal views on mechanisms of hypertension. In:

Genest J, Koiw E, Kuchel O, eds. *Hypertension Pathophysiology and Treatment.* New York: McGraw-Hill; 566:1977.

55. Lohmeier TE, Cowley AW, Trippodo NC, Hall JE, Guyton AC. Effects of endogenous angiotensin II on renal sodium excretion and renal hemodynamics. *Am J Physiol* 233:F368, 1977.

56. Davis JO. Regulation of aldosterone secretion. In: Blashko H, Sayers G, Smith AD, eds. *Handbook of Physiology, Section 7.* Washington, DC: American Physiology Society; 77:1975.

57. Lohmeier TE, Cowley AW, DeClue JW, Guyton AC. Failure of chronic aldosterone infusion to increase arterial pressure in dogs with angiotensin-induced hypertension. *Circ Res* 43:381, 1978.

58. Lohmeier TE, Cowley AW, Hall JE, Young DB. The renin-angiotensin system: its effects on renal retention of sodium and on long-term servocontrol of arterial pressure. In: Guyton AC: *Arterial Pressure and Hypertension.* Philadelphia: WB Saunders Co; 180:1980.

59. Blythe WB. Captopril and renal autoregulation. *N Engl J Med* 308:390, 1983. Editorial.

60. McCaa RE, Young DB, Lohmeier TE, Cowley AW, DeClue JW, Pan YP. The aldosterone system: its role in determining the set-point for long-term pressure control by the kidney blood volume servo system. In: Guyton AC. *Arterial Pressure and Hypertension.* Philadelphia: WB Saunders; 205:1980.

61. Conn JW. The evolution of primary aldosteronism: 1954-1967. *Harvey Lect* 62:257, 1986.

62. Reid IA, Ganong WF. Control of aldosterone secretion. In: Genest J, Koiw E, Kuchel O, eds. *Hypertension Pathophysiology and Treatment.* New York: McGraw-Hill; 265:1977.

63. Capponi AM, Auilere G, Fakunding JL, Catt KJ. Angiotensin: receptors and mechanisms of action. In: Soffer RL, ed. *Biochemical Regulation of Blood Pressure.* New York: John Wiley and Sons; 205:1981.

64. Van Ackee KJ, Scharpe SL, Deprettere AKR, Neels HM. Renin-angiotensin-aldosterone system in the healthy infant and child. *Kidney Int* 16:196, 1979.

65. Kowarski A, Katz H, Migeon CJ. Plasma aldosterone concentration in normal subjects from infancy to adulthood. *J Clin Endocrinol Metab* 38:489, 1974.

66. McGiff JC. Prostaglandins and blood pressure control. In: Soffer RL, ed. *Biochemical Regulation of Blood Pressure.* New York: John Wiley and Sons; 359:1989.

67. Dunn MJ, Hood VL. Prostaglandins and the kidney. *Am J Physiol* 233:F169, 1977.

68. Moncada S, Higgs EA, Vane JR. Human arterial and venous tissues generate prostacyclin (prostaglandin x), a potent inhibitor of platelet aggregation. *Lancet* 1:18, 1977.

69. McGiff JC, Nasjletti A. Kinins, renal function, and blood pressure regulation. *Fed Proc* 351:172, 1976.

70. Sun FF, Taylor BM, McGuire JC, Wong PYK. Metabolism of prostaglandins in the kidney. *Kidney Int* 19:760, 1981.
71. Ylitalo P, Pikajarvi T, Metsa-Ketela T, Vapaatalo H. The effect of inhibition of prostaglandin synthesis on plasma renin activity and blood pressure in essential hypertension. *Prostaglandins Leukotrienes Med* 1:479, 1978.
72. McGiff JC, Quilley J. Prostaglandins, kinins and the regulation of blood pressure. *Clin Exp Hypertens* 2 (3 & 4):729, 1980.
73. Godard C, Vollotton MB, Favre L. Urinary prostaglandins, vasopressin and kallikrein excretion in healthy children from birth to adolescence. *J Pediatr* 100:898, 1982.
74. Colman RW, Schmaier AH, Wong PY. The kallikrein-kinin system. In: Soffer RL, ed. *Biochemical Regulation of Blood Pressure*. New York: John Wiley and Sons; 321:1981.
75. Alving BM, Hajima T, Pisano JT, Mason BL, Buckingham RE, Mozen MM, Finlayuson JS. Hypotension associated with pre-kallikrein activator (Hageman factor fragments) in plasma protein fraction. *N Engl J Med* 299:66, 1978.
76. Sealey JWE, Atlas SA, Laragh JH, Silverberg M, Kaplan AP. Initiation of plasma prorenin activation by Hegeman factor-dependent conversion of plasma prekallikrein to kallikrein. *Pro Natl Acad Sci* 76:5914, 1979.
77. Thurston H, Swales JD. Converting enzyme inhibitor and saralasin infusion in rats: evidence for an additional vasodepressor property of converting enzyme inhibitor. *Circ Res* 42:588, 1978.
78. Wong PY, Talano RC, Williams GH, Colman RW. Response of the kallikrein-kinin and renin-angiotensin systems to saline infusion and upright posture. *J Clin Invest* 55:691, 1975.
79. Ng KKF, Vane JR. Some properties of angiotensin converting enzyme in the lung in vivo. *Nature* 225:1142, 1970.
80. McGiff JC, Terragno DA, Terragno NA, Colina J, Nasjletti A. Chemistry and biology of the kallikrein-kinin system in health and disease. In: Pisano JJ, Austen KF, eds. Washington, DC: US Government Printing Office, DHEW Publication No NIH 76-791, 267:1976.
81. Levinsky NG. The renal kallikrein-kinin system. *Circ Res* 44:441, 1979.
82. Nasjletti A, Colina-Chourio J. Interaction of mineralocorticoids, renal prostaglandins and the renal kallikrein-kinin system. *Fed Proc* 35:189, 1976.
83. Margolius HS, Horwitz D, Pisano JJ, Keiser HR. Relationship among urinary kallikrein, mineralocorticoids and human hypertensive disease. *Fed Proc* 35:203, 1976.
84. Warren SE, O'Connor DT. Does a renal vasodilator system mediate racial differences in essential hypertension? *Am J Med* 69:425, 1980.
85. Zinner SH, Margolius HS, Rosner B, Kass EH. Stability of blood pressure tank and urinary kallikrein concentration in childhood: an eight year follow-up. *Circulation* 58:908, 1978.

86. Sinaiko AR, Glasser RJ, Gillium RF, Prineas RJ. Urinary kallikrein excretion in grade school children with high and low pressure. *J Pediatr* 100:938, 1982.

87. Hohn AR, Riopel DA, Keil JE, Loadholt CB, Margolius HS, Halushka PV, Privitara PJ, Webb JO, Medley ES, Schuman SH, Rubio MI, Pantell RH, Braunstein ML. Childhood familial and biochemical factors related to hypertension. *Hypertension* 5:56, 1983.

88. Phillips MI. Angiotensin in the brain. *Neuroendocrinology* 25:354, 1978.

89. Smith MJ, Cowley AW Jr, Guyton AC, Manning RD Jr. Acute and chronic effects of arginine vasopressin on blood pressure, electrolytes and fluid volumes of the dog. *Am J Physiol* 237:F232, 1979.

90. Cowley AW Jr, Switzer SJ, Guinn M. Evidence and quantification of the vasopressin arterial pressure controlsystem in the dog. *Circ Res* 46:58, 1980.

91. Schmid PG, Sharabi FM, Matsuguchi H, Schmitt-Davis J, Lund DD. Vasopressin and neurogenic control of the circulation. In:Iwai J, ed. *Salt and Hypertension.* New York: Igaku- Shoin; 203:1982.

92. Padfield PL, Brown JJ, Lever AF, Morton JJ, Robertson JIS. Blood pressure in acute and chronic vasopressin excess. *N Engl J Med* 304:1067, 1981.

93. Somlzo AP, Somlzo AV. Calcium and magnesium in vascular smooth muscle function. In: Genest J, Koiw E, Kuchel O, eds. *Hypertension Pathophysiology and Treatment.* New York: McGraw-Hill; 440:1977.

94. Constantopoulos G. Cations and norepinephrine content of arteries in hypertension. In: Genest J, Koiw E, Kuchel O, eds. *Hypertension Pathophysiology and Treatment.* New York: McGraw-Hill; 452:1977.

95. Lang S, Blaustein MP. The role of the sodium pump in the control of vascular tone in the rat. *Circ Res* 46:463, 1980.

96. Ingelfinger JR. *Pediatric Hypertension.* Philadelphia: WB Saunders; 1982.

97. Aoki K, Kondo S, Michizuke A, Yoshida T, Kato S, Kazuaki K,Takikown K. Antihypertensive effect of cardiovascular Ca^{2+}: antagonist in hypertensive patients in the absence and presence of β-adrenergic blockage. *Am Heart J* 96:218, 1978.

98. De Wardener HE. Natriuretic and sodium-transport inhibitory factors associated with volume control and hypertension. In: Mulrow PJ, Schrier R, eds. *Arterial Hormones and Other Natriuretic Factors.* Bethesda: American Physiologic Society; 1987.

99. Valdes R, Graves SW, Brown BA, Landt M. Endogenous substances in newborn infants cause false positive digoxin measurements. *J Pediatr* 102:947, 1983.

100. Adams SP. Structure and biological function of atrial natriuretic peptides. *Endocrinol Metabol Clin North Am* 16:1, 1988.

101. Rascher W, Tulassay T, Lang RE. Atrial natriuretic peptide in plasma of volume-overloaded children with chronic renal failure. *Lancet* 2:303, 1985.

102. Kikuchi K, Nishioka K, Ueda T, Shiomi M, Takahashi Y, Sugawar A, Nakaok Imura H, Mori C, Mikawa H. Plasma atrial natriuretic peptide in patients with congenital heart disease. *J Pediatr* 111:335, 1987.

103. Panza JA, Quyyumi AA, Rush JE, Epstein SE. Abnormal endothelium-dependent vascular relaxation in patients with essential hypertension. *N Engl J Med* 323:22, 1990.

104. Furchgott RF, Vanhoutte PM. Endothelium-derived relaxing and contracting factors. *FASEB* 3:2007, 1989.

105. Ribeiro MO, Antunes E, de Nucci G, Lovisolo SM, Zatz R. Chronic inhibition of nitric oxide synthesis. A new model of arterial hypertension. *Hypertension* 20:298, 1992.

106. Yanagisawa M, Kurihara S, Kumura S, Kobayashi M, Mitsui Y, Yazake Y, Toto K, Masaki T. A novel potent vasoconstrictor peptide produced by vascular endothelial cells. *Nature* 322:411, 1988.

107. Yokokawa K, Tahara H, Murakawa K, Yasunari K, Nakagawa K, Hamada T, Otani S, Yanagisawa M, Takeda T. Hypertension associated with endothelin-secreting malignant hemangioendothelioma. *Ann Intern Med* 114:213, 1991.

108. Luscher TF, Rubanyi GM. Endothelium as a regulator of vascular tone and growth. *Circulation* 87(Suppl 5):V1-V81, 1993.

Chapter 2

Blood Pressure Measurements and Normal Pressure Values

Introduction

Considerable emphasis has been placed on including blood pressure measurements in the physical assessment of every young individual. Yet providers are faced with constraints of time and equipment. Often they are uncertain as to technique and need for the recording. These problems combine to make blood pressure measurements for all children an unattained goal. Despite these obstacles, it remains imperative that blood pressures be taken. Hypertensive tendencies in young patients must be discovered in order to prevent the ravages of this "silent slayer". Otherwise, the patient will suffer needlessly and the practitioner may find that he or she is called to account for not detecting the illness.

Blood pressure recording is serious business. Consider that pressure reflects cardiovascular dynamics. Heart pump function interacts with blood vessel resistance to produce blood flow needed for tissue viability. Derangements of blood pressure can, therefore, result from (or in) abnormalities in many systems. Discovery of a blood pressure outside the normal range signals a search for the cause, which may require the expenditure of significant resources. Inherent in the detection of altered pressure is accuracy of the determination. Not only is it necessary to find the child at risk from blood pressure problems, but also it is important not to label him or her as having a problem when in reality none exists. False-positives are to be condemned for needless cost of time and money.

37

Because so many factors affect the actual recording of the blood pressure, great care must be taken in the interpretation of the readings. Position, activity, fear, time of day, and comfort all can change the blood pressure. Thus, it behooves the observer not to add technical inaccuracies to the mix. Adherence to the listed protocol should be helpful in this regard.

Technique of Blood Pressure Recording

"K" Phases

Most blood pressures are taken using some type of indirect recording method. Properly done, the measurement will usually come within 10 mm Hg of directly measured intra-arterial pressure. With few exceptions, indirect recordings are made using a compression cuff. When compression over an artery is released, waves or sounds are generated which may then be detected by a Doppler or by a listening device. These waves were described by Korotkoff in 1905.[1] The "K" phases are named after those he described. K_1 begins when the first sound is heard. It is generated by arterial flow initiated when the compression cuff pressure is reduced. General agreement exists that this sound is a measure of systolic pressure. The K_4 phase is recognized as a muffling of the sounds with further reduction in cuff pressure while the K_5 phase is a disappearance of the sounds. In pediatric practice, it is common for sounds to persist until the cuff is completely deflated. That is why it is advocated to use the K_4 phase as the diastolic pressure.[2] Since some recommend the K_5 phase for routine measurement[3] and many studies are based on the K_5 phase, a number of authorities[4,5] recommend recording both K_4 and K_5 diastolic pressures in children.

In our practice, K_1 and K_5 are recorded except when K_5 is unclear because of persistent sounds. Then K_4 is used, recognizing that a slightly higher diastolic pressure will result. On the other hand, false-negatives are avoided. False-positives are dealt with by avoiding labeling an individual as having high pressure until a full evaluation protocol is carried out (see Chapter 9).

The Compression Cuff

Selection of the compression cuff is an important technical consideration. Should too small a cuff be used, falsely high readings will result from higher pressure needed to compress the artery.[6] When the cuff is too large, lower readings may occur from loss of arterial pulsation due to increased resistance in the long course under the cuff. The compression cuff achieves its effects through an inflatable bladder. Official American Heart Association policy advises that the cuff bladder be at least 40% of the mid-arm circumference and the length twice the width or 80% of the circumference.[7] Some debate exists on the appropriate bladder measurements.[8,9] Actual practice dictates use of the largest cuff which can be applied to the arm without encroaching on the axillary or antecubital fossae. In large or obese individuals, this may necessitate the use of a large adult cuff or even the so-called thigh cuff. For measurements in the lower extremities, the thigh cuff is used because it is the largest available. However, the accuracy of these readings may be less than optimal. Arm and leg pressures should be similar. The previously held belief that lower extremity pressure is higher has been shown to be in error, perhaps due to use of relatively small cuffs.[10]

Instrumentation

The standard device for biologic pressure measurements is the mercury gravity manometer, the instrument of choice for blood pressure measurement. Mercury manometers serve to calibrate all other systems for pressure recording such as aneroid manometers or strain gauges. Aneroid manometers are subject to mechanical error and must be calibrated at least yearly. Ultrasound measurement methods employing Doppler techniques use manometers which, if not mercury, must be calibrated against the mercury manometer. The Y-connector described in the American Heart Association 1980 Committee report is very satisfactory for all calibrations.[7] Of course, the mercury manometer must be kept vertical and also be checked periodically for clean filters, loss of mercury, and leveling of the mercury column at zero when open to atmospheric pressure.

The attachment of a manometer to the compression cuff and inflation-deflation device constitutes a sphygmomanometer system. It is important that the tubing in the system be monitored for leaks by exposing the secured, rolled cuff to a constant inflation pressure of over 200 mm Hg. The observed pressure should not vary more than a few mm Hg over the next 10 to 15 seconds. The cuff inflation mechanisms should likewise be inspected periodically for smooth function. Sticky valves should be relieved.

A number of instruments in addition to the mercury and aneroid sphygmomanometer are available for pressure measurement. Some are used mainly to measure blood pressure in infants and young children and are detailed in Chapter 8. However, for ease of reference, brief descriptions of them are included among the instruments listed below.

Ultrasound-Doppler Systems

Ultrasound-Doppler systems are based on reflecting sound waves from the pulsating artery.[11] The pulsatile movement changes the frequency of the Doppler signals that, in turn, can be perceived as K_1 when pulsations begin and K_4 when flow becomes more constant. The Doppler signal may be expressed as sound or as digital readout. Systolic Doppler measurements are accurate, but diastolic pressure recordings may not be exact.[12] The Doppler is especially useful in newborns and infants, as well as those in whom auscultation is difficult.

Oscillometric Devices

Oscillometric devices such as those manufactured by the Dinamap-Critikan (Tampa FL), are now widely used to measure pressures in patients in whom conventional methods of recording pressures are not feasible. Such devices have become the mainstay of noninvasive measurements for newborn and infants, and have been found to correlate well with direct arterial measurements.[13]

Strain-Gauge Plethysmography

Strain-gauge plethysmography uses volume changes with each heart pulsation in digits or distal extremities to signal systolic pressure, as the compression cuff is deflated.[14] *Photoelectric plethysmography* can be used to detect skin systolic pressure.[15] *Isotope clearance* can be used to measure muscle systolic pressure by observing isotope washout following pressure cuff release.[16]

Recording Protocol (Table 1.)

Children's Pressures

Blood pressure in children, is generally recorded after the child has been weighed and measured and has relaxed in the exam room

Table 1.

Childhood Blood Pressure Recording Protocol

1. Place patient relaxed in supine position
      arm at level of heart
      older child may be seated with right arm supported
2. Use mercury sphygmomanometer
      in good repair
      mercury column vertical
      meniscus at examiner eye level
3. Proper-sized compression cuff applied snugly to bare right arm
      free of leaks
      occupies entire arm leaving axillary and antecubital fossae free
      bladder encircles 80% of arm *over* artery with width 40% of
      circumference
4. Rapid inflation of cuff to 30 mm Hg above palpated radial pulse
      disappearance
5. Single measurement made by auscultation through gently applied
      stethoscope head over brachial artery in antecubital fossa
6. Cuff deflated 2 to 5 mm Hg/s.
      K_1 (sound appearance) taken as systolic pressure
      K_5 (sound disappearance) taken as diastolic pressure
7. If pressure is greater than 90th percentile or if weak or absent lower
      extremity pulses, take lower extremity pressure
      use a cuff as described in 3, substituting thigh for arm and popliteal for
      antecubital fossa
      use a large "thigh" cuff for large individuals
8. If pressure is similarly "high" in both extremities, arrange for follow-up
      measurement at later date (per Task Force recommendation)
      Avoid labeling patient as hypertensive
9. If blood pressure is greater than 10% above 95th percentile or if an arm
      or leg difference found, begin workup for hypertension

for a few moments. Every effort is made to have the patient seated quietly and comfortably or lying supine because anxiety or activity will elevate the pressure. A compression cuff ofappropriate size for the patient is placed snugly on the right arm, unless reasons compel otherwise. The arm is supported at the level of the heart. Care is taken to ensure that the antecubital fossa is open so the stethoscope head can be applied over the brachial artery without interference from the cuff. The cuff is then inflated while the examiner palpates the brachial pulse and notes its disappearance at a point roughly marking the systolic pressure. The bell stethoscope head is then *gently* applied over the brachial artery in the antecubital fossa. Cuff inflation is then carried out to a point about 20 or 30 mm Hg above the palpated systolic pressure. With the examiner comfortably seated, the cuff is deflated slowly at a rate of 2 to 5 mm Hg per second. Rapid deflation will induce errors. The meniscus of the manometer is kept at the examiner's eye level. Efforts are made to avoid digit preference, that is, mainly recording certain numbers such as those ending in zero or five.

The number of recordings needed to determine a child's blood pressure is a matter of debate. Some authorities advocate taking three pressures and using the average of the three readings or of the last two readings for the patient's pressure measurement.[17-19] Others recommend one recording only.[20,21] The truth is that 24-hour recordings[22] or frequent home blood pressure measurements[23] probably more accurately represent the individual patient's blood pressure status. However, since pediatric experience and data are not widely available, these techniques usually are not used in the young. The most practical solution is to take a single reading in the general examination situation. Our own data indicate little difference between the first reading and subsequent readings (Table 2) in either black or white children. Among the white patients, only the seated systolic pressure readings differed between the first and subsequent recordings. Among

Table 2.
Comparisons of Resting Blood Pressures

Systolic Blood Pressures

1st BP Taken				Mean of All 3 BPs		Mean of 2nd & 3rd BPs		
	Mean	SD	$(p)^1$	Mean	SD	Mean	SD	$(p)^2$
All Subjects (N = 168)								
Seated	103.5 ± 11.2		NS	103.7 ± 10.8		103.9 ± 10.8		NS
Supine	106.4 ± 10.3		(.03)	107.0 ± 10.8		107.2 ± 11.3		(.03)

Diastolic Blood Pressures

1st BP Taken				Mean of All 3 BPs		Mean of 2nd & 3rd BPs		
All Subjects (N = 168)								
Seated	70.9 ± 10.0		NS	70.9 ± 9.9		71.0 ± 9.9		NS
Supine	72.2 ± 9.2		NS	71.9 ± 9.0		71.8 ± 9.0		NS

$(p)^1$ = "p" values for comparison of 1st blood pressure taken with mean of all 3 blood pressures.
$(p)^2$ = "p" values for comparison of 1st blood pressure taken with mean of 2nd and 3rd blood pressures taken.

the blacks, only the standing pressure differed. Thus, it is our advice that, initially, a single blood pressure measurement be made.[24] In a busy practice this can save considerable time.

If the initial blood pressure is at or above the 90th percentile for age (Table 3), pressure is then recorded with a large cuff on one lower extremity. If this second initial pressure measurement remains outside the expected range for the patient, arrangements are made to sample the pressure further at another time, as recommended by the report of the Task Force on Blood Pressure Control.[2] If a discrepancy is found between upper and lower extremity pressure, steps must be taken to confirm or deny the existence of coarctation of the aorta. Should the pressure persist above the 95th percentile, a hypertensive workup should be initiated as recommended in Chapter 9. Where possible, one should avoid labeling an individual as hypertensive, for emotional, school, insurance, military, and employment consequences are great. Most elevated pressures will regress on subsequent readings. The protocol for recording blood pressure in children is summarized in Table 1.

Measuring Pressure in Newborns and Infants

Technical difficulties with auscultatory methods and frustrations with the crying baby preclude routine measurement of blood pressure in this age group. Yet, there are a number of clinical situations, particularly in the sick infant with circulatory impair-

Table 3.
Blood Pressure Values for the 90th Percentile
(Task Force Report) [2]
(Lowest Value for Either Boys or Girls Given)

Age Group (yr)	Systolic BP (mm Hg)	Diastolic BP (mm Hg)
Newborn (8–30 d)	98	65
Infant (<2)	105	68
Child (2–5)	109	68
Child (6–9)	115	74
Child (10–12)	121	77
Adoles (13–15)	125	79
Adoles (16–18)	127	84

adoles = adolescent.

ment, where measurement of the blood pressure provides vital information. In other circumstances, hypertension from renal, cerebral, or other causes must be detected and treated. It behooves the clinician, therefore, to take the blood pressure when any of the situations listed in Table 4 are present. As previously noted, a number of techniques and instruments can aid in noninvasive pressure measurement in the very young.

Ultrasound-Doppler

Formerly, the most widely used technique for infant blood pressure recording ultrasound- Doppler methods remains an accurate way to record infant blood pressure.[25-27] As mentioned, many Doppler systems, like oscillometric devices, give a digital readout. All that is necessary is to select and properly apply the appropriate compression cuff. A variety of very adequate Doppler systems have been marketed. Cost has become a factor in instrument selection. However, relatively inexpensive Doppler probes, which generate sounds equivalent to the K sounds of a stethoscope, are available and can be used in conjunction with a conventional mercury manometer system.

Flush Technique

A less expensive alternative is the flush technique of measuring infant blood pressures. Although less accurate and furnishing a

Table 4.
Conditions in Which Taking the Blood
Pressure is Advisable[2]

Presence of a heart murmur
Presence of heart failure
Finding weak or absent distal pulses
History of umbilical artery catheterization
Finding of tumors or neurofibromatosis
History of seizures
Failure to thrive
Finding gonadal abnormalities
Finding electrolyte abnormalities
Presence of major fracture or burns
Therapy with steroids

rough mean pressure reading only, it is nonetheless satisfactory for ambulatory clinical practice.[28] The flush method works best with two examiners. The first wraps the distal limb (hand or foot) with a pressure bandage to drain the extremity of blood. Simple hand compression of an infant's hand may suffice. The second examiner applies an inflated infant blood pressure cuff to around 160 mm Hg. The pressure cuff is then deflated while monitoring the pressure. The first observer removes the bandage and watches the blanched limb. When circulation returns to the extremity, a ruddy "flush" is seen. This event is marked by recording the blood pressure at that moment. The method is particularly useful in recording simultaneous upper and lower extremity pressure with both cuffs connected to the same manometer by a Y-tube. Having a third person available to watch for flushing of one of the limbs is helpful. Use of the flush technique presupposes an adequate circulation in the extremity. Anemia and excessive skin pigmentation make the method difficult.

Oscillometric Method

As already mentioned, the technique of oscillometry has been refined for measuring blood pressure in newborns.[13] With instruments such as the Dinamap pulsatile oscillations of the manometer corresponding to the onset of systole are magnified and can be recorded as the pressure. The accuracy and lower cost of these devices have largely replaced ultrasound-Doppler methods for general recording of blood pressure, but Doppler devices survive for use in intensive care settings and in some peripheral vascular work.

Ambulatory Blood Pressure Monitoring

Improved devices are available for recording blood pressures up to longer than 24 hours. Such instruments use auscultatory, oscillometric, or fingertip pulse technology.[29,30] Recordings are reasonably accurate, but about 10% to 20% must be discarded because of technical imperfections. Carefully recorded ambulatory blood pressures show good agreement with those obtained by conventional auscultatory methods[31] and are reasonably reproducible.[32] While pediatric data are relatively sparse,[33] increasing information regarding adults is becoming available.[34] Major uses of the ambulatory blood pressure monitoring (ABPM) are for epidemiologic studies, establishing individual patient drug-action duration, avoidance of "white coat hypertension," and cardiovascular risk assessment. At present, there are no long-term studies showing that ABPM is superior to carefully taken office or home blood pressures.[35]

Normal Blood Pressures

Resting Pressures

It is a generally held notion that blood pressure increases with age through childhood and that adults have higher blood pressures than children. Yet argument exists whether this should be so.[36] Evidence favoring minimal blood pressure change with age centers about studies in primitive peoples.[37] In adult circles, there is also ongoing debate as to the definition of hypertension. The World Health Organization defines normotension as pressure less than 140 mm Hg systolic and less than 90 mm Hg diastolic, and hypertension as greater than 160 mm Hg systolic and greater than 95 mm Hg diastolic. Pressures in between are considered borderline. However, these criteria do not vary with age or sex and are felt to be too high.[38] Pickering has disagreed with the concept of an arbitrary separation marking hypertension.[39] He believed that "there is no dividing line" rather, the process must be taken in context.

When examining the blood pressures of young people, most authorities accept the "dividing line" as pressures above the 95th percentile for age as indicating high blood pressure. The problem is that of the variability of the 95th percentile found in different studies of blood pressures from young people, especially for the diastolic readings.[40] The discrepancies may be explainable partially by technical differences such as the degree of relaxation of the subjects, the recording device used, and the use of the K_4 phase which may overestimate or the K_5 phase which underestimates diastolic pressure.[41] Fixler has examined these differences in detail and concludes that the variability in protocols made comparisons difficult.[42]

The 1987 publication of the Second Task Force Report presented "normal" blood pressure distribution grids based on data from several geographic areas and from several racial groups.[2] Blood pressure values were assessed by age, as well as by height. From this information, an algorithm was proposed to judge normal blood pressure. The pressures, sampled by differing protocols, were taken from various study populations some of whom perhaps became anxious as they stood in line waiting to have their pressures measured. Nevertheless, the Task Force "normal" blood pressure distribution grids furnish useful levels on which to base decisions such as the need for follow-up measurements or workup. The pressures are felt to represent situations found in ambulatory clinical practice, rather than "basal" survey type measurements.[43]

In our hypertensive progeny study, when the first seated blood pressure measurements from children aged 10 to 18 of hypertensive parents and their age-matched controls[44] were plotted on the Task Force grids, both the mean (50th percentile) and 95th percentile measurements for systole and diastole in males and females were lower than the corresponding Task Force grid values. It was felt that this represented our study protocol effort to allay anxiety and perhaps is a geographic influence. At any rate, these data give further credence to the use of the Task Force grids as high "normal" levels. The admonition of the Task Force to repeat the measurement of the blood pressure of anyone at or above the 95th percentile on two other separate occasions still holds, as noted in the reproduction of the Task Force algorithm in Figure 1.

With the Task Force standards expressed as percentiles for age, the familiar pattern found in growth grids is followed. This is easy for primary health-care providers to adopt. It should, however, be noted that the blood pressures are correlated with height and that tall individuals with blood pressures above the 90th percentile are probably normal as noted in the Second Task Force on Blood Pressure Control.[2] Other workers have developed percentile grids using such parameters to relate to blood pressure.[45] Mention must also be made that blood pressures should *not* be expected to "track" in channel on the grid as do height and weight. More will be said of the tracking, but the grid should be used to screen out those who are repeatedly above the 95th percentile only. Another note should be made of the effort to express blood pressure in "Systeme International" (SI) units, that is, the kiloPascals (kPa), using the formula kPa = mm Hg/7.5. The American Heart Association currently advises against using the kPa.[46]

Exercise Blood Pressures

More and more emphasis is being placed on physical fitness. At the same time, an awareness of testing exercising young

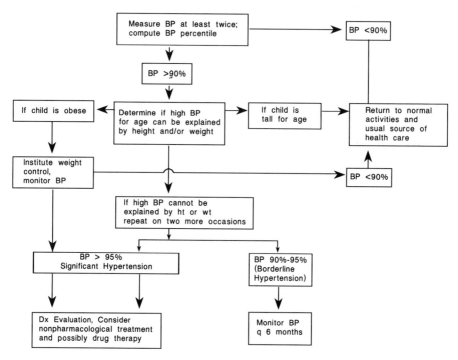

Figure 1: This algorithm has been modified from the United States Task Force Report[2] to aid the practitioner in patient blood pressure surveillance and management. Additional algorithms using these concepts are presented in Figure 1 of Chapter 10.

individuals has developed. The exercise test permits assessment of physical capabilities as well as the impact of training and treatments on these capabilities. Blood pressure ranks high among the measurements made during exercise testing. Normal data are being accumulated, again, for the most part, expressed as percentile for age. While exercise testing is best left to the specialized laboratory, it behooves the practitioner to be acquainted with the values obtained. The pediatric stress exercise laboratory at the Medical University of South Carolina has established "norms" for selected size groups using the treadmill (Fig. 2).[47] Others have established "norms" for the bicycle ergometer.[48] In either method, maximum exercise blood pressures in excess of 215 mm Hg are suspect for hypertensive tendencies.

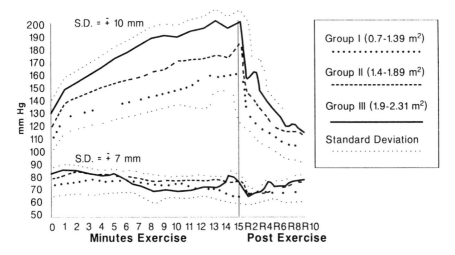

Figure 2: The exercise and recovery blood pressure data, summarized by size group in this figure,[47] indicate that adolescents may normally have systolic pressures of about 200 mm Hg with maximum treadmill exercise. Diastolic pressure usually declines or changes little. Those patients who respond with pressures +2 SD (97th percentile) above the plotted information may have hypertensive tendencies.

Summary

Measurement of blood pressure is a most important component of the physical assessment of infants, children, and young people. A variety of instruments are available for this task. While oscillometric instruments are best for infants, the mercury sphygmomanometer is advocated for children and young people. Selection of a proper blood pressure cuff cannot be over emphasized. Care should be taken to have the patient relaxed for the recording. A single, carefully made resting reading from the right arm as outlined in the recording protocol is satisfactory for most individuals (Table 1). Task Force percentile grids furnish useful comparisons for pediatric pressure measurements. Those outside the 95th percentile deserve further consideration, but labeling an infant or child as hypertensive should be avoided, at least initially.

References

1. Geddes LA, Hoff HE, Gadger AS. Introduction of the auscultatory method of measuring blood pressure: including a translation of Korotkoff's original paper. *Cardiovasc Res Cent Bull* 5:557-74, 1966.

2. National Heart, Lung, and Blood Institute's Task Force on Blood Pressure Control in Children. Report of the second task force on blood pressure control in children. *Pediatrics* 79:1-25, 1987.

3. Moser M. Report of the Joint National Committee on detection, evaluation, and treatment of high blood pressure: a cooperative study. *J Am Med Asssoc* 237:255-261, 1977.

4. Lieberman E. Blood pressure and primary hypertension in childhood and adolescence. *Curr Problems Pediatr* 10:1-35,1980.

5. Ingelfinger JR. *Pediatric Hypertension*. Philadelphia: WB Saunders; 1982.

6. Moss AJ, Adams FH. Auscultatory and intra-arterial pressure: a comparison in children with special reference to cuff width. *J Pediatr* 66:1094-1097, 1965.

7. Kirkendall WM, Feinleib M, Freis ED, Mark AL. Recommendations for human blood pressure determination by sphygmomanometers (American Heart Association Committee Report). *Circulation* 62:1147A, 1980.

8. Burch GE, Shewey L. Sphygmomanometric cuff size and blood pressure recordings. *JAMA* 3;225:1215-1218, 1973.

9. Steinfeld L, Alexander H, Cohen ML. Updating sphygmomanometry. *Am J Cardiol* 33:107-110, 1974.

10. Park MK, Guntheroth WC. Direct blood pressure measurements in brachial and femoral arteries in children. *Circulation* 41:231-237, 1970.

11. Stegall HF, Kardon HB, Kemmerer WT. Indirect measurement of arterial pressure by Doppler-ultrasonic sphygmomanometry. *J Appl Physiol* 25:793-798, 1968.

12. Lieberman E. Hypertension in childhood and adolescence. In: Kaplan NM. *Clinical Hypertension, 3rd ed.* Baltimore: Williams & Wilkins; 413:1982.

13. Colan SD, Fujii A, Borow KM, MacPherson D, Sanders SP. Noninvasive determination of systolic, diastolic and end-systolic blood pressure in neonates, infants and young children: comparison with central aortic pressure measurements. *Am J Cardiol* 52:867-870, 1983.

14. Nielsen PE, Bell G, Lassen NA. The measurement of digital systolic blood pressure by strain-gauge technique. *Scand J Clin Lab Invest* 29:371-379, 1972.

15. Nielsen PE, Poulsen NI, Gynteberg F. Arterial blood pressure in the skin measured by photoelectric probe and external counter pressure. *Vasa* 2:65-74, 1973.

16. Dahn I, Lassen NA, Westling H. Blood flow in human muscles during external pressure or venous stasis. *Clin Sci* 32:467- 473, 1967.

17. Goldring D, Londe S, Sivakoff M, Hernandez A, Britton C, Choi S. Blood pressure in a high school population: standards for blood pressure and the relation of age, sex, weight, height,and race to blood pressure in children 14 to 18 years of age.*J Pediatr* 91:884-889, 1977.

18. Moss AJ. Indirect methods of blood pressure measurement.*Pediatr Clin North Am* 25:3-14, 1978.

19. Prineas RJ, Gillum RF, Horibe H, Hannan PJ. The Minneapolis Children's Blood Pressure Study, Part I: Standards of measurement for children's blood pressure. *Hypertension* 2:I18-24, 1980.
20. Lauer RM, Connor WE, Leaverton PE, Reiter MA, Clarke WR. Coronary heart disease risk factors in school children: the Muscatine study. *J Pediatr* 86:697-706, 1975.
21. Fixler DE, Laird WP, Fitzgerald V, Steed S, Adams R. Hypertension screening in schools: results of the Dallas study. *Pediatrics* 63:32-36, 1979.
22. Sokolow M, Perloff D, Cowar R. Contribution of ambulatory blood pressure to the assessment of patients with mild to moderate elevation of office blood pressure. *Cardiovasc Rev Rep* 1:295, 1980.
23. Loggie JMH. Hypertension in children and adolescents. *Hosp Pract* 10:81, 1975.
24. Hohn AR, Riopel DA, Loadhold CD. Which blood pressure? *J Pediatr* 104:89-91, 1984.
25. Hernandez A, Goldring D, Hartmann AF Jr. Measurement of blood pressure in infants and children by Doppler ultrasonic technique. *Pediatrics* 48:788-794, 1971.
26. Black IFS, Kotrapu N, Massie H. Application of Doppler ultrasound to blood pressure measurements in small infants. *J Pediatr* 81:932-935, 1972.
27. Gordon LS, Johnson PE Jr, Penido JR, Printup CA Jr, Dietrick WR, Buggs H. Systolic and diastolic blood pressure measurements by transcutaneous Doppler ultrasound in premature infants in critical care nurseries and at closed heart surgery. *Anesth Analg* 53:914-918, 1974.
28. Moss AJ, Liebling W, Austin WO, Adams FH. An evaluation of the flush method for determining blood pressures in infants. *Pediatrics* 20:53, 1957.
29. The National High Blood Pressure Education Program Working Group report on ambulatory blood pressure monitoring. *Arch Intern Med* 150:2270-2280, 1990.
30. Imholz BPM, Langewouters GJ, van Montfrans GA, Parati G, van Goudoever J, Wesseling KH, Wieling W, Mancia G. Feasibility of ambulatory, continuous 24-hour finger arterial pressure recording. *Hypertension* 21:65-73, 1993.
31. Berglund G, DeFaire U, Castenfors J, Anderson G, Hartford M, Liedholm H, Ljungman S, Thulin T, Wikstrand J. Monitoring 24-hour blood pressure in a drug trial: evaluation of a noninvasive device. *Hypertension* 7:688-694, 1985.
32. Weber M, Drayer J, Nakamurs DK, Wyle FA. The circadian blood pressure pattern in ambulatory normal subjects. *Am J Cardiol* 54:115-119, 1984.
33. Fixler DE, Wallace JM, Thornton WE, Dimmitt P. Ambulatory blood pressure monitoring in hypertensive adolescents. *Am J Hypertens* 3:288-292, 1990.

34. Brunner HR, Waeber B. *Ambulatory Blood Pressure Recording.* New York: Raven Press; 1992.
35. Moser M. Ambulatory BP monitoring: a useful procedure or an unnecessary expense? *Hosp Pract* 27:12-15, 1992. Editorial.
36. Adams FH. Blood pressure of children in the United States. *Pediatrics* 61:931-932, 1978.
37. Beaglehole R, Salmond CE, Eyles EF. A longitudinal study of blood pressure in Polynesian children. *Am J Epidemiol* 105:87-89, 1977.
38. Kaplan NM. *Clinical Hypertension, 3rd ed.* Baltimore: Williams & Wilkins; 2:1982.
39. Pickering G. Hypertension: definitions, natural histories, and consequences. *Am J Med* 52:570-583, 1972.
40. Leumann EP. Blood pressure and hypertension in childhood and adolescence. *Ergeb Inn Med Inderheilkd* 43:109-183, 1979.
41. Ibsen KK. Normal and abnormal blood pressure in childhood. *Child Nephrol Urol* 12:90-95, 1992.
42. Fixler DE, Kautz JA, Dana K. Systolic blood pressure differences among pediatric epidemiologic studies. *Hypertension* 2:13-17, 1980.
43. Blumenthal S, Lauer RM. Where are children's blood pressures headed? *Hypertension* 3:46-47, 1981. Editorial.
44. Hohn AR, Riopel DA, Keil JE, Loadholt CB, Margolius HS, Halushka PV, Privitera PJ, Ebee JG, Medley ES, Schuman SH, Rubin MI, Pantell RH, Braunstein ML. Childhood familial and racial differences in physiologic and biochemical factors related to hypertension. *Hypertension* 5:56-70, 1983.
45. Voors AW, Webber LS, Berenson GS. Epidemiology of essential hypertension in youth: implications for clinical practice. *Pediatr Clin North Am* 25:15-27, 1978.
46. Ingelfinger JR. *Pediatric Hypertension.* Philadelphia: WB Saunders; 108:1982.
47. Riopel DA, Taylor AB, Hohn AR. Blood pressure, heart rate, pressure: rate product and electrocardiographic changes in healthy children during treadmill exercise. *Am J Cardiol* 44:697-704, 1979.
48. James FW, Kaplan S, Glueck CJ, Tsay JY, Knight MJ, Sarwar CJ. Responses of normal children and young adults to controlled bicycle exercise. *Circulation* 61:902-912, 1980.

Chapter 3

The Epidemiology of Hypertension in Young People

Introduction

Epidemiology has been defined as the science that deals with the incidence, distribution, and control of a disease in a population. It considers the many factors which control the presence or absence of a pathologic process.[1] Thus, considerations of the epidemiology of hypertension must focus on the influences of the disorder and the population in which the influences are found. In young people, the problem is complicated by the difficulty of defining hypertension. As noted in Chapter 2, no unanimity of opinion exists. However, it has become customary to define pediatric hypertension when the blood pressure is greater than the 95th percentile on three separate occasions. This definition may overestimate the presence of the disorder by including some children who are normal but have pressures at the upper end of the spectrum incidence.[2] Indeed, the vast majority of children with blood pressures outside the usual range will be asymptomatic. Some young people will be labeled as hypertensive solely on the basis of a persistent elevation of blood pressure. However, based on extrapolation from adult studies such as the Framingham,[3] and from limited information available from young people followed over time,[4] such individuals appear to be at risk for catastrophic events in later life and therefore justify the label.

53

Prevalence

Hypertension has been classified as primary (essential) where no etiology is obvious, and secondary when a cause can be found. As more large surveys are reported, it is becoming clear that primary hypertension is far more common than other forms of the disorder. The survey of Dallas school children found that 1.6% of 10,641 children were hypertensive after three screens.[5] In the Muscatine study, 41 of 6622 children were hypertensive after four screens.[6] Kilcoyne found 1.2% of 3537 Harlem youths who had systolic hypertension on repeated screens.[7] From these and other studies,[8,9] the prevalence of primary hypertension is estimated to be 0.5% to 2.0% of the school age population. Involved individuals generally do not have symptoms and may be considered to have mild, but significant hypertension.[10]

In contrast, the child with secondary hypertension most often will have symptoms such as headaches, nausea and vomiting, and convulsions. Generally, the level of pressure elevation is much higher in secondary than primary hypertension during childhood. Contrary to previous opinions, secondary hypertension is less common in an epidemiologic sense than is primary hypertension. Leumann estimated the prevalence of secondary hypertension to be 0.1% on the basis of data from five surveys.[2] Information assembled in his review found 74% of secondary hypertension was due to renal disorders (with 7% from renovascular causes). Nineteen percent were from coarctation of the aorta, and all other causes comprised 7%, among which were 1% to 2% with endocrine-caused hypertension. When considering the causes of secondary hypertension it is best to group them by relation to age. For example, coarctation of the aorta and thrombosis-induced renovascular hypertension are more common in newborns whereas renal causes predominate in children and adolescents.

Individuals with secondary hypertension frequently have required medical attention in childhood whereas those with primary hypertension often have not. Thus, the true prevalence of the different etiologies of hypertension has been obscured. The data from the Muscatine study,[6] as well as studies by Gill,[11] Briedigkeit,[12] Pistulkova,[13] and Strunge and Trostmann[14] all suggest that the prevalence of secondary hypertension is less than one-fifth that of primary hypertension. Accordingly, the major portion of this chapter will be devoted to the epidemiologic factors related to primary hypertension. Factors related to secondary hypertension will be covered in ensuing chapters.

Age

Blood pressure is known to increase with age in a nonlinear fashion. In the newborn, systolic pressure increases until about 1 month of age, when a plateau begins.[15] At about age 6 years, blood pressure again gradually increases,[10] but then tapers somewhat during late adolescence and early adulthood. Thereafter, a steady increase again occurs.[16] With the use of percentile criteria, a segment of each population will be listed as hypertensive. This, however, can be reduced by taking blood pressure readings on three separate occasions prior to labeling an individual as hypertensive. While primary hypertension has been reported in the first decade of life,[10,17] it is the adolescent who has received the focus of pediatric attention with respect to blood pressure. A number of surveys have been carried out in this age group.[5,7,8,18,19] The identification of a number of young people as hypertensive, on the basis of three separate blood pressure recordings, may indicate a group requiring treatment.[20] However, this has not yet been proven.[21] It is thought that primary hypertension is commonly detected from the ages of 20 to 40 years, and such individuals may not develop symptoms for another 10 to 15 years.[22] The summary in Figure 1 indicates the general sequence. Whether those who will develop the disorder in later years can be detected in childhood is a question of great consequence which has yet to be answered.[23]

Tracking

Perhaps the best single predictor for blood pressure level in later years is an individual's current or previous blood pressure.[24] Considerable effort has been used to determine whether a young person's blood pressure will maintain the same percentile rank or "track" over time. Adult studies from Framingham show a correlation coefficient of 0.6 for two measurements taken 2 years apart. This indicates a 36% chance of predicting blood pressure 2 years hence ($[0.6]^2 \times 100$).[25] The blood pressure data from the children of Bogalusa, Louisiana, after statistical manipulation, revealed similar

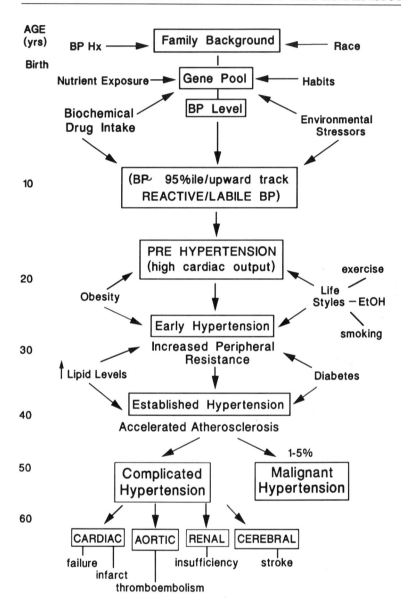

Figure 1: The natural history of hypertension (in the boxes) and the epidemiologic factors associated with it (impact arrows). Age, in log scale, is given at the left vertical margin beginning with birth. However, it can be seen that preconception factors are important as well. The epidemiologic factors offer points at which the disorder may be modified.

correlations.[26] In a study of children moving across cultures, Beagle-hole was able to demonstrate tracking of systolic blood pressure.[27] In contrast, the Muscatine study found 0.3 systolic and 0.18 diastolic correlation for school children followed over a 6-year period.[28] Our own information is similar (Table 1). About half of those who had blood pressures in the top one-fourth of their group again had blood pressures in the top one-fourth when another measurement was made 2 years later.[29] Position and activity did not make much difference. This information appears to indicate that, while tracking does occur in childhood, its usefulness in predicting later primary hypertension may be limited to certain groups. Nonetheless, if an individual's pressure is repeatedly in the upper percentiles or tending upward that person should be suspect for adult onset primary hypertension.[30]

Familial and Genetic Influences

Relationship between heredity and hypertension was first sum-marized by Ayman in 1934.[31] He noted that hereditary factors had been known since 1876. Subsequent workers have added consider-able additional information,[32,33] but it is clear that we still lack a full understanding of the nature of hereditary influences.

Animal studies, mainly in rats, demonstrate definite genetic factors in hypertension, but transposing this information to humans is difficult.[34] Platt has suggested an incompletely dominant autoso-mal inheritance,[35] while Pickering[36] in 1967, and Loggie[24] in 1982,

Table 1.
Two-Year Blood Pressure Comparisons*

BP Measured	% Still in Top ¼
Seated	60
Supine	52
Standing	63
Max exercise	51
Postexercise	56

*Comparisons of blood pressures taken 2 years apart in 35 adolescents who were in the top quar-ter of the blood pressure distribution at the time of the first measurement.[29]

favored a polygenic inheritance. It is now generally accepted that numerically defined blood pressure (e.g., 95th percentile) is not caused by disorder of a single gene).[33] Rather, there are genetic determinants of blood pressure. Most evidence for the hereditary influence of hypertension centers on family studies as reported early by Ayman[31] and more recently by a number of workers,[2,3,26,34-40] and studies in twins.[35,41]

The classic study of Zinner and colleagues found blood pressure comparisons of siblings with their parents to vary less than when compared with other children.[38] This familial aggregation of pressures was found as early as age 2 years and remained constant over the 8 years of their study. In another landmark study, the Montreal group noted that blood pressures found in adopted children of the same racial and ethnic background did not correlate with their adoptive parents whereas those of natural children did.[42] The pressures of adoptive and natural siblings had some degree of correlation, but this was thought to be on the basis of similar weight. Feinleib and coworkers[41] summarized parent-offspring blood pressure correlation coefficients as 0.24 and 0.27 for systolic and diastolic pressures respectively, whereas parent-adoptive child was 0.003 and 0.009. Sibling-sibling coefficients were 0.24 and 0.23, which was similar to those found in dizygotic twins (0.27 to 0.40). However, in monozygotic twins, the coefficients were 0.54. The summary encompassed both adults and childhood age groups and was felt to indicate a genetic contribution to the determination of blood pressure between 30% and 50%.

Thus, there is nearly universal agreement that a family history of hypertension indicates a signal to follow the concerned family member(s) for the disorder. In our own biracial hypertensive progeny study, black children of hypertensive parents had higher pressures than black children of normotensive parents. Among the whites, however, this separation was not clear.[43]

Racial Considerations

About 27% of black adults have hypertension. This known prevalence of black adult hypertension is almost twice as great as in white adults.[44] Yet, in children and young people, the picture of racial prevalence is not so clear. In older studies from Evans County,

Georgia, McDonough and coworkers noted in 1964 that black youths aged 15-24 had higher pressures than whites.[45] Likewise, Kilcoyne and colleagues[7] found among inner city youths that black males had a higher prevalence of persistent diastolic hypertension. In contrast, Goldring and his associates found higher pressures in white high school students in St. Louis,[46] while Zinner and colleagues found no racial differences.[47] In Dallas adolescents, Fixler's group found only minor differences in the persistence of pressure elevations among three ethnic groups.[5] In the Bogalusa study, blacks were found to have slightly, but consistently higherblood pressures than whites. However, this difference was only significant in those at or above the upper-fifth percentile of the blood pressure stratum.[48] Harshfield and coworkers found a reduced nocturnal blood pressure decline among young blacks.[49] This suggested that possible alterations in the renin-angiotensin-aldosterone system, as well as in renal sodium excretion, were the basis for the differences. In our study of hypertensive progeny, black children of hypertensive parents had higher pressures than black children of normotensive parents and higher pressures than corresponding white children.[43] These differences persisted even after weight adjustments. However, pressures of black children of normotensive parents did not differ from corresponding white children (Table 2). Racial differences in humoral substances were also found.

At about age 25, higher blood pressures are found in blacks ascompared to whites. Because African blacks do not have a high frequency of hypertension, environmental influences have been postulated to play a major role in the hypertension found in American blacks.[50] The early mechanisms of hypertension in blacks may be different from those in whites.[51] Blacks as a group have lower plasma-renin activity, higher sodium, and lower potassium excretion, lower kallikrein excretion, and tend to have lower heart rates, especially in the higher blood pressure stratum.[43,52] A renal mechanism may be operational in blacks, whereas whites as a group have higher plasma-renin activity, tend to have higher norepinephrine values, and higher heart rates. They may have an overactive sympathetic nervous system mechanism which may be a precursor to hypertension.[53] Blacks in the United States may handle sodium and potassium differently than whites.

From this information, certain implications are suggested.First, the subgroup of blacks from hypertensive families may have a greater tendency to develop hypertension in later life than other

Table 2.
Blood Pressure (mm Hg) and Sodium Excretion (mEq/2h) Comparisons[†]

Hypertensive Black Progeny (B-HBP)

Subjects	Number	Seated	Supine	Max Ex	Na Excrete
		vs Normotensive Black Progeny (B-NBP)			
B-HBP	42	108/75	111/77	175/93	23.8
significance:		**/*	**/*	NS/*	NS
B-NBP	20	99/70	104/72	174/88	21.7
		vs Hypertensive White Progeny (W-HBP)			
W-HBP	34	104/69	107/70	161/87	15.3
significance:		NS/**	*/**	*/**	**
		vs Normotensive White Progeny (W-NBP)			
W-NBP	45	102/70	104/70	160/89	14.6
significance:		*/*	**/**	**/NS	**

* = $P < 0.05$; ** = $P < 0.005$; NS = P; not significant; Max Ex = maximum exercise BP.
†Data from Charleston, S.C. Hypertensive Progeny Study[43]

blacks, as well as whites. Second, both the black children of hypertensive parents and those black youths in high blood pressure strata need to be evaluated and followed carefully. Lastly, should overt hypertension develop, early intervention based on the particular mechanisms involved may be indicated. This may be especially true for diabetic blacks. There is an increased susceptibility to end-stage renal disease in blacks affected with noninsulin-dependent diabetes, as compared with whites.[54]

Obesity

In young people, body weight correlates with blood pressure.[55,56] Weight reflects both growth or physiologic maturity and adipose tissue. Whereas normal skeletal muscle growth (lean body mass) is physiologic, increased body fatness is not. Therefore, it is important to separate these components when assessing their impact on blood pressure.[55] In primitive societies, weight and blood pressure increase with maturation. However, once adult status is reached, weight and pressure remain constant.[57,58] Triceps skin-fold thickness may be considered a measure of fatness. Since weight/height^2 (Quetelet's index) correlates in a similar manner to skin-fold thickness with blood pressure, it may be substituted for the skin-fold measurements. These measures are often used when speaking of obesity or fatness.

Data from the Tecumseh study revealed that the prevalence of all forms of hypertension were highest in those who were in the top quintile for fatness, 15 years earlier.[59] Correlations were found between blood pressure and both fatness and change in fatness. Others report similar findings.[60] In primitive peoples, weight decreases with age after maturity and blood pressure does not rise.[61]

Obesity appears to have a limited, although definite, contribution to blood pressure. If weights were reduced in everyone to less than 20% above desired weight, it is estimated there would be a decrease in the prevalence of hypertension of 30% to 50%.[59] Dallas adolescents with blood pressures above the 95th percentile who weighed 40% more than their group median weight (based on their age, height, and sex) were found to have a 28% chance of having their blood pressure remain elevated on subsequent checks.[62] Those with similar pressures, but lower weights, had a much lower prevalence of persistent hypertension. Obese children from obese families may form a special group that requires continued observation for blood pressure elevation.[63] Weight control in young people may be beneficial in such individuals for its preventive effect on hypertension.

Dietary Influence

Sodium

While numerous animal studies confirm the relationship of sodium intake to blood pressure in animals,[64-66] the relationship in humans is less clear. In societies with known low blood pressure, low sodium intake is the rule and hypertension is almost nonexistent. When people from these traditional, non-Western cultures migrate to the Western world, blood pressure rises with the acculturation.[67] High sodium intake societies appear to favor a high incidence of hypertension. Thus, in Akita, Japan, very heavy salt ingestion is related to hypertension.[68] On the other hand, not all societies with high sodium intake have a high incidence of hypertension. For example, Thailand farmers are reported to have relatively low blood pressure in spite of high salt intake.[69] Many of the studies cited in these reports were poorly executed, as they were based on *estimates* of dietary intake of sodium. More recently, workers in Framingham found no relationship between blood pressure and sodium excretion. The latter is felt to be the most acceptable measure of sodium intake.[70] Simpson was skeptical of the relationship of salt to hypertension,[71] as were Holden and coworkers in a study of 2.1 million Connecticut residents.[72] McCarron and colleagues analyzed data from 10,372 persons over age 18 years and found that those with higher sodium intakes actually had lower blood pressures.[73] These inconsistencies led to a large international cooperative study of blood pressure and electrolyte excretion involving both high- and low-salt intake cultures: the Intersalt Study.[74] Fifty-two centers in 32 countries studied10,079 adult subjects. Both sodium excretion (= intake) and sodium-potassium ratio and systolic blood pressure were positively related significantly. Diastolic relationships were weak and, in certain subgroups, for example women aged 20 to 39 years, the relationships were not significant. The four low-salt cultures included all had low blood pressures with virtually absent hypertension.

The case for sodium influence on blood pressure is even more tenuous in children. Dietary manipulation of salt intake by Gillum and coworkers in children with blood pressures over the 95th percentile failed to lower the pressures.[75] Likewise, feeding black infants a low sodium diet failed to change blood pressure with respect to another group which was fed higher sodium diets.[76] Lauer's group could not find significant correlation between salt preference and blood pressure.[77] However, Zinner found that babies who were more responsive to salt-taste stimuli had higher blood pressures.[78] Hoffman, Hazebroke, and Valkenburg compared newborn infants fed a low-sodium formula with those on a regular formula. Those on the low-sodium formula had lower blood pressures than those fed the "normal" sodium formula over the first 6 months of life.[79] At age 4, no differences in the blood pressures of the two groups were found.[80] The reasons for these desperate findings are not clear, but methodologic problems have been cited.[81]

Several workers have proposed that, as in animals, individuals may be salt sensitive.[82,83] With salt loading, black adults were found to have a greater increase in blood pressures than did whites.[84] Voors and coworkers found a positive correlation between sodium excretion and blood pressure in black Bogalusa children in the high blood pressure stratum.[52] In our studies of Charleston, South Carolina children from hypertensive families, blacks were found to have higher pressures than the black children from normotensive families and the white children from both normo- and hypertensive parents (Table 2). The black progeny of both normo- and hypertensive parents excreted larger amounts of sodium than the white children.[43] The finding that all of the black progeny studied had high-sodium intake (excretion = intake), but only the children of hypertensive parents had higher blood pressures, is compatible with the idea that black children from hypertensive families may be salt sensitive. Thus, while high levels of sodium intake may not have a general causal relationship to hypertension,[62] it may be well to seek subsets of the young population who are salt sensitive for whom the preventive measure of reduced sodium intake would be beneficial. However, other cations must also be considered (see below).

Potassium

A number of investigators have noted a relationship of potassium intake to blood pressure both in animals and humans.[66,73,85-88] Enhanced potassium intake was found to correlate with lower blood pressure or to prevent excessive pressure rise with sodium load. However, despite the fact that potassium is the major cellular cation, little knowledge exists of its role in blood pressure regulation. Indeed, some authors have largely overlooked potassium in their considerations of diet and blood pressure in infants and children.[77,78,89]

Paller and Linas found vasodilator effects from excess potassium.[90] Fujita, Noda, and Ando suggested that potassium has a natriuretic effect.[87] McCarron and coworkers felt that potassium-influenced cell membrane and intracellular mechanisms contributing to vascular smooth muscle cell regulation.[73] They also suggested that potassium contributed to humoral and volume factors functioning for cardiovascular regulation. In addition, others have noted that potassium ions are involved in carbohydrate metabolism with the uptake of glucose by cells being associated with a shift of potassium into cells.[66]

Regardless of the mechanism involved, data linking potassium intake to blood pressure level cannot be ignored. First, information from animal models demonstrates that a large intake of potassium protects the "subject" from expected effects of hypertension caused by excessive dietary sodium.[66] Similarly, humans living in Japan who consumed large amounts of both sodium and potassium did not develop hypertension.[91,92] Further consideration needs to be given to the fact that, in primitive societies, blood pressure does not rise with age. In particular, the Yanomamo Indians of South America, whose blood pressures remain about 107/69 mm/Hg past the age of 20 years, excrete (and therefore consume) about 152 mEq potassium in 24 hours but only 1.0 mEq of sodium.[58] The low ratio of sodium to potassium in the diet of these Indians is not unlike that found in raw foods available to accultured societies. The much higher urinary sodium-potassium ratios found in present-day cultures results from food preparation which adds sodium and leaches out potassium.[66] McQuarrie found, in the acute situation, that potassium was useful in lowering the blood pressure of diabetic children.[93] Fujita, Noda, and Ando found that in young adult patients with borderline hypertension, dietary supplementation with potassium attenuated the rise in blood pressure that occurs with a sodium load.[87] Finally, McCarron, and coworkers found that potassium intake of less than 900 mg per day was associated with a 12% to 14% risk of hypertension in their analysis of adult data from the National Center for Health Statistics, Health and Nutrition Examination Survey I (Hanes I).[73]

Racial differences in blood pressures of adults were found to correlate with ingestion of potassium but not sodium, by Grim and colleagues.[86] Generally, blacks have been found to excrete and therefore ingest less potassium than whites,[94] even in childhood,[52] and, as a group to have more hypertension. Similar findings were noted in our study of South Carolina children.[43] However, in the latter study, the black children of normotensive parents had lower blood pressures than the black children of hypertensive parents, indicating that while the level of potassium appears to be important when concerned with blood pressure, heredity (and probably other factors) may modify the effects of potassium. Nonetheless, provision of adequate potassium in the diet (i.e., greater than 900 mg per day), may be considered of prime importance in the nutritional management of those with or predisposed to hypertension.

Calcium and Other Divalent Cations

An increasing body of knowledge indicates a strong role for divalent cations, especially calcium, in the regulation of blood pressure.[95-101] Studies have cited the reduced incidence of cardiovascular disease, presumably due to lower blood pressure in those drinking "hard water" (with high calcium content).[102,103] An inverse relationship between dietary calcium consumption and eclampsia during pregnancy has been described.[104] McCarron also found that subjects with essential hypertension reported less daily calcium ingestion.[98] When Belizan and coworkers conducted a random population study of young adults who took calcium supplements and those receiving a placebo, found that the supplemented group had more than a 5% lower blood pressure as compared to the placebo group.[104]

In contrast, Earll and coworkers related hypercalcemia to hypertension and noted that hypertension was present in about one-third of those with hyperparathyroidism.[96] Others have also reported acute positive relationships between serum calcium and blood pressure.[105,106] Kesteloot and Geboers found direct correlation between serum level of total calcium and both systolic and diastolic pressure in a study of a large population of normotensive men.[97]

Pediatric information concerning calcium and other divalent cations is sparse. However, in a population study of five 14-year-olds, those in the higher blood stratum tended to have higher calcium levels in the serum and in the urine.[105] Whites were found to excrete more calcium than blacks. Gruskin and colleagues found serum calcium and phosphorus levels higher in hypertensive adolescents than normotensive in controls, but calcium excretion, phosphate reabsorption, and serum parathormone levels were similar.[108]

There is no clear explanation for the conflicting reportswhich appear to link both high levels of calcium and calcium deficiency to hypertension. It is, however, accepted that membrane permeability is altered in hypertension, resulting in an increase in intracellular calcium concentration. The entry of calcium into the smooth muscle cell may stimulate calcium release from the sarcoplasmic reticulum leading to the actual mechanical contraction[107,108] and increased vascular resistance. In the laboratory, increased calcium concentration has been found toeither depress or augment the contractile response of vascular smooth muscle depending on whether its membrane-stabilizing effect or its effect on the coupling reaction is dominant.[87] This change in membrane permeability to calcium may be mediated by parathormone or natriuretic hormone.[100,101]

The effect of calcium entry blockers is thought to be felt at the plasma membrane level whereby intracellular calcium is reduced-with resultant vascular smooth muscle relaxation. Altered membrane permeability to calcium is proposed to account for low renin hypertension by leading to decreased extracellular calcium and increased intracellular calcium.[99] The latter would result in arteriolar vasoconstriction and reduce renin secretion as well as a decrease in the release of parahormone. On the other hand, the increased renin found in high renin hypertension may initiate a chain of events through increased angiotensin II to release intracellular stores of calcium leading to the high serum calcium levels associated with high renin primary hypertension. Serum magnesium levels correlate inversely with calcium, perhaps through an aldosterone mechanism.

The net to be gained from this information is that calcium and other divalent cation metabolism are intertwined with hypertension. While incompletely understood, important considerations for treatment and prevention may result from unraveling the mysteries of the divalent cations. For the present, only the usual recommendations for good mineral nutrition seem indicated.

Other Nutritional Influences

A brief further note is warranted on the analysis of McCarron concerning the relationship of 17 nutrients to blood pressure.[73] In addition to potassium and calcium, these workers found lowconsumption of vitamin C and vitamin A to signal those at risk for hypertension. The vitamins appear to be associated with the cations previously described; that is, potassium with vitamin C and calcium with vitamin A. Thus, they may constitute adjuncts to the nutritional support recommended and as such, deserve further study.

Summary

When hypertension is defined by three separate blood pressure readings outside the 95th percentile, about 0.4 to 2.0% of the high-school-age population will be found to have the disorder. About one-tenth of these will have secondary forms of hypertension, likely associated with symptoms. The other 90+% will be found to have primary hypertension and will usually be free of symptoms. While primary hypertension often goes undetected until the fifth or later decades, discovery of those at risk is a pediatric challenge. Detection of latent hypertension in youth is best done by considering such predictors as tracking. This concept suggests that one's present blood pressure is related to past pressure levels and one's current blood pressure is the best single predictor of future blood pressure level. At present, tracking is useful epidemiologically, but clinical application requires caution. Most agree that there is familial aggregation of blood pressure levels. When elevated blood pressure is discovered in association with a family history of hypertension, early treatment of the disease may be undertaken without extensive workup. Black children from hypertensive families may be especially prone to hypertension. In blacks, hypertension is likely to be related to renal mechanisms, whereas in whites a sympathetic nervous mechanism may be a major contributor to the disorder. Obesity is another predictor for hypertension. It may be assessed by Quetelet's index (weight over height²) of ponderosity. Obese children from obese families may constitute a group especially prone to hypertension. Nutrients, in addition to those pertaining to weight, have received much attention. Great controversy exists over the role of sodium in hypertension. In those who are salt sensitive, sodium restriction may be beneficial. Increased potassium in the diet may also be beneficial. Such a diet is found in primitive people who, as a group, have lower blood pressures with advancing age than a civilized population. Likewise, additional calcium in the diet may lower the pressure depending on the nutritional state of the individual. Thus, judicious calorie control and attention to dietary cations in young hypertensives, especially in those likely to have a subclinical deficiency, may provide alternatives or additions to the treatment of hypertension. Such measures may prevent or delay the onset of primary hypertension as young people mature into adulthood.

References

1. Webster's Third New International Dictionary. Chicago: G & C Merriam; 1971.
2. Leumann EP. Blood pressure and hypertension in childhood and adolescence. In: Frick P, Von Harnack GA, Martini GA, Prader A, Schoen R, Wolff HP, eds. *Advances in Internal Medicine and Pediatrics*. Berlin: Springer-Verlag; 111-183:1979.
3. Kannel WB. Importance of hypertension as a major risk factor in cardiovascular disease. In: Genest J, Koiw E, Kuchel O, eds. *Hypertension: Pathophysiology and Treatment*. New York: McGraw-Hill; 888-970:1977.

4. Heyde S, Barel AG, Hames CG, McDonough JR. Elevated blood pressure levels in adolescents, Evans County, Georgia: seven- year follow-up of 30 patients and 30 controls. *J Am Med Assoc* 209:1683-1689, 1969.

5. Fixler DE, Laird WP, Fitzgerald V, Stead S, Adams R. Hypertension screening in schools: results of the Dallas study. *Pediatrics* 63:32-36, 1979.

6. Rames LK, Clarke WR, Connor WE, Reiter MA, Lauer RM. Normal blood pressure elevation in childhood: The Muscatine Study. *Pediatrics* 61:245-251, 1978.

7. Kilcoyne MM, Richter RW, Alsup PA. Adolescent hypertension 1: detection and prevalence, *Circulation* 50:758-764, 1974.

8. Miller RA, Shekelle RB. Blood pressure in tenth-gradestudents. *Circulation* 54:993-1000, 1976.

9. Reichman LB, Cooper BM, Blumenthal S. Hypertension testing among high school students. I: surveillance procedures and results. *J Chron Dis* 28:161-171, 1975.

10. Task Force on Blood Pressure Control in Children. Report of the Second Task Force on Blood Pressure Control in Children. *Pediatrics* 79:1-25, 1987.

11. Gill DG. Blood pressure in Dublin school children. *Ir Med J* 146:255-259, 1977.

12. Briedigkeit W. Die pravention von Herz-Kreislau-Krankheiten in Kindes und Jugendalter. Theoretiche Voraussetzuner, gegenwartige Moglichkeiten und proxisbezogene Schlussfolgercingen Am Beispiel einer Modellstudie. Dissertation, Universitat, Berlin: GDR, 1978.

13. Pistulkova H, Blaha J, Skodova I. Prevalence of hypertension in children and adolescents. *Cor Vasa* 18:237-240, 1976.

14. Strunge P, Trostmann AF. Serum lipids, blood pressure, skinfolds, height and weight in 580 Danish school children. *Dan Med Bull* 25:166-171, 1978.

15. Levine RS, Hennekens CH, Kelin B, Goutrley J, Briese FW, Hokenson J, Gelband H, Jessie MJ. Tracking correlations of blood pressure levels in infancy. *Pediatrics* 61:121-125, 1978.

16. Voors A, Webber LS, Berenson GS. Epidemiology of essential hypertension in youth: implications for clinical practice. *Pediatr Clin North Am* 25:1:15-28, 1978.

17. Londe S, Bourgoignie JJ, Robson AM, Goldrink D. Hypertension in apparently normal children. *J Pediatr* 78:569-577, 1971.

18. Cornoni-Huntley J, Harlan WR, Leaverton PE. Blood pressure in adolescence: The National Health Examination Survey. *Hypertension* I:566-571, 1979.

19. Alpert BS, Fox ME. Racial aspects of blood pressure in children and adolescents. *Pediatr Clin North Am* 40:13-22, 1993.

20. Berenson GS, Voors AW, Webber LS, Frank GC, Farris RP, Tobian L, Aristmuno GG. A model of intervention for prevention of early essential hypertension in the 1980s. *Hypertension* 5:41-54, 1983.

21. Jessie MJ. Commentary. "Early" essential hypertension, prevention, intervention. *Hypertension* 5:54-55, 1983.

22. Kaplan NM. *Clinical Hypertension*: 3rd ed. Baltimore: Williams and Wilkins; 80-81:1982.

23. Loggie JMH, Horan MJ, Hohn AR, Gruskin AB, Dunbar JB, Havlik RJ. Juvenile hypertension: highlights of a workshop. *J Pediatr* 104:657-663, 1984.

24. Loggie JMH. Systemic Hypertension. In: Adams RH, Emmanoullides GC, ed. *Moss Heart Disease in Infants, Childrenand Adolescents, 3rd ed.* Baltimore: Williams and Wilkins; 697-707:1983.

25. Jessie MJ. Essential hypertension in children. *Hosp Prac* 81-88, 1982.

26. Berenson GS, McMahan CA, Voors AW, Webber LS, Srinivasan SR, Franki GC, Foster TA, Blonde CV. *Cardiovascular Risk Factors in Childhood.* New York: Oxford University Press; 1980.

27. Beaglehole R, Salmond CE, Yelkes EF. A longitudinal study of blood pressures in Polynesian children. *Am J Epidemiol* 105:87-89, 1977.

28. Clarke WR, Shrott HG, Leaverton PE, Connor WE, Lauer RM. Tracking of blood lipids and blood pressures in school age children: The Muscatine Study. *Circulation* 58:626-634, 1978.

29. Hohn A. Hypertensive progeny study. Unpublished data, 1982.

30. Lauer RM, Clarke WR, Beaglehole R. Level, trend, and variability of blood pressure during childhood. The Muscatine Study. *Circulation* 69:242-249, 1984.

31. Ayman D. Heredity in arteriolar (essential) hypertension: a clinical study of the blood pressure of 1524 members of 277families. *Arch Intern Med* 53:792-802, 1934.

32. Schieken RM. Genetic factors that predispose the child to develop hypertension. *Pediatr Clin North Am* 40:1-11, 1993.

33. Kurtz TW. Review: Genetics of essential hypertension. *Am J Med* 94:77-84, 1993.

34. Thomas CB. Genetic pattern of hypertension in man. In: Onesti G, Kin KE, Moyer JH, eds. *Hypertension: Mechanisms and Management.* The Twenty-sixth Hahnemann Symposium. New York: Grune and Stratton; 67-73, 1973.

35. Platt R. The influence of heredity. In: Stamler J, Stamler R, Pullman TN, eds. *The Epidemiology of Hypertension.* New York: Grune and Stratton; 9-15:1967.

36. Pickering G. The inheritance of arterial pressure. In:Stamler J, Stamler R, Pullman TN, eds. *The Epidemiology of Hypertension.* New York: Grune and Stratton; 18-25:1967.

37. Zinner SH, Levy PS, Kass EH. Familial aggregation of blood pressure in children. *N Engl J Med* 284:401-404, 1971.

38. Biron P, Mongeau JG. Familial aggregation of blood pressure and its components. *Pediatr Clin North Am* 25:29-35, 1978.

39. Londe S, Goldring D, Gollub SW, Hernandez A. Blood pressure and hypertension in children: studies, problems and perspectives. In: New MI, Levine LS, eds. *Juvenile Hypertension.* New York: Raven Press; 13-24:1977.

40. Hennekens CH, Jessie MJ, Klein BE, Gourley JA, Blumenthal S. Aggregation of blood pressure in infants and their siblings. *Am J Epidemiol* 103:457-463, 1976.
41. Feinleib M, Garrison RJ, Havlik RJ. Environmental and genetic factors affecting the distribution of blood pressure in children. In: Lauer RM, Shakelle RB, eds. *Childhood Prevention of Atherosclerosis and Hypertension.* New York: Raven Press; 271-279:1980.
42. Biron P, Mongeau JG, Bertrand D. Familial aggregation of blood pressure in 558 adopted children. *Can Med Assoc J* 115:773-774, 1976.
43. Hohn AR, Riopel DA, Keil JE, Loadhold DB, Margolius HS, Halushka PV, Privitera PJ, Webb JG, Medley ES, Schuman SH, Ruybin MI, Pantell RH, Braunstein ML. Childhood familial and racial differences in physiologic and biochemical factors related to hypertension. *Hypertension* 5:56-70, 1983.
44. National Health Survey: *Hypertension and hypertensive heart disease in adults, U.S. 1960-1962.* Washington, DC: US Dept of Health, Education and Welfare: Vital and Health Statistics Series 11:No 13:1966.
45. McDonough JR, Garrison GE, Hames CG. Blood pressure and hypertensive disease among negroes and whites. *Ann Intern Med* 61:208, 1964.
46. Goldring D, Londe S, Sivakoff M, Hernandez A, Britton C, Choi S. Blood pressure in a high school population. *J Pediatr* 91:884-889, 1977.
47. Zinner SH, Margolius HS, Rosner B, Kass EH. Stability of blood pressure rank and urinary kallikrein concentration in childhood: an eight-year follow-up. *Circulation* 58:908-915, 1978.
48. Voors AW, Foster TA, Fredrichs RR, Webber LS, Berenson GS. Studies of blood pressures in children, ages 5–14 years, in a total biracial community: The Bogalusa Heart Study. *Circulation* 54:319-327, 1976.
49. Harshfield GA, Alpert BS, Willey ES, Somes GW, Murphy JK, Dupaul LM. Race and gender influence ambulatory blood pressure patterns of adolescents. *Hypertension* 14:598-603, 1989.
50. Ingelfinger JR. *Pediatric Hypertension.* Philadelphia: WB Saunders; 86-76:1982.
51. Voors AWS, Berenson GS, Dalferes ER, Webber LS, Shuler SE. Racial differences in blood pressure control. *Science* 204:1091-1094, 1979.
52. Voors AW, Webber LS, Berenson GS. Racial contrasts in cardiovascular response tests for children from a total community. *Hypertension* 2:686-694, 1980.
53. Sever PS, Peart WS, Meade TW, Davies IB, Gortdfon D, Tunbridge RDG. Are racial differences in essential hypertension due to different pathogenetic mechanisms? *Clin Sci* 55:3835-3865, 1978.
54. Brancati FL, Whittle JC, Whelton PK, Seidler AJ, Klag MJ. The excess incidence of diabetic end-stage renal disease among blacks: a population-based study of potential explanatory factors. *JAMA* 268:3079-3084, 1992.

55. Harlan WR, Cornoni-Huntley J, Leaverton PE. Blood pressure in childhood: the national survey. *Hypertension* I:559-565, 1979.
56. Falkner B, Kushner H, Onesti G, Angelakos ET. Cardiovascular characteristics in adolescents who develop essential hypertension. *Hypertension* 3:521-527, 1981.
57. Pickering CT. *High Blood Pressure.* London: J & A Churchill; 223:1968.
58. Oliver WJ, Cohen EL, Neel JV. Blood pressure, sodium intake and sodium related hormones in the Yanomamo indians: a "no-salt" culture. *Circulation* 52:146-151, 1977.
59. Higgins MW, Hinton PC, Keller JB. Weight and obesity as a predictor of blood pressure and hypertension. In: Loggie JMH, Horan MJ, Gruskin AB, Hohn AR, Dunbar JB, Havlik RJ, eds. *NHLBI: Workshop on Juvenile Hypertension: Proceedings from aSymposium.* New York: Biomedical Information Corp; 125-144:1984.
60. Katz SH, Hediger ML, Schall JI, Valleroy LA. Growth and blood pressure. In: Kotchen TA, Kotchen JM, eds. *Clinical Approaches to High Blood Pressure in the Young.* Boston: John Wright PSG; 91-131:1983.
61. Dustan HP: quoted In: Loggie JMH, Horan MJ, Hohn AR, Gruskin AB, Dunbar JB, Havlik RJ, eds. Juvenile hypertension: highlights of a workshop. *J Pediatr* 104:657-663, 1984.
62. Fixler DE. Epidemiology of childhood hypertension. In: Strong WB, ed. *Atherosclerosis: Pediatrics Aspects.* New York: Grune & Stratton; 978.
63. Prineas RJ, Giullum RF, Gomez-Marin O. The determinants of blood pressure levels in children: the Minneapolis children's blood pressure study. In: Loggie JMH, Horan MJ, Gruskin AB, Hohn AR, Dunbar JB, Havlik RK, eds. *NHLBI: Workshop on Juvenile Hypertension: Proceedings from a Symposium.* New York: Biomedical Information Corp; 21-36:1984.
64. Dahl LK. Salt and hypertension. *Am J Clin Nutr* 25:231- 244:1972.
65. Cherchovich GM, Copek K, Jefremova Z, Pohlova I, Jelinek J. High salt intake and blood pressure in lower primates (papio hamadryas). *J Appl Physiol* 40:601-604, 1976.
66. Meneely GR, Battarbee HD. High sodium-low potassium, environment and hypertension. *Am J Cardiol* 38:768-784, 1976.
67. Page LB. Dietary sodium and blood pressure: evidence from human studies. In: Lauer RM, Shekelle RB, eds. *Childhood Prevention of Atherosclerosis and Hypertension.* New York: Raven Press; 291-303:1980.
68. Takahashi EN, Sasaki JT. The geographic distribution of cerebral hemorrhage and hypertension in Japan. *Hum Biol* 29:139, 1957.
69. Thailand. *Nutritional Survey of the Armed Forces. A report by the Interdepartmental Committee on Nutrition for the National Defense.* Washington DC: US Gov't Printing Office; 1960.
70. Watson RL, Langford HG. Usefulness of overnight urines in population groups. *Am J Clin Nutr* 23:290-304, 1970.

71. Simpson FO. Salt and hypertension: a skeptical review of the evidence. *Clin Sci* 57(suppl 5):463, 1979.
72. Holden RA, Adrian MO, Freeman DH, Hellenbrand KG, D'Atri DA. Dietary salt intake and blood pressure. *JAMA* 250:365-369, 1983.
73. McCarron DA, Morris CD, Henry HJ, Stanton JL. Blood pressure and nutrient intake in the United States. *Science* 224:1392-1398, 1984.
74. Stamler J, Rose R, Elliott P, Dyer A, Marmot M, Kesteloot H, Stamler R, for the INTERSALT Cooperative Research Group. Findings of the International Cooperative INTERSALT Study. *Hypertension* 17(suppl I):I-9–I-15, 1991.
75. Gillum RF, Elmer PJ, Prineas RJ, Subrey D. Changing sodium intake in children. *Hypertension* 3:698-703, 1981.
76. Whitten CF, Steward RA. The effects of dietary sodium in infancy on blood pressure and related factors. *Acta Paedtr Scand Suppl* 279(suppl):3, 1980.
77. Lauer RM, Filer LJ, Recter MA, Clarke WR. Blood pressure, salt preference, salt threshold, and relative weight. *Am J Dis Child* 130:493-497, 1976.
78. Zinner SH, Kass EH. Epidemiology of blood pressure in infants and children. In: Loggie JMH, Horan MJ, Gruskin AB, Hohn AR, Dunbar JB, Havlik RK, eds. *NHLBI: Workshop on Juvenile Hypertension. Proceedings from a Symposium.* New York: Biomedical Information Corp; 93-106, 1984.
79. Hoffman A, Hazebroek A, Valkenburg HA. A randomized trial of sodium intake and blood pressure in newborn infants. *JAMA* 250:370-373, 1983.
80. Grobbee DE, Bak AAA. Electrolyte intake and hypertension in children. In: Rettig R, Ganten D, Luft F, eds. *Salt and Hypertension.* Heidelberg: Springer-Verlag; 283-292:1989.
81. Liu K, Cooper R, McKeever J, McKeever P, Byinton R, Soltero I, Stamler R, Gosch F, Stevens E, and Stamler J. Assessment of the association between habitual salt intake and high blood pressure: methodological problems. *Am J Epidemiol* 110:219-226, 1979.
82. Luft FC, Weinberger MH. Sodium intake and essentialhypertension. *Hypertension* 4 Part II:III-14-III- 19, 1982.
83. Scribner BH. Salt and hypertension. *JAMA* 250:388-389, 1983. Editorial.
84. Luft FC, Rankin LI, Bloch R, Weyman AE, Willis LR, Murray RH, Grim CE, Weinberger MH. Cardiovascular and humoral responsesto extremes of sodium intake in normal black and white men.*Circulation* 60:697-705, 1979.
85. Addison W. The use of sodium chloride, potassium chloride, sodium bromide and potassium bromide in cases of arterial hypertension which are amenable to potassium chloride. *Can Med Assoc J* 18:281-285, 1928.
86. Grim CE, Luft FC, Miller JZ, Meneely GR, Battarbee HD, Hames CG, Dahl LK. Racial differences in blood pressure in Evans County, Georgia: relationship to sodium and potassium intake in plasma renin activity. *J Chron Dis* 33:87-94, 1980.

87. Fujita T, Noda H, Ando K. Sodium susceptibility and potassium effects in young patients with borderline hypertension.*Circulation* 69:468-476, 1984.
88. Hoffman A. Blood pressure in childhood: an epidemiological approach to the etiology of hypertension. *J Hypertension* 2:323-328, 1984.
89. Ellison RC. Relationship of low salt intake in infancy tolower blood pressures. In: Blumenthal S, ed. *Hypertension: Prevention, Diet and Treatment in Infancy and Childhood. Proceedings from a Symposium.* New York: Biomedical Information Corp. 1 4-7:1983.
90. Paller MS, Linas SL. Hemodynamic effects of alterations in potassium. *Hypertension* 4 Suppl III: 20-26:1982.
91. Sasaki N, Mitsuhashi T, Fukushi S. Effects of the ingestion of large amounts of apples on blood pressure in farmers in Akita prefecture. *Igaku to Seibut-Sugaku* 51:103-105, 1959.
92. Sasaki N. High blood pressure and salt intake of the Japanese. *Jpn Heart J* 3:313-324, 1962.
93. McQuarrie I, Flipse MJ, Gofman JW. A discussion of Chapman CB. Some effects of the rice-fruit diet in patients with essential hypertension. In: *Hypertension.* Minneapolis: University of Minnesota Press; 517-523:1950.
94. Watson RL, Langford HG, Abernathy J, Barnes TY, Watson MJ.Urinary electrolytes, body weight, and blood pressure. *Hypertension* 2(suppl I):93-98, 1980.
95. Bohr DF. Vascular smooth muscle: dual effect of calcium *Science* 139:597-599, 1963.
96. Earll JM, Kurtzman NA, Moser RH. Hypercalcemia and hypertension. *Ann Intern Med* 64:378-381, 1966.
97. Kesteloot H, Geboers J. Calcium and blood pressure. *Lancet* I:813-815, 1982.
98. McCarron DA, Morris CD, Cole C. Dietary calcium and human hypertension. *Science* 217:267-269, 1982.
99. McCarron DA. Calcium, magnesium and phosphorus balance in human and experimental hypertension. *Hypertension* 4 (Suppl III):27-33, 1982.
100. Belizan JM, Vilar J, Pineda O, Gonzales AE, Sainz E, Garrera G, Sibrian R. Reduction of blood pressure with calcium supplementation in young adults. *JAMA* 249:1161-1165, 1983.
101. Resnick LM, Laragh JH, Sealey JE, Alderman MH. Divalent cations in hypertension: relations between serum ionized calcium, magnesium, and plasma renin activity. *N Engl J Med* 309:888- 891, 1983.
102. Neri LC, Mandel JS, Hewitt D. Relation between mortality and water hardness in Canada. *Lancet* I:932-934, 1972.
103. Shaper E. Soft water, heart attacks, and stroke. *JAMA* 230:130-131, 1974.
104. Belizan JM, Villar J. The relationship between calcium intake and edema-proteinuria and hypertension gestosis: a hypothesis. *Am J Clin Nutr* 33:2202-2210, 1980.

105. Weidmann P, Massry SG, Coburn WJ, Maxwell MH, Atleson J, Kleeman CR. Blood pressure effects of acute hypercalcemia: studies in patients with chronic renal failure. *Ann Intern Med* 76:741-745, 1972.
106. Clowes GHA Jr, Simeone FA. Acute hypocalcemia in surgical patients. *Ann Surg* 146:530-540, 1957.
107. Berenson GS, Voors AW, Dalferes ER Jr, Webber LS, Shuler SE. Creatinine clearance, electrolytes, and plasma renin activity related to the blood pressure of white and black children: The Bogalusa Heart Study. *J Lab Clin Med* 93:535-548, 1979.
108. Gruskin AB, Perlman SA, Baluarte HJ, Morgenstern BZ, Polinsky MS, Kaiser BA. Primary hypertension in the adolescent: facts and unresolved issues. In: Loggie JMH, Horan MJ, Gruskin AB, Hohn AR, Dunbar JB, Havlik RJ, eds. *NHLBI: Workshop on Juvenile Hypertension: Proceedings from a Symposium.* New York: Biomedical Information Corp; 125-144:1984.
109. Blaustein MP. Sodium concentration, calcium concentration, blood pressure regulation and hypertension: a reassessment and a hypothesis. *Am J Physiol* 232:165-173, 1977.
110. Frank GB. The current view of the source of trigger calcium in excitation-contraction coupling in vertebrae skeletal muscle. *Biochem Pharmacol* 29:2399-2407, 1980.

Chapter 4

Risk Factors in the Young for Adult Onset Hypertension

Introduction

The detrimental effects of hypertension in adults are well known. Stroke and coronary heart disease are common in older persons with high systolic and/or diastolic blood pressure.[1] Lowering the pressure may prevent or delay these morbid or fatal events. Similarly, extremely high systolic and/or diastolic blood pressure in children is dangerous. For example, the marked hypertension with renal disorders may cause seizures or heart failure. In such cases reduction of the blood pressure elevation usually controls or eliminates the noxious complication. However, in those young people with less extreme pressure elevation and no associated underlying disorder, it is not clear that treatment is necessary. On the other hand, it is known that from 15% to 25% of young people will become hypertensive in later life. Logic dictates that if those destined to have hypertension can be found prior to the onset of their disorder, the likelihood is that morbidity can be lessened or avoided. The challenge is to find those at risk. Then preventive programs can be instituted.

Current knowledge allows the detection of approximately one in five of the 15% of young people who are prone to adult onset hypertension. The question then is how to find the others (roughly 12% of the population) who will develop this "silent killer" disease in later life. Attention to known risk factors for hypertension may

75

increase the chances for discovery of those who will be afflicted with the disorder. This chapter will summarize present thinking about risk factors for hypertension (Table 1). Application of this information may be made to single out those who need help to avoid adult onset hypertension and its ensuing complications.

Blood Pressure

A person's blood pressure at any point in time is generally felt to be the best predictor of future blood pressure levels.[2] That is, blood pressure tracks or maintains relative rank order over time, particularly in adults but also in a number of children.[3] Elevated blood pressure in older individuals is considered to be an important risk for future disease.[1] Recent evidence has shown that the same may be true for children. Despite low tracking coefficients for blood pressure, Lauer and Clarke found that 24% of children who had at least one systolic pressure recorded above the 90th percentile had high systolic blood pressure as young adults.[4,5] In other words, a single childhood high systolic blood pressure (> the 90th percentile) equated to a twofold risk increase for adult onset high blood pressure. While not true for a single diastolic pressure elevation, multiple high diastolic blood pressure recordings similarly indicated increased risk for high adult diastolic pressure.

This information is based on population data, and their application to an individual child may result in more variability. Nevertheless the discovery of systolic or diastolic blood pressure above the 90th percentile in a young person is cause for evaluation and follow-up. For this purpose, the recommendations in the task force report on blood pressure control in children are useful.[6] Attention

---

Table 1.
Childhood Risk Factors for Later-Life Hypertension

1. Blood pressure	7. Smoking
2. Heredity	8. Alcohol and drugs
3. Obesity	9. Maternal and newborn
4. Race	10. Diabetes
5. Dietary cations	11. Uric acid
6. Exercise, stress, and anxiety	12. LV mass (by echo)

LV = left ventricular.

should be given to annual blood pressure readings or even obtaining an ambulatory 24-hour blood pressure study. Fortunately more than 60% of children with systolic pressures over the 90th percentile will have systolic pressures below the 80th percentile in adult life.[5]

Plotting blood pressures on the task force percentile grids, similar to the familiar growth chart plots, may offer additional insight as to what a child's future blood pressure may be.[7] About 25% of those with high systolic pressures will consistently have pressures in the upper deciles of the blood pressure distribution (around or above the 90th percentile). Another group will have pressures below this level, but over time will track or move into higher deciles. The trend to higher pressures over time is also thought to indicate risk for adult onset hypertension. Still others with irregular blood pressure plots, none of which are in the upper deciles, will have an overall upward trend. They too may be at risk. However, in children with marked variability in blood pressure levels, trends should be interpreted with great caution. Finally, those with level or declining blood pressure trends are probably not at risk. Overall, blood pressure grid plots should be used with care, recognizing predictive accuracy in the order of 30%, hardly favorable gambling odds.

Heredity

It is appealing to believe that altered interplay between hereditary and environmental factors results in primary hypertension. Indeed, numerous reports indicate that genetic predisposition reacts with environment to produce changes in the blood pressure level.[8] While direct proof is lacking, a large portion of hypertension is felt to be genetically determined. Genetic animal models have been constructed to show that the propensity for hypertension is most likely polygenic.[9] Schieken recently summarized data suggesting that childhood high blood pressure was controlled by either a major gene effect or the polygenic expression of genes.[10] In all probability, many genetic loci are involved. However, specific genes cosegregating with hypertension have not been identified. Certain HLA antigens have been noted to be increased in a small number of individuals with primary hypertension.[11] However, at present, this information is inconclusive evidence for the genetic origin of hypertension.

Despite the lack of specific gene proof, twin studies have consistently shown the heritability of blood pressure. The relationship of blood pressures is particularly strong among monozygotic twins, even if living apart.[12,13] Correlation coefficients for systolic blood pressure are about 0.55 for monozygotic and 0.25 for dizygotic adult twins. Correlation coefficients for diastolic pressure are similar (Fig. 1). [14] Like findings are noted in childhood, both at rest and during activity.[15]

On a more clinical level in young people over 12 years of age, a family history of hypertension, stroke, or ischemic heart disease is the second strongest risk factor for adult onset hypertension. Nearly 13% of adults with positive family histories for the disorders just listed had high blood pressure. In comparison, 9.5% of those with negative family histories had high blood pressure.[5] Individuals with a positive family history have a risk for developing hypertension prior to age 50, nearly fourfold that of those with a negative

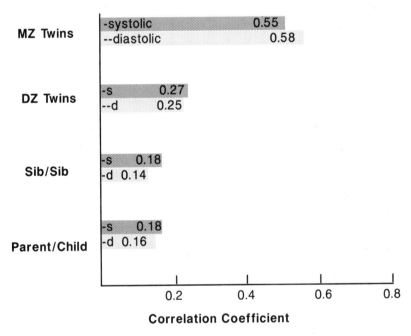

Figure 1: Blood Pressure Correlations Between Related Individuals. MZ = monozygotic; DZ = dizygotic; SIB = sibling. (Modified from Williams[14]).

history.[8] Likewise, about 75% of the siblings of adults whose hypertension began prior to age 50 will be found to have the disorder. In contrast, minimal correlation has been noted between spouses or their adopted children.[16]

Hereditary influences may act through the renin-angiotensin (RA) system or through metabolic channels, especially those of cation and lipid metabolism. Unfortunately, markers in the RA system for future hypertension are not available. Likewise sodium-lithium countertransport markers, although suggestive for hypertension risk, are not yet clinically useful for this purpose.[17] Other biochemical substances, such as urinary kallikrein level, are also of little help. In certain instances, particular lipid patterns in families may be suspect and deserve elicitation, but again are not widely applicable for clinical use.

Thus, it comes down to searching for evidence of hereditary propensities for hypertension through a careful history (Chapter 9). False-negative histories may be avoided by specific questions about medications used by relatives, most specifically antihypertension therapy. This information can then be interpreted in the light of the above considerations and a risk assessment made. Generally speaking, any positive historical information denotes two- to fourfold increased risk for later- life blood pressure elevation. For those at risk, it is reasonable to consider some kind of program to reduce the tendency to hypertension.

Obesity

Body fatness has long been considered to have a positive relationship with blood pressure. Obesity has been described as a major independent risk factor for hypertension.[18] Over half of hypertensive children are obese.[19] Obesity may be defined as a weight that exceeds the average for a given height by 20% or more. A number of indices relate weight to height. One commonly used body mass index (BMI) is the Quetelet index (weight in kilograms/height in meters^2 = BMI). In the Tecumseh Community Health Study, measures of body fatness (weight and Quetelet) were consistently correlated with blood pressure.[20] Lauer and colleagues, analyzing their Muscatine, Iowa study data with a genetic sense, found higher blood pressures in those homozygous for the high BMI gene than all other groups.[21] They suggested that variability in BMI was due 34% to genotype differences at a single recessive locus, 41% at polygenic loci, and 25% to nongenetic factors.

Rocchini has theorized that obesity hypertension is related to selective insulin resistance.[22] In turn, hyperinsulinemia leads to renal sodium retention. The latter effect may be dependent on antidiuretic hormone.[23]

Although there is consensus for the positive association of high BMI and both systolic and diastolic hypertension, it is to be recognized that as many as one-third of those with high BMI have normal pressures. In a similar sense, while weight reduction is advocated to decrease BMI in hypertensive individuals, the blood pressure will not be lowered in about one-third of those who lose significant weight.[24]

The evidence linking hypertension to obesity is compelling even in the first years of childhood.[25] Accordingly, it is important that weight counseling be given to parents of children from families wherein excess weight is a problem. Further, those children with BMI 20% above the median for age should have careful attention to diet to reduce weight gain velocity. Such children should be encouraged to exercise. Their parents and/or caretakers should be informed of the need to have the child's blood pressure followed carefully over time. Special efforts should focus on those with blood pressure over the 80th percentile and from families with a history of hypertension. Control of obesity is one of the most difficult tasks faced by the patient, caregivers, and involved physicians. The genetics of the problem make it enduringly difficult, requiring constant vigilance. Recidivism is an ever present threat to success.

Race

It is well known that the rate of hypertension is much higher for black people in the United States than for other races. This increased rate of hypertension begins to appear in young adulthood (age 18 to 24 years) and increases thereafter. In the over 65-year-old group the rate is 55.1/100 for blacks compared to 39.3/100 for whites, and 40.7/100 for all races.[26] Reports in the literature contain conflicting information concerning racial differences in blood pressure in young people.[27,28] The net outcome of these studies may be summed up into a consensus that there may be some, but no major racial population difference in blood pressure prior to adulthood.

On the other hand, certain subgroups of young black people have been found to have higher pressures than corresponding white subgroups. Thus, in our study of the progeny of hypertensive parents, black teenage children (mean age about 14 years) had higher pressures than their white counterparts and black children of normotensive parents even after adjustment for size.[27] Exercise testing in these groups revealed black hypertensive progeny to have higher pressures at all levels of activity. Racial differences were also found in humeral substances influencing blood pressure. Others have found humeral substance differences between the races in young people in the upper strata of the blood pressure distribution.[29] It has also been noted that cardiovascular reactivity to video-game stress is greater among black children.[30] However, in older individuals, hypertensive blacks and whites were found to have similar levels of autonomic function.[31] This finding is consistent with the thought that mechanisms for hypertension may be set in earlier life, then become fixed and similar for all groups.

More recently we found that the number of high school students with blood pressure above the 95th percentile was higher among Asian females than in other racial groups including Asian males, blacks, Latinos, and whites.[32] The reason for these findings remains unclear. Perhaps it is from a nutrient etiology, since those of Asian heritage, like blacks, tend to suffer from lactase deficiency.[33] Salt sensitivity is found in blacks,[34] but is not a major factor in childhood populations, although the low potassium and high sodium diet of many blacks may manifest itself in higher blood pressure.[27,35]

From the foregoing, it is apparent that young black people from families with a history of hypertension have an increased risk of developing hypertension in adulthood. This may be true especially if the individual under question is obese. Hypertension, though, is generally not a problem for such people until later life. The impact of hypertension on black adults is well documented in the literature.[36] Mortality is much higher in blacks than in whites as are complications like stroke and renal disease. Accordingly, close surveillance of black children from hypertensive families is urged. Such young people and their families should be encouraged to adopt nonpharmacologic measures, like diet and weight control, to contain blood pressure in the normal range. These measures should become a part of the involved individual's permanent lifestyle.

Dietary Cations

Salts of various kinds have long been used in the preparation of foods. In recent decades, they have become known to be associated with hypertension. Whether or not these dietary substances, particularly the sodium cation, actually constitute risk factors for hypertension is a matter of debate. As can be seen from the following summary of the major monovalent (sodium and potassium) and the major divalent cations (calcium and magnesium) much is left to be learned especially for children.

Sodium

Of the dietary cations, sodium has received the most attention. A myriad of past and recent adult human studies have linked sodium-rich diets to hypertension.[37,38] The multinational, quality-controlled INTERSALT study of 10,079 adults confirmed the influence of sodium on blood pressure of previously reported works, many of which had procedural problems.[39] Other researchers have demonstrated that sodium restriction in adults with hypertension lowers blood pressure, even in those with less severe hypertension.[40] The effect of a 100 mmol/day dietary sodium reduction averages a 5.4 mm Hg decrease in systolic and 6.5 mm Hg in diastolic pressure.[41] Few studies of those in the pediatric age group have been carried out. One study revealed that infants who were fed a low sodium formula had lower systolic pressures than others on a normal sodium intake.[42] However, 4 years later, no differences were found between the groups.[43] Normotensive children who were fed low sodium diets had little change in their blood pressure.[44] In contrast, a study of a small group of hypertensive children found a fall in both systolic and diastolic pressure while on a short period of low sodium intake while a control group did not.[45]

When, in the course of a hypertension workup, the question of excessive sodium ingestion arises, some quantitative estimate of the amount of sodium consumed should be made. A dietary food-frequency history will, in most instances, furnish an estimate of sodium intake. Perhaps the best way to assess the amount of sodium that an individual ingests is to measure that person's 24-hour urinary sodium. In the United States, urinary sodium excretion of more than 255 mmol/day may be considered high.[46] If the intake is judged to be high, it may be reasonable to advise curtailment of sodium intake, although little benefit may accrue in children.

In some cultures, little dietary salt is available.[39] People from these populations excrete small amounts sodium and have minimal blood pressure increase postadolescence. Other dietary, environmental, and cultural factors may also influence their blood pressures. Their low sodium diets are apparently beneficial and, at the very least, do not seem detrimental.

Certain individuals respond to increased salt intake with elevation in blood pressure. They are termed "salt sensitive." Only a small percent of the population is salt sensitive and the phenomenon increases in frequency with age. Documentation of salt sensitivity in children is lacking, for most young people seem to be resistant to dietary salt alterations.[47] Thus, it appears that the amount of dietary sodium consumed by children is not, of itself, a significant risk factor. In the presence of childhood hypertension or perceived risk for the disorder, practical advice to avoid excessively salty foods will inflict no harm. At this time, however, a truly low sodium diet is not advisable and may not even be helpful for most hypertensive children.

Potassium

Considerable information exists on the inverse relationship of potassium intake and blood pressure.[48] There is debate as to why potassium should exert a lowering affect on blood pressure.[49] In normotensive young people, a high potassium diet may lower the diastolic blood pressure as much as 5 mm Hg, particularly if they have a family history of hypertension.[50] Teleologically, it has been recognized that in primitive societies diets are characteristically low in sodium and high in potassium content. Whether or not low potassium intake in children, as is found in the diet of our accultured society, constitutes a true risk factor for later-life hypertension is not known. Certainly, it is not high on anyone's list of risk factors. A high potassium diet of itself may be hard to achieve, for most foods do not have a high potassium content. However, it is generally felt that a return to a more unaccultured diet, lower in sodium and higher in potassium, is efficacious. The ratio of dietary sodium to potassium may be the important factor. It must also be noted that the ingestion of a potassium salt as a dietary supplement is of unproved benefit, and may not have any affect on blood pressure.[51] Unmonitored potassium supplementation may be dangerous, particularly if renal function is impaired.

Calcium

The divalent cation, calcium, is necessary for many of life's processes. Calcium plays an essential role in the excitation, coupling, contraction of all muscle cells. As such, increased calcium levels would be expected to increase smooth muscle contraction in blood vessels and therefore cause an elevation of blood pressure. Such is the case with the hypercalcemia of renal disease or when demineralization of bone occurs as a result of immobilization. In the same manner, calcium-channel blockers are commonly used in the treatment of hypertension. On the other hand, a number of epidemiologic studies have reported an inverse relationship of dietary calcium to hypertension.[52] Hyperactivity of the parathyroid gland with elevated levels of parathormone have been found in young persons with hypertension.[53] These findings have led some to feel that in certain hypertensives there is disturbed calcium metabolism. It has been further hypothesized that the intrinsic metabolic calcium disturbances occur at a young age, perhaps resetting calcium homeostasis at a lower level. A possible example could be the lactase deficiency found in black populations. The end result in such instances could be a relative calcium deficiency.

A number of mechanisms have been postulated to explain why an inverse relationship between calcium and blood pressure exists in some individuals. These include cell membrane stabilizing effects of elevated calcium levels; calcium-induced increased production by vascular tissue of the vasodilator, prostacyclin; direct calcium intracellular effects; calcium effects mediated through the central nervous system, or calcium-regulating hormones (parathormone/1, 25[OH]2 vitamin D); and calcium action through phosphate depletion of nonvascular mechanisms.[52] Multiple animal studies, primarily on spontaneously hypertensive rats, have been carried out to test these hypotheses. Regardless of the mechanism, a number of dietary calcium supplementation trials have been carried out in humans. Some have evidenced reduction in blood pressure.[54,55] Others report little if any calcium effect on blood pressure.[56,57]

Those likely to benefit from calcium supplementation include men with salt sensitivity,[58] older women,[59] pregnant women with hypertension,[60] those with insulin-resistant diabetes,[61] and people with alcohol-associated hypertension.[62] Information with regard to calcium supplementation in children is sparse. We carried out a trial of 1500 mg calcium supplementation per day in Pasadena black high school students from the upper deciles of the school blood pressure distribution. Initial results showed a marginally significant decrease in diastolic blood pressure of 2.5 mm Hg between the supplemented and placebo group.[63] The effect was more marked in those who consumed a low calcium diet. In addition, there was an increased calcium effect of lowering pressure in those who consumed less potassium and more sodium. Until further information becomes available, adequate intake of 800 to 1000 mg calcium per day through usual dietary sources (largely dairy products such as milk and cheese) should be assured. The use of calcium supplements is not advocated for the general childhood population.

Magnesium

Like calcium, magnesium is a divalent cation with dietary intake levels related to sociodemographic factors.[64] Magnesium is the second most common intracellular cation. In many instances, its actions are antagonistic to those of calcium. Maternal prenatal magnesium intake has a weak inverse relationship to infant blood pressure in the first year of life. This, however, may be related to the level of concomitant calcium intake. Indeed, magnesium is commonly considered, along with calcium, in reference to its influence on blood pressure. Blood levels of magnesium do not appear related to blood pressure,[65] but the relationship of low urinary excretion of magnesium to high blood pressure may be suggestive that greater dietary intake would be of benefit.[66] The few trials of magnesium supplementation have produced conflicting results.[67,68] With this evidence in mind, magnesium supplements to the diet are not yet recommended.[69]

Exercise, Stress, and Anxiety

Much has been written about the changes in the circulatory system in response to physical stress, both dynamic and isometric. Systolic pressure generally increases with acute exercise, whereas diastolic pressure either changes little or decreases. There are corresponding decreases in peripheral resistance and increases in catecholamine secretion. Such changes are more marked in hypertensive individuals,[70] who as a rule have increased cardiovascular reactivity. Whether or not the level of change can be used to predict hypertension may be debatable. However, in the evaluation of children and adolescents, Mahoney and colleagues felt systolic blood pressure was best predicted from initial resting and maximal exercise systolic blood pressure.[71] Fixler and coworkers also found exercise useful for predicting blood pressure trends in the young.[72] Likewise, studies in young adult men have suggested that exercise responses might predict future hypertension.[73]

While acute exercise unquestionably elevates blood pressure, chronic or repetitive exercise will lower blood pressure.[74] Indeed, an exercise program is a useful nonpharmacologic intervention for the treatment of hypertension. Exercise-induced decrease in sympathetic tone reduces systemic blood pressure. Weight loss from exercise is also beneficial. It appears that both dynamic exercise like endurance training and isometric exercise such as weight lifting (although not completely isometric) are useful for this purpose.[75]

Mental stress also evokes changes in blood pressure, by elevating systolic and diastolic blood pressure along with heart rate and catecholamines.[76] In the progeny of hypertensive parents these increases are more marked. Common techniques for testing mental stress include difficult arithmetic, reaction time tasks[77] and video games.[78] Again, the predictive usefulness of this information is open to debate. However, Falkner and coworkers followed individuals with increased cardiovascular reactivity and "high genetic risk" for periods up to 5 years. They found that about two thirds became hypertensive.[79] Measures of mental stress-induced cardiovascular reactivity are greater in blacks than in whites.[78,79] Consequently, such measures may be more predictive of future hypertension in black hyperreactors.

Anxiety from continual job-related mental stress in adults is thought to be a risk factor for hypertension. For example, a higher prevalence of hypertension has been noted among male bus drivers than in males in other occupations.[80] A number of strategies such as the "relaxation response" have been developed to overcome the risk[81] (Chapter 10).

Another test of cardiovascular reactivity is the cold pressor test. Immersion of the foot in a bucket of ice water may evoke excessive cardiovascular reactivity. Over 70% of hyperreactors to the test in childhood were shown by Wood to be hypertensive in adult life.[82]

It would appear that there is some usefulness in using stress (both physical and mental) testing to evaluate hypertensive tendencies. The combination of peak stress blood pressure with resting level may be a powerful predictor of future pressure.[83] Stress testing appears to be especially useful as a predictor for hypertension in blacks and in those with a family history of hypertension. Simple methods for this type of stress testing are outlined in Table 2.[79,84] Those in the upper deciles of the blood pressure distribution with excessive stress responses should be kept under surveillance. In addition, they should be encouraged to develop health habits consistent with blood pressure containment. In persons at risk for future high blood pressure, exercise programs are a useful adjunct to maintaining blood pressure at lower levels.

Smoking

In addition to the adverse health impact of smoking due to carcinogenesis, compromise of lung function, and promotion of atherosclerosis (including coronary artery disease), smoking also affects adult blood pressure unfavorably. Excessive smoking in-

---

Table 2.
Methods of Stress Testing

1. Exercise
   A. Dynamic (modified from [84]: Step test–requires one step (could be a stairway); test subject steps up, first with one then with the other foot, and down, similarly, repeatedly to the commands "step up", "step down" (said rapidly and regularly in approximately 1 s for the 4 words). Duration–3 min
   Results–The heart rate usually is < 160 and the blood pressure < 160/80.
   B. Isometric[79]: Hand grip–requires Smedley Hand Dynamometer Manufacturer: Stoelting Co., Chicago, IL Method:
      1. Establish MVC according to the Stoelting manual.
      2. Test subject squeezes the dynamometer for 5 min at 20% MVC.
      3. Blood pressure is recorded before and at 1-min intervals during the test.
      Results–Blood pressure usually is < 160/90.
2. Mental stress: (see Falkner).[76]

MVC = Maximum Voluntary Contraction.

creases systolic and diastolic blood pressure, probably as a result of norepinephrine released at nerve endings.[85] On a chronic basis, adult smokers have no more hypertension than nonsmokers. However, the ambulatory systolic blood pressure of smokers is higher in the daytime than in nonsmokers, especially in those over 50 years of age. Nighttime pressures are similar.[86] Smokers also have higher death rates from hypertension. The data for the hypertension detection and follow-up program (HDFP) revealed that smokers had twice the mortality rate of nonsmokers.[87] In addition, the incidence of malignant hypertension in smokers is five times that of nonsmokers.[88] These effects may be due to carbon monoxide and other toxins generated by smoking. Smokeless tobacco also results in elevation of blood pressure, possibly related to the high sodium content (3%) in the tobacco.[89]

Other adverse effects of smoking related to hypertension include the fact that smoking in the presence of hypertension causes higher blood viscosity, hematocrit, and pulse wave velocity.[90] Maternal smoking results in hypoxemia, in turn causing placental lesions and abruption.[91] Smoking also modifies the effects of alcohol on systolic and diastolic blood pressure.[92] The duration of smoking is a predictor of intracranial atherosclerosis.[93] Smokers are at increased risk for peripheral vascular disease,[94] as well as being at risk for carotid stenosis or occlusion.[95] In hypertensive adults, smoking cigarettes is a determinant risk factor for the occlusive disorder. Smoking in hypertensive individuals is a better predictor of carotid atherosclerosis than lipid level.[96] Low density lipoprotein (LDL) lipids cause carotid thickening, whereas smoking in hypertensives causes plaques.[97] Additionally, smoking with hypertension is a risk factor for fatal aortic aneurysm.[98]

Smoking may interfere with the treatment of hypertension.[99] For example, smoking decreases the bioavailability of propranolol through increased degradation of propranolol in the liver.[100] As a consequence, smokers on propranolol have an attenuated blood pressure response and no change in the incidence of strokes. On the other hand, nonsmokers given propranolol have a decrease in strokes.[101] Noncardioselective β-blockers such as propranolol have dyslipidemic effects in both smokers and nonsmokers. However, highly cardioselective β-blockers such as celiprolol minimize these dyslipidemic effects in smokers.[102]

Thus, it seems prudent to discourage smoking to decrease not only heart and lung disease risks but also to decrease the incidence of strokes.[103] Unfortunately, smoking cessation interventional programs do not produce self-sustaining results. Further, quitting smoking may result in higher blood pressure possibly due to weight gain.[104] Those who stop smoking have a 35% incidence of hypertension while those who continue to smoke have a hypertension incidence of 27%.[105]

The applicability of this information to young people and children is untested. While most are agreed that it is worthwhile to prevent smoking in young people, the number of student smokers is largely undefined. In our Pasadena study we found that 79% of the students claimed they never smoked (Table 3).[106] Yet Dwyer and colleagues found that only 63% of a comparable group of German students said they abstained from smoking (measures of carbon monoxide confirmed the German students' history of not smoking).[107] As in the Pasadena study, blood pressures in the young German smokers were lower than in the nonsmokers.[108] Many smoking avoidance programs are available for young people.[109] Their use is laudable but not under the guise of preventing hypertension.

Alcohol, Medications, Drugs

Alcohol use has been linked to hypertension in adults for many years.[110] It may be confounded by concomitant smoking.[92] However,

Table 3.
Smoking Habits (by gender)
1317 Pasadena High School 9th Grade Student in 1987[106]

	n	*%*	*K5*
Females			
Never smoked	533	79	70
Quit	62	9	69
Occasionally	49	7	70
Regularly	27	4	65
Males			
Never smoked	509	79	70
Quit	67	10	70
Occasionally	43	7	69
Regularly	27	4	68

the mechanism by which the use of alcohol causes blood pressure elevation remains obscure.[111] The coincident elevation of α-glutamyl-transpeptidase (a marker of alcohol consumption) and angiotensin-converting enzyme levels in drinkers with high blood pressure was felt to be a result of alcohol- induced hepatic cell destruction rather than an etiologic mechanism.[112] At the same time, reports of a number of questionnaire-type studies of adults who imbibe ethyl alcohol reveal that the incidence of hypertension in those who have three or more drinks per day is more than twice that of those who drink less or do not drink at all.[113,114] This effect is seen in both sexes and persists when the data are controlled for other factors such as weight, race, and smoking. Curiously, those who have one or two drinks may have lower pressures than nondrinkers.[115] Beer and wine appear to have the least affect on diastolic and systolic blood pressure, respectively. For those who are hypertensive, discontinuation of the drinking habit, an effective intervention, results in lowering the blood pressure.[116] Blood pressure elevations due to alcohol are more marked in older individuals.[117] In fact, young people who drink and those who do not seem to have no difference in blood pressure.

It is safe to conclude that the drinking of alcoholic beverages by young people is not, of itself, a significant risk factor for hypertension. However, the habit should be avoided because in later life, taking three or more drinks per day can cause all manner of difficulties, including high blood pressure. As of the present writing, it is still considered beneficial to take one or two drinks a day for "health purposes."

A variety of medications can cause elevation of blood pressure or even frank hypertension.[118] These include sympathomimetics (such as are contained in decongestants), oral contraceptives, cyclosporine,[119] and steroids. In our Pasadena high school blood pressure study, only oral contraceptives and anticonvulsants were linked with high blood pressure (Table 4).[119] It is best that patients be urged to use medications sold over the counter with care. Regardless of the source of the medication, if hypertension is found, withdrawal of the medication will generally relieve the pressure elevation. In situations where the medication cannot be withdrawn, as with immunosuppression therapy following organ transplantation, treatment of the hypertension often permits control of the pressure elevation. Thus, in cyclosporine-induced hypertension nifedipine appears especially useful.[120]

Table 4.
Medications Used by 827 Pasadena 9th Grade Students[119]

Medication	n	%
Antibiotic	37	4.4
Antiasthmatic	31	3.7
Analgesic-antiinflammatory	19	2.3
Vitamin-diet supplement	16	1.9
Decongestant	11	1.3
Birth control*	6	0.7
Antihistamine	4	0.5
Anticonvulsant*	2	0.2
Diuretic	2	0.2
Antacid	1	0.1
Other	15	1.8

*BP > 90th %ile

Certain "street drugs" are known to cause hypertension. Cocaine,[121] amphetamines, and phencyclidine (PCP or "angel dust")[122] are especially known to cause transient hypertension. On occasion a hypertensive "crisis" may ensue which will respond to antihypertensive treatment. Avoidance remains the best philosophy.

Maternal and Newborn Factors

Because teen pregnancy is now common, it has become an important health supervision issue. "Risk factors" for pregnancy-related hypertension must be considered by those caring for young people. Between 5% and 10% of pregnancies are complicated by hypertension.[123] Four major categories of hypertension in pregnancy are recognized. The first is preexistent hypertension, either primary or secondary. It is usually distinguishable by history. The second is the late or transient variety in which the pressure elevation is the sole finding and rapidly returns to normal postpartum. Women so afflicted may be destined for hypertension in later life.[124] The third and fourth types are preeclampsia and/or eclampsia with or without preexisting hypertension. The latter types of hypertension are more common and the pressure elevation is pathophysiologic.

Preeclampsia is heralded by edema and proteinuria and followed by hypertension at about the twentieth week of pregnancy.

Cardiac output is decreased and peripheral resistance markedly increased.[125] Prior to the onset of the disorder, there is increased responsiveness to angiotensin in contrast to the usual angiotensin resistance in normal pregnancy. Preeclampsia may be complicated by hemolysis, elevated liver enzymes, and low platelets (the HELLP syndrome) with the necessity of treatment by termination of the pregnancy.[126] Preeclampsia is most common in first pregnancies,[125] especially in teenagers. Thus, a primary preventive strategy must be developed to avoid teenage pregnancies. Preeclampsia may lead to the convulsive and potentially lethal disorder, eclampsia. Fetal difficulties are frequent with preeclampsia, as are premature delivery (either by necessity for treatment or spontaneously induced by the preeclampsia).[127]

Diastolic blood pressure greater than or equal to 84 mm Hg is considered a signal for concern and requires close monitoring. At this point, low-dose aspirin,[128] or calcium supplementation[129] may be effective in preventing preeclampsia. Should diastolic pressures reach 100 mm Hg, methyldopa is recommended as safe therapy with no late adverse effects on the infants of mothers so treated.[125] β-blockers are also used. Diuretic use is generally discouraged during pregnancy while channel blockers have been used favorably. Angiotensin-converting enzyme inhibitors cause newborn renal problems, and are contraindicated in pregnant women. Hydralazine and magnesium sulfate may be efficacious treatment for diastolic pressures over 110 mm Hg, particularly at the time of delivery. Those who suffer from preeclampsia or eclampsia do not appear to have an increased risk for hypertensive disorders in later life.

On the other hand, the hypertensive diseases of pregnancy may increase the risk of hypertension in later life for the infant issue of the pregnancy. However, in the neonatal period hypotension may be a problem for such babies.[127] Also, they are often small for gestational age and have small head size. These and other low-birth-weight infants may have blood pressure regulation difficulty and are at risk for renal artery thrombosis if the umbilical artery is cannulated (as noted in Chapter 8).Additionally, low birth weight of itself may be a risk factor for later-life hypertension.[130]

Another concern is the development of hypertension in those infants requiring extracorporeal membrane oxygenation (ECMO) for survival. In one series, the systolic blood pressure of 38 of 41 newborns managed with ECMO was elevated to over 90 mm Hg, and

18 had intracranial hemorrhage (ICH).[131] The cause of the high blood pressure is unknown at this time, but there was elevation of a number of humeral substances, including plasma-renin activity. Treatment with captopril (0.1 mg/kg per dose every 8 hours) was recommended to prevent ICH.

Diabetes Mellitus

Children with diabetes mellitus seldom have hypertension. In those few individuals with juvenile diabetes and hypertension, the elevation of blood pressure is likely to be the result of a coexisting disorder. Yet many juvenile diabetics are destined to develop hypertension as adults. It is in that sense that diabetes mellitus is listed as a risk factor for future hypertension. Interestingly, a family history of diabetes does not appear to relate to blood pressure in children and adolescents.[132] However, in a study of Framingham offspring aged 20 to 49 years, blood sugar was related to hypertension.[133]

Insulin-dependent (type I) diabetics develop microvascular complications leading to renal malfunction and hypertension. Evaluation of normotensive adults has disclosed over half to have either incipient or frank nephropathy as evidenced by urinary albumen excretion (> 30 or > 300 mg/day, respectively).[134] Retinal lesions were also found. Thus control of juveniles with diabetes, especially for those with blood pressure in the upper deciles, is most important to delay onset of these lesions. Early treatment of those with higher blood pressures may be necessary.[135]

Uric Acid

Elevated serum uric acid levels have been found in children and young people with hypertension.[136] Some hypertensives have high-normal uric acid levels while others have significant elevations. The reason for the high uric acid levels is uncertain, but it may be related to decreased tubular transport of uric acid. In reality, elevation of uric acid in the serum is a marker for hypertension and not a risk factor, and has been recognized as such in adults.[137] In the hypertensive youngster with significant uric acid elevation, the levels appear to correlate positively with plasma-renin activity.[136] No treatment is required for the hyperuricemia in the young.

Left Ventricular Hypertrophy

Echocardiographic studies (ECHO) performed over the last 2 decades have verified previous anatomical, pathologic. and electrocardiographic findings of left ventricular hypertrophy (LVH) in hypertensive adults.[138] Left ventricular hypertrophy can be detected earlier by ECHO than by other means. The finding of LVH represents target-organ damage and carries an ominous prognosis.[139] Because elevated blood pressure is a premorbid event in children and adolescents it usually is not associated with any outward physical sign of disease. Thus it becomes necessary to search for subtle signs of organ involvement. The retinal fundoscopic examination is one approach. However, with minimal blood pressure elevation, even though for a good portion of each day, fundoscopic examination maybe unrevealing. In contrast, providing other causes of LVH in young people can be excluded, ECHO may indicate the existence of significant periods of blood pressure elevation in those with that finding.[140]

A number of echocardiographic techniques can be used to search for LVH as a mirror of high blood pressure. Of the available ECHO M-mode determinations, calculated left ventricular mass (LV mass) appears to be the most useful indicator of pressure elevation and may even be predictive of future hypertension.[71] However, data confirming the predictive value of the LV-mass calculation are not presently available. This fact not withstanding, an LV-mass determination should be obtained in any pediatric patient with persistently high blood pressure, as well as in those who have other risk factors and/or illness leading to hypertension. If the LV mass is outside of usual limits, measures are indicated to avoid later-life hypertension. Adult studies have shown that the occurrence of hypertension can be more than halved by nutritional-hygienic means.[141] There is reason to believe that similar measures would work in young people as well.

Summary

Most predictive of the known risk factors for hypertension in children are current blood pressure, family history, body size, and race. Each impacts on blood pressure independently. In combination, these risk factors are very threatening for disease in later life.

The first, current blood pressure, thought to be the single most predictive factor for future elevated pressure, must be used with some caution as a risk factor. The percentage of individuals whose pressures maintain the same rank order or percentile over time ("track") is relatively low. Heredity is second only to blood pressure as an independent risk factor for hypertension. A family history of hypertension may indicate up to a fourfold increase in hypertension risk. Obesity is the third most common risk factor for hypertension. It has a large genetic component. Over half of the hypertensive children are obese. Unfortunately, weight reduction does not always reduce pressure. About one-third of those who successfully lose weight remain hypertensive.

Hypertension is more common in older black people than in those of other races. However, blood pressure levels are similar in children and adolescents of all races. Black people have a tendency for high sodium and low potassium diets. They may also have a relative calcium deficiency due to lactose intolerance. The cations, sodium, potassium, and calcium along with magnesium, have importance in blood pressure regulation. Yet, at present, they are not recognized risks for hypertension in the young. Other than prudent dietary recommendations and avoidance of excesses, there are no general limitations or supplementations advocated for blacks or the public at large.

While alcohol, smoking, and diabetic disorders ultimately cause severe disease and affect blood pressure adversely, these problems cause little in the way of hypertensive difficulty in pediatric age groups. On the other hand, certain medications like cyclosporine and street drugs like PCP, may result in hypertension requiring treatment. Likewise pregnancy, now a not uncommon teenage condition, will be associated with hypertension in a significant number of instances.

Various types of stress, both physical and mental, are used to test for cardiovascular reactivity. While there are reported suggestive trends, the predictive accuracy of such stress testing remains to be confirmed. Nevertheless, it may be worthwhile to assess blood pressure response to exercise or to cold, especially in those with other risk factors such as a family history of hypertension. Other measures, such as blood uric acid level and echocardiographic LV mass, can be of further help in evaluating the risk for hypertension. While lacking in documentation, they are believed to be useful tests.

A window of opportunity exists to reduce the incidence of the disorder in the youth of our population by careful health advice to receptive young people. For them, knowledge of the just elaborated risk factors for hypertension could be a great benefit.

References

1. Stamler J. Blood pressure and high blood pressure: aspects of risk. *Hypertension* 18(suppl I):I-95-107, 1991.
2. Loggie JMH. Systemic hypertension. In: Adams FH, Emmanoulides GC, eds. *Moss' Heart Disease in Infants, Children and Adolescents, 3rd ed.* Baltimore: Williams & Wilkins; 1983:692-707.
3. Shear CL, Burke GL, Freedman DS, Berenson GS. Value of childhood blood pressure measurements and family history in predicting future blood pressure status: results from 8 years of follow-up in the Bogalusa Heart Study. *Pediatrics* 77:862- 869, 1986.
4. Clarke WR, Schrott HG, Weaverton PE, Connor WE, Lauer RM. Tracking of blood lipids and blood pressures in school-age children: The Muscatine study. *Circulation* 58: 626-634, 1978.
5. Lauer RM, Clarke WR. Childhood risk factors for high adult blood pressure: the Muscatine study. *Pediatrics* 84:633-641, 1989.
6. National Heart, Lung, and Blood Institute's Task Force on Blood Pressure Control in Children. Report of the second task force on blood pressure control in children. *Pediatrics* 79:1-25, 1987.
7. Lauer RM, Clarke WR, Beaglehole R. Level, trend and variability of blood pressure during childhood: The Muscatine Study. *Circulation* 69:242-249, 1984.
8. Williams RR, Hunt SC, Hasstedt SJ, Hopkins PN, Wu LL, Berry TD, Stults BM, Barlow GK, Schumacher MC, Lifton RP, Lalouel JM. Are there interactions and relations between genetic and environmental factors predisposing to high blood pressure? *Hypertension* 18(suppl I):I-29-37, 1991.
9. Rapp JP. Dissecting the primary causes of genetic hypertension in rats. *Hypertension* 18(suppl I):I-18-28, 1991.
10. Schieken RM. Genetic factors that predispose the child to develop hypertension. *Pediatr Clin North Am* 40:1-11, 1993.
11. Svejgaard A, Platz P, Ryder LP. HLA and disease 1982: a survey. *Immunol Rev* 70:193-218, 1983.
12. Feinleib M, Garrison RJ, Fabsitz R, Christian, JC, Hrubec, Borhani NO, Kannel WB, Rosenman R, Schwartz JT, Wagner JO. The NHLBI twin study of cardiovascular risk factors: methodology and summary of results. *Am J Epidemiol* 106:284-295, 1977.
13. Hunt SC, Hasstedt SJ, Kuida H, Stults BM, Hopkins PN, Williams RR. Genetic heritability and common environmental components of resting and stressed blood pressures, lipids, and body mass index in Utah pedigrees and twins. *Am J Epidemiol* 129:625-638, 1989.

14. Williams RR, Hunt SC, Hasstedt LB, Jorde LB, Wu LL, Barlow GK, Ash KO, Stults BM, Kuida H. The genetics of hypertension: an unsolved puzzle with many pieces. In: Vogel F, Sperling K, eds. *Human Genetics.* Berlin: Springer Verlag; 1987:311-325.

15. McIlhany ML, Shaffer JW, Hines EA. The heritability of blood pressure: an investigation of 200 pairs of twins using the cold pressor test. *Johns Hopkins Med J* 136:57-64, 1975.

16. Havlik RJ, Garrison RJ, Feinleib M, Katz HH, Kamnel WN, Castelli WP, McNamara PM. Blood pressure aggregation in families. *Am J Epidemiol* 110:304-312, 1979.

17. Leong GM, Gad K. Diet, salt, anthropological, and hereditary factors in hypertension. *Child Nephrol Urol* 12:96-105, 1992.

18. Havlik RJ, Feinleib M. The influence of federal programs on research on high blood pressure in the young. In: Kotchen TA, Kotchen JM, eds. *Clinical Approaches to High Blood Pressure in the Young.* Boston: John Wright; 1983:335-351.

19. Londe S, Bourgoignie JJ, Robson AM, Goldring D. Hypertension in apparently normal children. *J Pediatr* 78:569-577, 1978.

20. Higgins MW, Hinton PC, Keller JB. Weight and obesity as predictors of blood pressure and hypertension. In: Loggie MH, Horan MJ, Gruskin AB, Hohn AR, Dunbar JB, Havlick RJ, eds.*NHLBI Workshop on Juvenile Hypertension, Proceedings from a Symposium.* New York: Biomedical Information Corp; 1984: 125-143.

21. Lauer RM, Burns TL, Clarke WR, Mahoney LT. Childhood predictors of future blood pressure. *Hypertension* 18(suppl I):I-74-81, 1991.

22. Rocchini AP. Adolescent obesity and hypertension. *Pediatr Clin North Am* 40:81-92, 1993.

23. Gupta AR, Clark RV, Kirchner, KA. Effects of insulin on sodium excretion. *Hypertension* 19(suppl I):I-78-I-82, 1992.

24. Maruyama F. Nutritional modification in the young patient with hypertension. In: Kotchen TA, Kotchen JM, eds. *Clinical Approaches to High Blood Pressure in the Young.* Boston: John Wright; 1983:301-311.

25. Schachter J, Kuller L, Perfetti C. Blood pressure during the first two years of life. *Am J Epidemiol* 116:29-41, 1982.

26. *Blood Pressure Levels of Persons 6–74 Years, United States, 1971-1974.* Washington, DC: National Health Survey, National Center for Health Statistics. US Department of Health, Education, and Welfare, 1977.

27. Hohn AR, Riopel DA, Keil JE, Loadholt CB, Margolius HS, Halushka PV, Privitera PJ, Webb JG, Medley ES, Schuman SH, Rubin MI, Pantell RH, Braunstein ML. Childhood familial and racial differences in physiologic and biochemical factors related to hypertension. *Hypertension* 5:56-70, 1983.

28. Alpert BS, Fox ME. Racial aspects of blood pressure in children and adolescents. *Pediatr Clin North Am* 40: 13-22, 1993.

29. Berenson GS, Sprinivasan SR, Hunter SM, Nicklaus TA, Freedman DS, Shear CL, Webber LS. Risk factors in early life as predictors of

adult heart disease: The Bogalusa Heart Study. *Am J Med Sci* 298:141-151, 1989.

30. Murphy JK, Alpert BS, Walker SS, Willey ES. Race and cardiovascular reactivity: a replication. *Hypertension* 11:308-311, 1988.

31. Parmer GJ, Cervenka JH, Stone RA, O'Connor DT. Autonomic function in hypertension: are there racial differences? *Circulation* 81:1305-1311, 1990.

32. Hohn AR, Dwyer JH, Dwyer K. Blood pressure in four young racial groups: the Pasadena study. Submitted for publication, 1993.

33. Greenberger NJ, Isselbacher KJ. Disorders of absorption. In: Isselbacher KJ, ed. *Harrison's Principles of Internal Medicine, 9th ed.* New York: McGraw-Hill; 1980:1406-1407.

34. Sowers JR, Zemel MB, Zemel P, Beck FWJ, Walsh MF, Zawada ET. Salt sensitivity in blacks: salt intake and natriuretic substances. *Hypertension* 12:485-490, 1988.

35. Frisancho AS, Leonard WE, Bollettino LA. Blood pressure in blacks and whites and its relationship to dietary sodium and potassium intake. *J Chronic Dis* 37: 515-519, 1984.

36. Cook CA. Pathophysiologic and pharmacotherapy considerations in the management of the black hypertensive patient. *Am Heart J* 116:288-295, 1988.

37. Ruskin A. *Classics in Arterial Hypertension.* Springfield: Charles C Thomas; 1956:x-xii.

38. Stamler J. Blood pressure and high blood pressure: aspects of risk. *Hypertension* 18(suppl 1):1-95-107, 1991.

39. Stamler J, Rose G, Elliott P, Dyer A, Marmot M, Kesteloot H, Stamler R, for the INTERSALT Cooperative Research Group. Findings of the international cooperative INTERSALT Study. *Hypertension* 17(Suppl I):I-9-15, 1991.

40. Grobbee DE, Hofman A. Does sodium restriction lower blood pressure? *Br Med J* 293:27-29, 1986.

41. Kaplan NM. Long-term effectiveness of nonpharmacological treatment of hypertension. *Hypertension* 18(suppl I):I-153-160, 1991.

42. Hofman A, Hazebrook A, Valkenburg HA. A randomized trial of sodium intake and blood pressure in newborn infants. *JAMA* 250:370-374, 1983.

43. Grobbee DE, Bak AAA. Electrolyte intake and hypertension in children. In: Rettig R, Ganten D, Luft F, eds. *Salt and Hypertension.* Heidelberg: Springer-Verlag; 1989:283-292.

44. Miller JZ, Weinberger MH, Daugherty SA, Fineberg NS, Christian JC, Grim C. Blood pressure response to dietary sodium restriction in healthy normotensive children. *Am J Clin Nutr* 47:113-119, 1988.

45. Rauh W, Levine LS, New MI. The role of dietary salt in juvenile hypertension. In: Giovanelli G, New MI, Gorini S, eds.*Hypertension in Children and Adolescents.* New York: Raven Press; 1981:34-44.

46. Life Science Research Office, Federation of American Societies for Experimental Biology. *Evaluation of the health aspects of sodium*

chloride and potassium chloride as food ingredients. Contract No FDA 223-75-2004, 1979. Washington, DC: Bureau of Foods, Food and Drug Administration.

47. Howe PRC, Cobiac L, Smith RM. Lack of effect on short-term changes in sodium intake on blood pressure in adolescent school children. *J Hypertens* 9:181-186, 1991.

48. Treasure J, Ploth S. Role of dietary potassium in the treatment of hypertension. *Hypertension* 5: 864-872, 1983.

49. Fujito T, Ando K. Hemodynamic and endocrine changes associated with potassium supplementation in sodium loaded hypertensives. *Hypertension* 6:184-192, 1984.

50. Skrabal F, Aubock J, Hortnagi H. Low sodium-high potassium diet for prevention of hypertension: probable mechanisms of action. *Lancet* 2 (8252):895-900, 1981.

51. Miller JZ, Weinberger MH, Christian JC. Blood pressure response to potassium supplementation in normotensive adults and children. *Hypertension* 10:437-442, 1987.

52. McCarron DA, Calcium metabolism and hypertension. In: Cohen JJ, Harrington JT, Kassierer JP, Madias NE, eds. *Nephrology Forum.* Kidney Int 35:717-736, 1989.

53. Grobbee DE, Hackeng WHL, Birkenhager JC, Hofman A. Raised plasma intact parathyroid hormone concentrations in young people with mildly raised blood pressure. *Br Med J* 296:814-816, 1988.

54. Grobbee DE, Hofman A. Effect of calcium supplementation on diastolic blood pressure in young people with mild hypertension. *Lancet* 2:703-706, 1986.

55. Lyle RM, Melby CL, Hyner GC, Edmondson JW, Miller JZ, Weinberger MH. Blood pressure and metabolic effects of calcium supplementation in normotensive white and black men. *JAMA* 257:1772-1776, 1987.

56. Meese RB, Gonzales DG, Casparian JM, Ram CV, Pak CM, Kaplan NM. The inconsistent effects of calcium supplements upon blood pressure in primary hypertension. *Am J Med Sci* 294:219-224, 1987.

57. Nowson C, Morgan T. Effect of calcium carbonate on blood pressure in normotensive and hypertensive people. *Hypertension* 13:630-639, 1989.

58. Kurta TW, Al-Bander HA, Morris RC. "Salt-sensitive" essential hypertension in men. *N Engl J Med* 317:1043-1048, 1987.

59. Johnson NE, Smith EL, Freudenheim JL. Effects on blood pressure of calcium supplementation of women. *Am J Clin Nutr* 42:12-17, 1985.

60. Taufield PA, Ales KL, Resnick LM, Gertner JM, Laragh JH. Hypocalciuria in preeclampsia. *N Engl J Med* 316:715-718, 1987.

61. Heath H, Lambert PW, Service FJ, Arnaud SB. Calcium homeostasis in diabetes mellitus. *J Clin Endocrinol Metab* 49:462-466, 1979.

62. Criqui MH, Langer RD, Reed DM. Dietary alcohol, calcium and potassium. Independent and combined effects on blood pressure. *Circulation* 80:609-614, 1989.

63. Dwyer JH, Scribner R, Hohn A, Dwyer KM. Effect of calcium supplementation on blood pressure in African-American youth. *33rd Annual Conference on Cardiovascular Epidemiology* Santa Fe, NM: 1993. Abstract.

64. McGarvey ST, Zinner SH, Willett WC, Rosner B. Maternal prenatal dietary potassium, calcium, magnesium, and infant blood pressure. *Hypertension* 17:218-224, 1991.

65. Rinner MD, Spliet-van Laar L, Kromhout D. Serum sodium, potassium, calcium, and magnesium and blood pressure in a Dutch population. *J Hypertens* 7:977-981, 1989.

66. Tillman DM, Semple PF. Calcium and magnesium in essential hypertension. *Clin Sci* 75:395-402, 1988.

67. Saiato K, Hattori K, Omatsu T, Hirouchi H, Sano H. Effects of oral magnesium on blood pressure and red cell sodium transport in patients receiving long-term thiazide diuretics for hypertension. *Am J Hypertens* 1:71S-74S, 1988.

68. Murphy MB, Zebrauskas D, Schutte S, Wood G, Geiser R, Douglas FL, Elliott WJ. Oral magnesium supplementation in diuretic treated patients. *Am J Hypertens* 2:43A, 1989. Abstract.

69. Kaplan NM. Comment. In: Schlant RC, Collins JJ Jr, Engle MA, Frye RE, Kaplan NM, O'Rourke RA, eds. *Yearbook of Cardiology*. Chicago: Year Book Medical Pub; 1989:305.

70. Jose PA, Martin GR, Felder RA. Cardiovascular and autonomic influences on blood pressure. In: Loggie JMH, ed. *Pediatric and Adolescent Hypertension*. Boston: Blackwell Scientific Pub; 1992:44-48.

71. Mahoney LT, Schieken RM, Clarke WR, Lauer, RM. Left ventricular mass and exercise responses predict future blood pressure. The Muscatine study. *Hypertension* 12:206-213, 1988.

72. Fixler DE, Laird WP, Dana K. Usefulness of exercise stress testing for prediction of blood pressure trends. *Pediatrics* 75:1071-1075, 1985.

73. Wilson MF, Sung BH, Pincomb GA, Lovallo WR. Exaggerated pressure response to exercise in men at risk for systemic hypertension. *Am J Cardiol* 66:731-736, 1990.

74. Hammond HK, Fjroelicher VF. The physiologic sequelae of chronic dynamic exercise. *Med Clin North Am* 69:21-39, 1985.

75. Hagberg JM, Ehsani AA, Goldring D, Hernandez A, Sinacore DR, Holloszy JO. Effect of weight training on blood pressure and hemodynamics in hypertensive adolescents. *J Pediatr* 104:147-151, 1984.

76. Falkner B, Onesti G, Angelakos ET, Fernandez M, Langman C. Cardiovascular response to mental stress in normal adolescents with hypertensive parents. *Hypertension* 1:23-30, 1979.

77. Light KC, Obrist PA, Sherwood A, James SA, Strogatz DS. Effects of race and marginally elevated blood pressure on responses to stress. *Hypertension* 10:555-563, 1987.

78. Murphy JK, Alpert BS, Walker SS, Willey ES. Race and cardiovascular reactivity: A replication. *Hypertension* 11:308-311, 1988.

79. Falkner B, Onesti G, Hamstra B. Stress response characteristics of

adolescents with high genetic risk for essential hypertension: a five year follow-up. *Clin Exp Hypertens* 3:583-591, 1981.

80. Ragland DR, Winkleby MA, Schwalbe J, Holman BL, Morse L, Syme SL, Fisher JM. Prevalence of hypertension in bus drivers. *Int J Epidemiol* 16:208-214, 1987.

81. Hoffman JW, Benson H, Arns PA, Stainbrook GL, Landsberg L, Young JB, Gill A. Reduced sympathetic nervous system responsivity associated with the relaxation response. *Science* 215:190-192, 1982.

82. Wood DL, Sheps SG, Elveback LR, Schirger A. Cold pressor test as a predictor of hypertension. *Hypertension* 6:301-306, 1984.

83. Parker FC, Croft JB, Cresanta JL, Freedman DS, Burke GL, Webber LS. The association between cardiovascular response tasks and future blood pressures levels in children: Bogalusa Heart Study. *Am Heart J* 113:1174-1179, 1987.

84. Dwyer K. Modified Pawtucket step test: grant manual for the Pasadena prevention project (personal communication), 1992.

85. Benowitz NL, Kuyt F, Jacob P III: Influence of nicotine on cardiovascular and hormonal effects of cigarette smoking. *Clin Pharmacol Ther* 36:74-81, 1984.

86. Mann SJ, James GD, Wang RS, Pickering TG. Elevation of ambulatory systolic blood pressure in hypertensive smokers: A case-control study. *JAMA* 265:2226-2228, 1991.

87. Heydon S, Schneider KA, Fodor JG. Smoking habits and antihypertensive treatment. *Nephron* 47:99-103, 1987.

88. Isles C, Brown JJ, Cumming AMM, Lever AF, McAreavey D, Robertson JIS, Hawthorne VM, Stewart GM, Robertson JWK, Wapshaw J. Excess smoking in malignant-phase hypertension. *Br Med J* 1:579-581, 1979.

89. Hampson NB. Correspondence: Smokeless is not saltless. *N Engl J Med* 312:919-920, 1985.

90. Levenson J, Simon AC, Cambien FA, Beretti C. Cigarette smoking and hypertension: factors independently associated with blood hyperviscosity and arterial rigidity. *Arteriosclerosis* 7:572-577, 1987.

91. Williams MA, Mittendorf R, Monson RR. Chronic hypertension, cigarette smoking, and abruptio placentae. *Epidemiology* 2:450-453, 1991.

92. Keil U, Chambless L, Filipiak B, Haertel U. Alcohol and blood pressure and its interaction with smoking and other behavioral variables: results from the MONICA Augsburg Survey 1984-1985. *J Hypertens* 9:491-498, 1991.

93. Ingall TJ, Homer D, Baker HL Jr, Kottke BA, O'Fallon WM, Whisnant JP. Predictors of intracranial carotid artery atherosclerosis: duration of cigarette smoking and hypertension are more powerful than serum lipid levels. *Arch Neurol* 48:687-691, 1991.

94. Fowkes FG, Housley E, Riemersma RA, MacIntyre CC, Cawood EH, Prescott RJ, Ruckley CV. Smoking, lipids, glucose intolerance, and blood pressure as risk factors for peripheral atherosclerosis compared

with ischemic heart disease in the Edinburgh Artery Study. *Am J Epidemiol* 135:331-440, 1992.

95. Mueller HR, Buser MW. Smoking and hypertension: risk factors for carotid stenosis. *J Neurol* 238:97-102, 1991.

96. Homer D, Ingall TJ, Baker HL Jr, O'Fallon WM, Kottke BA, Whisnant JP. Serum lipids and lipoproteins are less powerful predictors of extracranial carotid artery atherosclerosis than are cigarette smoking and hypertension. *Mayo Clin Proc* 66:259-267, 1991.

97. Salonen JT, Salonen R. Association of serum low density lipoprotein cholesterol, smoking, and hypertension with different manifestations of atherosclerosis. *Int J Epidemiol* 19:911-917, 1990.

98. Strachan DP. Predictors of death from aortic aneurysm among middle-aged men: the Whitehall study. *Br J Surg* 78:401-414, 1991.

99. Materson BJ, Reda D, Freis ED, Henderson WD. Cigarette smoking interferes with treatment of hypertension. *Arch Intern Med* 148:2116-2119, 1988.

100. Feely J, Crookes J, Stevernson IH. The influence of age, smoking, and hyperthyroidism on plasma propranolol steady state concentration. *Br J Clin Pharmacol* 12:73-78, 1981.

101. Medical Research Council (MRC) Working Party: Stroke and coronary heart disease in mild hypertension: risk factors and the value of treatment. *Br Med J* 296:1565-1570, 1988.

102. Vyssoulis GP, Karpanou EA, Pitsavos CE, Toutouzas MA, Paleologos AA, Toutouzas PK. Dyslipidemic effects of cigarette smoking on β-blocker-induced serum lipid changes in systemic hypertension. *Am J Cardiol* 67:987-992, 1991.

103. Ballantyne D, Devine BL, Fife R. Interrelation of age, obesity, cigarette smoking, and blood pressure in hypertensive patients. *Br Med J* 1:880-881, 1978.

104. Seltzer CC. Effect of smoking on blood pressure. *Am Heart J* 87:558-564, 1974.

105. Gerace TA, Hollis J, Ockene JK, Svendsen K. Smoking cessation and change in diastolic blood pressure, body weight, and plasma lipids. MRFIT Research Group. *Prevent Med* 20:602-620, 1991.

106. Hohn AR. The Pasadena Study: Unpublished data, 1987.

107. Dwyer JH, Lippert P, Rieger-Ndakorerwa GE, Semmer NK. Some chronic disease risk factors and cigarette smoking inadolescents: the Berlin-Bremen Study. *MMWR* 36(suppl 4):36S-40S, 1988.

108. Dwyer JH. The Berlin-Bremen Study. Unpublished data: (personal communication). 1992.

109. Wilson JF, Straus R. Behavioral considerations in high blood pressure in the young. In: Kotchen TA, Kotchen JM, eds. *Clinical Approaches to High Blood Pressure in the Young.* Boston: John Wright; 1983:288-289.

110. Lian C. L'alcoholisme, cause d'hypertension arterielle. *Bull Acad Natl Med* (Paris) 74:525-528, 1915.

111. Mori TA, Puddey IB, Wilkinson SP, Beilin LJ, Vandongen R. Urinary

steroid profiles and alcohol-related blood pressure elevation. *Clin Exp Pharm Physiol* 18:287-290, 1991.
112. Yamada Y, Ishizaki M, Kido T, Honda R, Tsuritani I, Ikai E, Yamaya H. Elevations of serum angiotensin-converting enzyme and α-glutamyl-transpeptidase activities in hypertensive drinkers. *J Human Hypertens* 5:183-188, 1991.
113. Klatsky AL, Friedman GD, Siegelaub AB, Gerard MJ. Alcohol consumption and blood pressure. *N Engl J Med* 296:1194-1200, 1977.
114. Criqui MH, Wallace RB, Mishkel M, Barrett-Conner E, Heiss G. Alcohol consumption and blood pressure: the Lipid Research Clinics Prevalence Study. *Hypertension* 1:557-565, 1981.
115. Kannel WB, Sorlie P. Hypertension in Framingham. In: Paul O, ed. *Epidemiology and Control of Hypertension*. New York: Straton Intercontinental Medical Book 1975;553-581.
116. Maheswaran R, Beevers M, Beevers DG. Effectiveness of advice to reduce alcohol consumption in hypertensive patients. *Hypertension* 19:79-84, 1992.
117. Klatsky AL, Friedman GD, Armstrong MA. The relationships of alcoholic beverage use and other traits to blood pressure: a new Kaiser Permanente Study. *Circulation* 73:628-636, 1986.
118. Bradley JG. Nonprescription drugs and hypertension. Which ones affect blood pressure? *Postgraduate Med* 89:195-197, 201-202, 1991.
119. Hohn AR. The Pasadena Study, Unpublished data, 1985.
120. Porter GA, Bennett WM, Sheps SG, for the National High Blood Pressure Education Program. Cyclosporine-associated hypertension. *Arch Intern Med* 150:180-283, 1990.
121. Cregler LL, Mark H. Medical complications of cocaine abuse.*N Engl J Med* 315:1495-1500, 1986.
122. McCarron MM, Schulze BW, Thompson GA, Conder MC, Goetz WA. Acute phencyclidine intoxication: clinical patterns, complications and treatment. *Ann Emerg Med* 10:290-297, 1981.
123. Barron WM, Murphy MB, Lindheimer MD. Management of hypertension during pregnancy. In: Laragh JH, Brenner BM, eds. *Hypertension: Pathophysiology, Diagnosis, and Management*. New York: Raven Press; 1990:1809-1827.
124. Fisher KA, Luger A, Spargo BH, Lindheimer MD. Hypertension in pregnancy: clinical-pathological correlations and remote prognosis. *Medicine* 60:267-276, 1981.
125. Cunningham FG, Lindheimer MD. Hypertension in pregnancy. In: Desforges JF, eds. Current concepts. *N Engl J Med* 326:927- 932, 1992.
126. Van Dam PA, Renier M, Baekelandt M, Baytaert P, Uyttenbroeck F. Disseminated intravascular coagulation and the syndrome of hemolysis, elevated liver enzymes, and low platelets in severe preeclampsia. *Obstet Gynecol* 73:97-102, 1989.
127. Brazy JE, Grim JK, Little VA. Neonatal manifestations of severe maternal hypertension occurring before the thirty-sixth week of pregnancy. *J Pediatr* 100:265-271, 1982.

128. Imperiale TF, Petrulis AS. A meta-analysis of low-dose aspirin for the prevention of pregnancy-induced hypertensive disease. *JAMA* 266:260-264, 1991.

129. Belizan JM, Villar J, Gonzalez L, Campodonico L, Bergel E. Calcium supplementation to prevent hypertensive disorders of pregnancy. *N Engl J Med* 325:1399-1405, 1991.

130. Gennser G, Rymark P, Isberg PE. Low birth weight and risk of high blood pressure in adulthood. *Br Med J* 296:1498-1500, 1988.

131. Sell LL, Cullen ML, Lerner GL, Whittlesey GC, Shanley CJ, Klein MD. Hypertension during extracorporeal membrane oxygenation: cause, effect, and management. *Surgery* 102:724-730, 1987.

132. Ibsen KK. Factors influencing blood pressure in children and adolescents. *Acta Paediatr Scand* 74:416-422, 1985.

133. Garrison RJ, Kannel WB, Stokes J III, Castelle WP. Incidence and precursors of hypertension in young adults: the Framingham Offspring Study. *Prevent Med* 16:235-251, 1987.

134. Le Floch JP, Christin S, Bertherat J, Perlemuter L, Hazard J. Blood pressure and microvascular complications in type I (insulin-dependent) diabetic patients without hypertension.*Diabetes Metab* 16:26-29, 1990.

135. Christlieb AR. Treatment selection considerations for the hypertensive diabetic patient. *Arch Intern Med* 150:1167- 1174, 1990.

136. Prebis JW, Gruskin AB, Polinsky MS, Baluarte HJ. Uric acid in childhood essential hypertension. *J Pediatr* 98:702-707, 1981.

137. Fessel JW. High uric acid as an indicator of cardiovascular disease: independence from obesity. *Am J Med* 68:401-404, 1980.

138. Devereux RB. Detection of left ventricular hypertrophy by M- mode echocardiography: anatomic validation, standardization and comparison to other methods. *Hypertension* 9(suppl II): II-19-II-26, 1987.

139. Casale PN, Devereux RB, Milner M, Zullo G, Harshfield GA, Pickering TG, Laragh JH. Value of echocardiographic measurement of left ventricular mass in predicting cardiovascular morbid events in hypertensive men. *Ann InternMed* 105:173-178, 1986.

140. Culpepper WA III. Cardiac risk factors in juvenile hypertension. *Hosp Pract* 51-60, 1985.

141. Stamler R, Stamler J, Gosch FC, Civinelli J, Fishman J, McKeever P, McDonald A, Dyer AR. Primary prevention of hypertension by nutritional-hygienic means: final report of a randomized, controlled trial. *JAMA* 262:1801-1807, 1989.

Chapter 5

Cardiac Hypertension

Introduction

The heart has a vital role in all hypertensive disorders. Indeed the physiologic adjustments of the heart to systemic hypertension can be readily assessed by noninvasive testing. While the electrocardiogram may indicate severe cardiac involvement, the response of the heart to pressure overload can best be evaluated using echocardiography or magnetic resonance imaging. Left ventricular wall thickness as quantitatively determined by these modalities is a measure of how much pressure must be generated by the heart over time. In other words, if the left ventricular wall thickness is increased in a hypertensive individual, that person has a significant disorder. Conversely, if wall thickness is normal, the hypertension noted is probably intermittent in nature. The latter findings are common with early or labile hypertension.

The type of left ventricular response found in systemic hypertension, i.e., left ventricular hypertension, can also be seen with ventricular outflow obstruction. Some of the highest left ventricular pressures are found with aortic stenosis. Yet such disorders are not considered hypertensive because there are no systemic manifestations of the elevated pressure. However, with coarctation of the aorta, a unique set of circumstances affecting left ventricular pressure pertain. Not only are there contrasting blood pressures proximal and distal to the coarctation, but there are contrasts pre- and postinterventional treatment. Thus, a fertile clinical setting is provided to study certain hypertensive mechanisms.

Today, as a result of modern diagnostic technology, coarctation of the aorta is largely a disorder of infants and young children. In that age group it may account for as much as 20% of those found hypertensive from a known cause.[1] On occasion, coarctation may escape detection until later ages so that all initial clinical examinations for hypertension must include palpation of upper and lower extremity pulses and, preferably, blood pressure sampling from those sites. Those providing health care for the young must take their young patient's blood pressure. If it is high, pressures from the other three limbs must be obtained. Once a discrepancy is found, echo-Doppler study can be used to seal the diagnosis in most cases.

Coarctation, Embryology, and Anatomy

Embryologic theories provide certain insights into the cause of hypertension found in coarctation of the aorta. Of the explanatory hypotheses, faulty union of the aortic arches with the descending aorta is no longer accepted as a valid cause. While constriction of ductal tissue in the aorta has been found to cause aortic constriction after palliation for the hypoplastic left heart syndrome, this mechanism generally is not felt to fully account for aortic coarctations.[2] Most hold that fetal hemodynamic forces mold the disorder.[3] It is thought that decreased antegrade aortic blood flow develops. This leads to a proportionate increase in fetal right heart-main pulmonary artery blood flow. In turn, there is increased flow through the ductus arteriosus into the descending aorta. A posterior aortic shelf forms and may deflect ductal flow proximally into the left subclavian artery and distally into the descending aorta. Ductal constriction may impact on this process after birth. Although sufficient fetal ascending aorta flow exists to supply the first arch branches, there is reduced isthmic flow. Tubular hypoplasia of the isthmus results from this process. In extreme cases, isthmic atresia occurs, causing interrupted aortic arch. Anomalies, such as malalignment ventricular septal defects which divert blood from the aorta, promote the process described. However, defects like tetralogy of Fallot, which increase ascending aortic flow are seldom associated with coarctation of the aorta.

Current anatomical classifications of aortic coarctation are based on the elaborated embryologic concepts. Thus, in the young, coarctations are labeled as "periductal" in recognition of the fact

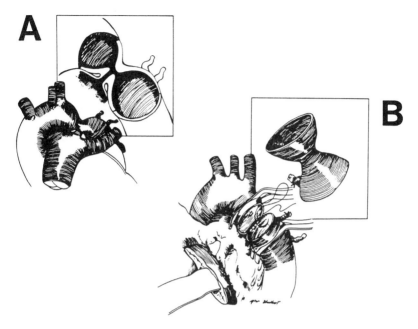

Figure 1: (A) Aortic arch with periductal coarctation. Inset showing entry of a patent ductus at the site of the coarctation. (B) Excision of the aortic coarctation and ductal stump (inset) with repair of the aorta by end-to-end anastomosis. (Modified from drawings provided through the courtesy of Winfield Wells, M. D.).

that the aortic constriction may be at, above, or below the site of ductal entry (Fig. 1A). In older individuals, where the site of coarctation generally is distal to the ligamentum arteriosum, the terminology of "adult coarctation" is in common usage.

Pathophysiology

Mechanical Factors

Over the years it has become increasingly clear that the hypertension found in coarctation of the aorta is not simply the result of the anatomical aortic narrowing. Indeed, mechanical factors as a cause of coarctation hypertension have been discredited by arguments such as infrarenal coarctation, which fails to produce hypertension, and the fact that the proximally transplanted kidney relieves hypertension in coarctation.[4] Yet, such statements do not take into account that renal depressor mechanisms could normalize blood pressure in infrarenal coarctation. Nor do they consider that the cervical kidney adds a low-resistance circuit to the proximal circulation, which could also lower blood pressure. Certainly, hypertension follows immediately in experimental narrowing of the aorta, and the embryologic considerations previously cited make it likely that a chain of events is initiated by mechanical factors of aortic narrowing.

Renal Mechanisms

Beginning with Goldblatt's studies in 1939 of aortic constriction and the studies of cervical renal autotransplantation by Scott and colleagues in 1951, renal factors in the hypertension of coarctation of the aorta have received considerable attention.[4,5] Investigations of the renin-angiotensin (RA) system have led many to conclude that the RA system has an important role in the hypertension of coarctation. Findings such as greater elevation of plasma renin following exercise in those with unoperated coarctations than in those without coarctation, and excessive RA activity by saralasin testing pre- and postoperative repair of coarctation gives credibility to the involvement of the RA system.[6] The inverse relationship of angiotensin II to volume has been shown experimentally to be true for acutely induced aortic constriction. On the other hand, with chronic experimental coarctation the relationship is less clear. Accordingly, other workers have postulated mechanisms not involving angiotensin II and/or volume retention. Renal sympathetic nerves also have been felt to play a role in the hypertension of coarctation, for removal of these nerves in animals with coarctation reduces their hypertension by about half.

Nonrenal Neural Mechanisms

Neural mechanisms like baroreceptor-mediated responses have been demonstrated to play a role in the hypertension of acute experimental aortic constriction. In chronic animal models there is a resetting of the baroreceptors and little of the changes seen with the acute response can be found. But subtle changes in sympathetic nervous system activity do exist. There are alterations in vascular resistance and decreased levels of plasma norepinephrine.

Regional Vascular Factors

Reactivity of various regional vascular beds are thought to be altered in coarctation of the aorta and thus contribute to the pathophysiology. However, conflicting information has been reported with respect to regional vascular factors such as degree and location of "waterlogged" arterial walls. Therefore, further and more controlled studies are required to determine the significance of regional vascular factors in coarctation.

Clinical Patterns

Age has a profound bearing on the expressed features of aortic coarctation.[7] The sick infant with symptomatic coarctation has a clinical picture characteristically different from the asymptomatic child or older individual and will be discussed separately.

Infantile Coarctation Syndrome

Associated cardiovascular anomalies are the rule in infants with symptomatic coarctation. Only 10% have isolated aortic narrowing. Most common associations include arch hypoplasia (in 75%), patent ductus arteriosus (in 67%), and bicuspid aortic valve.[8-11] Fifty percent are found to have ventricular septal defects. Multiple left-sided lesions may be present with the coarctation, such as combinations of mitral valve, supramitral, and aortic valve abnormalities (the Shone complex).[8,9] The left subclavian artery, with its proximity to the site of coarctation, may be underdeveloped as well. As would be anticipated, the clinical picture in these patients depends on the interaction of the pathophysiologies of the various associated lesions with the degree of aortic narrowing and collateral formation.

Most infants with the coarctation syndrome present with symptoms of congestive heart failure. Historically, there is tachypnea or dyspnea, especially with feeding, excessive perspiration, and poor weight gain. Evidences of these features are seen on examination along with tachycardia and hepatomegaly. Heart murmurs reflecting both the coarctation and associated defects are heard. Pulses may be diminished or absent in the lower extremities with corresponding lower blood pressures. In severe cases, an infant's critical condition is evidenced by a general absence of pulses. On the other hand, with a widely patent ductus arteriosus, pulses and blood pressures may be similar in all limbs. In the latter instance, spontaneous sudden closure of the ductus may result in rapid onset of a shock syndrome.

Roentgenographic studies show cardiomegaly and increased pulmonary vascularity. Right ventricular hypertrophy, the result of increased intrauterine stress on the right ventricle, is found on the electrocardiogram (ECG). Two-dimensional echocardiography is so effective in identifying not only the coarctation but also associated defects that cardiac catheterization may not be necessary.[12] Doppler studies, especially with color, confirm the expected flow patterns and aid in visualizing the defects.

Childhood Coarctation

Coarctation in those outside the infant age group is generally an asymptomatic condition and often occurs as an isolated situation. However, in two thirds of cases there is an associated bicuspid aortic valve. Usually the diagnosis is made by a careful physician noting pulse or blood pressure differences between upper and lower limbs on an examination for a heart murmur or in the course of a workup for hypertension.[13] However, blood pressure may be normal if there are large collaterals around the coarctation. In occasional instances, there may be complaints of fatigability, leg weakness, or pain. Cardiac failure is very uncommon. Typically a grade 1–2/6 long systolic murmur, from turbulence at the coarctation site, is heard at the cardiac apex as well as along the left lower sternal border and left axilla. In addition, the basal ejection murmur of a bicuspid aortic valve or a posterior continuous murmur in the scapular area from collaterals may be heard. In these cases the proximal aorta may be dilated but the ductus is most often closed.

Normal heart size and pulmonary vascularity on chest radiograph is the rule. On occasion, an indentation of the descending aortic coarctation may be seen. Rib notching is infrequent, being found only in those who escape detection until they are over 5 years of age. Although often normal, the ECG may indicate left ventricular hypertrophy. An incomplete right bundle branch block is found in about 10% of children with coarctation. Echo-color-flow Doppler studies are usually diagnostic. In a few large children, there may be some difficulty in obtaining adequate transthoracic echo- Doppler studies due to size. In equivocal cases, when diagnostic echo studies cannot be obtained, aortography may resolve any doubts about location and aortic collaterals. Magnetic resonance imaging of the area will also provide such information.

Protocol for Diagnosis

While clinical criteria suffice for diagnosis in all but a few infants and older individuals, it is likely that catheter verification of the diagnosis will continue at many centers in conjunction with the catheter interventional treatment to be described. The diagnostic protocol listed below must be modified according to local philosophy.

1. Diagnosis of coarctation is suspected when one of the following is present: a) pulses diminished and or absent in lower extremities in contrast to the upper limbs; b) blood pressures are higher in the upper versus lower extremities; generally, there is a difference of about 40 mm Hg between the limbs. Proximal hypertension may exist and be especially high among infants with poor collateral circulation; c) presence of the previously described coarctation or collateral murmur with (a) or (b); d) chest radiograph showing indentation of the proximal descending thoracic aorta with (a) or (b).

2. Confirmation of the diagnosis is by visualization of the coarctation by echocardiography, aortography, digital subtraction angiography, or magnetic resonance imaging along with echo-Doppler demonstration of variation of flow at the coarctation site.

3. When coarctation of the aorta has been confirmed by the above criteria, the status of collateral arterial circulation should be considered if there is either a high (over 50 mm Hg) or a low (below 20 mm Hg) blood pressure gradient between the upper and lower limbs. Detection of collateral vessels may require imaging studies such as aortography.

4. Assessment for the presence of associated defects by echocardiography and/or other suitable imaging techniques. Should the

patient be found to have associated defects, cardiac catheterization may be indicated.

Treatment

The currently accepted definitive treatment of aortic coarctation by surgery is being increasingly challenged by advocates of balloon aortoplasty. Initial results are encouraging, but this debate will only be settled by long-term follow-up studies. While many authorities use operative techniques to repair previously unoperated or native coarctation, consensus holds that balloon aortoplasty is usually the choice in discrete, recurrent, or residual coarctation. In any event, a symptomatic patient should first be treated medically. However, prolonged medical treatment of proximal hypertension should be avoided. These concepts are elaborated in the following sections.

Medical Measures

Coarctation of the aorta commonly results in congestive heart failure in early infancy. The cardiac decompensation may occur suddenly as a result of ductal closure and associated aortic narrowing. Alternatively, it may be the progressive result of one or more of the variety of defects in the coarctation complex. As is often the case, the failure is severe and requires medical therapy prior to definitive invasive treatment. In these cases, inotropic treatment is especially efficacious. Digoxin has been used for years for this purpose and may yield dramatic improvement. Antihypertensive measures are useful, particularly with high proximal pressures. Aggressive propranolol therapy (1 mg/kg per dose every 6 hours orally) can produce needed relief. Captopril also may be used for this purpose (0.1 to 0.4 mg/kg per dose every 8 hours orally). When sudden newborn ductal closure leads to a shock-like picture, prostaglandin E-1 infusion (0.05 to 0.1 μg/kg per minute) to reopen the ductus arteriosus may be life saving (Table 1).[14]

Unless symptoms are mild, the goal of medical measures is to prepare the patient for surgery or perhaps other interventional treatment. In those with minimal problems, intervention is generally carried out at age 1 to 3 years. In more symptomatic infants, it is unwise to delay definitive relief. Even with good initial response to

Table 1.
Pharmacologic Agents Useful in Coarctation of the Aorta

Agent	Dose/Frequency	Route of Adm.
Propranolol	1 mg/kg/dose q6h	P. O.
	(0.1–0.2 mg/kg per dose q4 to 6h)	I. V.
Captopril	1–6 mg/kg divided to 3 doses q8h	P. O.
	(for infants: 0.1–0.4 mg/dose q8h)	P. O.
Prostaglandin E:1	0.05–0.1 μg/kg per min (infusion)	I. V.
Hydralazine	0.15 mg/kg/4h	I. V.
Nitroprusside	0.5–1.0 μg/kg per min (infusion)	I. V.

a medical approach, such measures have limited value and myocardial damage may become severe.

Balloon Dilation Aortoplasty

Angioplastic techniques have seen increasing usage and success in pediatrics. Beginning around the early eighties, carefully sized balloon-dilation catheters have been introduced via the femoral artery route, commonly using percutaneous techniques, and passed in retrograde fashion to the site of aortic narrowing (Fig. 2 A&B).[15] Balloon aortoplasty was first used for recurrent coarctation. Catheter-balloon dilatation of the site of recurrent coarctationhas proven so successful that many consider it the procedure of choice. The attractiveness of the procedure is enhanced by the fact that the repeat surgical approach to these problems is difficult. Adhesions cause the operative anatomy to be distorted and greatly increase the effort of surgical access. Thus, the results of reoperation for aortic coarctation may not be completely satisfactory. With the support of cardiovascular surgeons, considerable experience has been gained with balloon aortoplasty for recurrent coarctation.[16] Aortoplasty has proven safe and effective. Residual gradients are generally reduced below 15 to 20 mm Hg and the aortic lumen size increased to three fourths of normal or larger. However, the procedure awaits long-term follow-up data to determine whether or not recoarctation, aneurysm formation, or other complications will develop as late sequelae.

Catheter-balloon dilatation of native coarctation is also used increasingly, even in neonates via the umbilical artery.[17] There is a distinct lack of enthusiasm on the part of cardiac surgeons for balloon dilation of native coarctations. Aneurysmal formation at the site of coarctation dilation has been reported and is of great concern.[18] Since surgical relief has been generally efficacious, operative intervention continues as the mainstay of native coarcta-

A

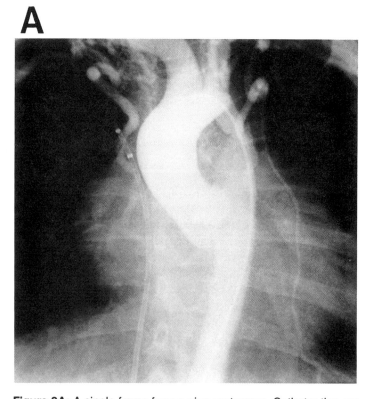

Figure 2A: A single frame from a cine aortogram. Catheter tips are in the ascending aorta (for injection) and superior vena cava (as a marker). An aortic coarctation is seen distal to the arch branches. A collateral artery arises just distal to the aortic narrowing. It overlays most of the obstructing "posterior shelf."

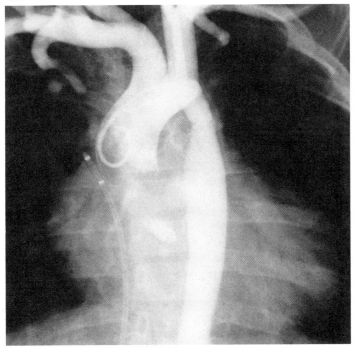

Figure 2B: Same case after a balloon aortoplasty. Most of the "posterior shelf" has been obliterated. Preballoon pressures were 170/95 in the ascending aorta and, 100/80 distal to the coarctation. Postballoon pressures were 157/80 and 135/85, respectively.

tion relief in most centers, particularly in the very young. However, aneurysms also occur following surgery, albeit rarely. Recent studies indicate that balloon dilation of native aortic coarctation is effective and safe.[19-21] The work is too current to know of late sequelae and should be regarded as preliminary.

Surgical Repair

The surgery for coarctation of the aorta has seen considerable change since it was first introduced by Crafoord and Gross in 1941.[22,23] Age for operation, excision versus relief of obstruction, and prosthetic materials used have all evolved. Current philosophy in many centers suggests that elective resection of the coarctation at 1 to 3 years of age is the approach of choice. Earlier operation is recommended if there is significant hypertension or symptoms. Operation at a young age is best to prevent late postoperative hypertension. In those over the age of 1 year, the aorta is of sufficient size that recoarctation is unlikely, and the use of interrupted sutures of strong, thin, new materials such as prolene allows for growth of the aortic lumen.

In the newborn or infant who does not respond rapidly to medical measures, surgery should be undertaken at once. In such instances, some form of aortoplasty has seen common usage. Of the two-patch aortoplasty techniques, synthetic patch or subclavian flap, the latter has found wide acceptance.[24] Many surgeons now use the subclavian flap aortoplasty for infants, and may employ the same technique for older patients as well. Late postoperative synthetic-patch aortoplasty aneurysms found in certain instances have lessened the use of the technique.[25] Similarly, subclavian flap enthusiasts point to studies showing late postoperative gradients across aortic resection repair sites as evidence for the superiority of their repair.[26,27] However, such studies compared cases done with suture methods no longer in use and may not be pertinent. Most recently, there has been a resurgence of interest in using resection and end-to-end aortic anastomosis for neonates and infants (Fig. 1B). In any event, final risk assessment of the flap repair method versus resection and anastomosis still requires further study over time to determine if late postoperative complications particularly recoarctation, hypertension, and aneurysm will be problems.

Postcoarctation Repair Syndromes

Paradoxical Hypertension

Hypertension may exacerbate instead of resolve following coarctation repair. This paradoxical situation may be found in the early (within 24 hours of operation) or in the late postoperative period (2 to 5 days later). It may even persist for an indefinite period (over 1-month after operation). At least two thirds of patients operated on for aortic coarctation experience some type of postoperative hypertension. Investigations concerning mechanisms responsible for these types of paradoxical hypertension are provocative in our understanding of blood pressure regulation and hypertension.

Early Postoperative Hypertension

Early postoperative hypertension is likely related to the intense response of the sympathetic nervous system to the repair. Plasma norepinephrine is markedly elevated after coarctation surgery as compared to other kinds of operations.[6,28-30] Occurring in the first hours after coarctation relief, it is probably the result of a vigorous baroreceptor response. The abrupt fall in proximal aortic pressure evokes a homeostatic sympathetic discharge aimed at maintaining the previous set point of pressure regulation. The baroreceptors then reset and the catecholamine response abates. An alternate explanation is that manipulation of the aortic isthmus stimulates the intra-aortic stretch receptors with the resultant catecholamine release. Support for the latter explanation is found in the fact that those undergoing surgery for thoracic aneurysms also may have a hypertensive response.[6]

With early postoperative hypertension, systolic pressure elevation is moderate to severe. Use of sympathetic antagonists such as intravenous propranolol (0.1 mg/kg per 6 hours), nitroprusside infusion (0.5 to 1.0 µg/kg per minute), or hydralazine (0.15 mg/kg per 4 hours, I.V.) generally effects relief. Aggressive treatment, advocated for persistent postoperative pressure elevation, may lead to the postcoarctectomy syndrome. Prevention of the paradoxical pressure elevation may be possible with oral propranolol 1.5 mg/kg per day divided in 6-hour doses beginning 2 weeks prior to surgery.[31] However, the impact on the total operative response of this prophylaxis remains to be fully assessed.

Late Postoperative Hypertension

Late postoperative hypertension is usually a continuation of early pressure elevation. It appears related to activation of the renin-angiotensin system. Plasma-renin concentrations have been found to be elevated in these patients[29] and angiotensin blockade results in a lowering of the blood pressure.[6] Several mechanisms have been proposed for these events. Direct catechol stimulation of the renin-angiotensin system may result from the previously mentioned increased sympathetic activity. The baroreceptors may also reflexively stimulate the renin-angiotensin system. With the onset of "normal" pulsatile renal arterial blood flow, humoral or neural mediators may be released. These in turn may stimulate renin-angiotensin production. A like effect has been ascribed to the redistribution of renal blood flow.

Diastolic blood pressure is mainly elevated in late postoperative hypertension in contrast to earlier systolic elevation. It is often less severe and responds to angiotensin blockade or sympatholytic treatments. In particular, propranolol and captopril have proven useful when cardiac function and rhythm are normal. Late postoperative hypertension usually resolves in about 2 weeks, but those with persistent high pressures are prone to develop the postcoarctectomy syndrome. For them vigorous treatment is necessary and may even involve intravenous nitroprusside (0.5 to 1.0 µg/kg per minute).

Postcoarctectomy Syndrome

Labeled as the "postcoarctectomy syndrome" by Sealy in 1953, this clinical problem is characterized by abdominal complaints, i.e., pain, tenderness, and fever.[32] These symptoms usually begin on the third postoperative day and are associated with hypertension, ileus, and melena resulting from mesenteric arteritis. The arteritis was discovered in the histology of the mesenteric vessels from some of these patients who required resection of a small bowel necrosis.

The explanation of the syndrome is that small blood vessel injury occurs distal to the site of coarctation repair. It results from pulsatile arterial flow permitted by the removal of the previous aortic obstruction in association with paradoxical hypertension from vasoconstriction. The relatively fragile arterioles have less than usual connective tissue support. These vessels are especially responsive to the vasoconstrictive effects of angiotensin released as a consequence of the coarctation repair. Accordingly, barotrauma-caused damage is seen. Blockage of the vasoconstriction by angiotensin inhibitors can prevent the syndrome or at least its damaging effects.

Previously a common problem, the postcoarctectomy syndrome is seldom seen. Early treatment of paradoxical hypertension and delay in oral postoperative feedings mainly obviates the syndrome. In the rare event the syndrome is found, intravenous nutrition rather than oral alimentation, along with antihypertensive therapy, are required. At the same time, the patient must be carefully observed for signs of intestinal necrosis.

Paraplegia

Paraplegia is a rare but devastating complication of surgical repair of coarctation of the aorta. Occurring in less than 1/100 operations, paraplegia probably results from compromise of spinal cord circulation during the period of aortic cross-clamping.[33] Despite its rarity, the risk of paraplegia must be considered in every operation for coarctation. Those with fever and poor collateral circulation about the aortic narrowing appear to be at special risk. Current reliance on noninvasive imaging (by echo or MRI) makes it more difficult to assess collaterals. Accordingly, those with large pressure differences across the coarctation should be suspect for having decreased collaterals. Further investigation should then be undertaken.

In all surgery for coarctation, euthermia must be maintained. When the spinal cord is in jeopardy, such as with minimal collateral circulation, the technique of surgery is generally altered. Rapid operation with attention to lower body perfusion are employed. Unfortunately, no operative technique, including cardiac bypass methods, prevents paraplegia. Thus, if the patient is found to be at risk because of poor collateral circulation, balloon aortoplasty should be considered in lieu of surgical repair.

Persistent Postoperative Hypertension

Persistent postoperative hypertension is dependent on age and anatomy. As many as 15% to 30% of those surgically treated for coarctation may remain hypertensive, particularly with exercise. Most have mild pressure elevation only and thus require no therapy. Others, however, may need further operative intervention. These patients require careful follow-up and evaluation, perhaps with cardiac catheterization and aortography. For some, treatment may prove less than optimal. They may ultimately be burdened with a lifetime of medical modification of their hypertension.

Hypertension from Residual or Recurrent Coarctation

Significant postoperative anatomical narrowing of the aorta at the site of repair or at a segment of aortic hypoplasia can be found in about two thirds of patients who have long-term persistent elevation of proximal blood pressure despite the previous repair. These individuals are found by examination to have a pulse disparity between upper and lower extremities, as well as a measurable pressure difference between these extremities. As a rule, postexercise pressures should be obtained in all patients after coarctation repair.[27,34] These postexercise pressure measurements will demonstrate whether a hypertensive response to exercise exists. Systolic pressures in excess of 215 mm Hg are deemed hypertensive. In addition, arm and/or leg pressure-gradient measurements can be made and may be needed in equivocal cases to decide on the relevance of a residual narrowing. A gradient of over 40 mm Hg following exercise is felt to be significant.

When a residual aortic obstruction is suspected, further evaluation is necessary. Echocardiography or other imaging techniques, such as magnetic resonance imaging or aortography, with or without digital subtraction, will permit description of the residual narrowing so that further treatment can be planned. Many such cases will respond to balloon aortoplasty but a few others will require reoperation and perhaps insertion of an aortic graft.

Postoperative Hypertension Persisting Without Anatomical Obstruction

In about one-third of those with long- term persistent postoperative hypertension, pulses and blood pressure will be equal in the upper and lower extremities. These individuals have no anatomical obstruction to aortic blood flow. While the reason for their hypertension is unknown, several mechanisms have been proposed as possible explanations.

1. There may be increased proximal aortic impedance: experimental animal studies of coarctation reveal altered proximal aortic impedance. The proximal aortic wall was less distensible than in controls and had abnormal muscular reactivity to catecholamines. In certain humans, when the coarctation is removed at older ages,

differential maximal muscle blood flow in the precoarctation versus distal vascular bed can be found.[29]

2. Baroreceptor set point may be increased with decreased sensitivity; baroreceptor responses initially tend to maintain precoarctation pressures.[35] A slow adjustment then ensues. However, in some, this adjustment may be markedly delayed or even absent. In these patients, there is an increase in baseline sympathetic tone along with the elevated baroreceptor set point.[32]

3. Abnormal renin-angiotensin system function may occur. The expected reset of the renin-angiotensin system to normal renal blood flow postcoarctation repair may not occur. The persistent hypertension has shown response to blockade of the renin-angiotensin system by saralasin.[6]

The three described mechanisms may produce long-term elevation of the blood pressure in the postoperative coarctation patient. Treatment for such individuals is anti the renin-angiotensin system or sympatholytic. Propranolol or captopril are generally effective and must be given over a prolonged period of time, in doses appropriate for age and size.

Abdominal Coarctation

Uncommonly, a patient will present with the pulse and blood pressure findings of aortic coarctation and yet be found to have normal intrathoracic anatomy with no evidence of thoracoaortic obstruction. In such individuals, the possibility of abdominal coarctation should be entertained, especially if there is an abdominal bruit. Because abdominal coarctation anatomy is more varied than in thoracic coarctation, aortography is required to visualize not only the coarctation but also to check for possible involvement of adjoining vessels.

Surgical relief of abdominal coarctation is dictated by the individual's anatomy and may involve widening branch aortic vessels as well, with special care given to the renal arteries.[36] Postoperative care for such patients is very similar to those with thoracic coarctation and the same concern for possible complications must be used.

Pseudocoarctation

When the thoracic aorta is incidentally found to be tortuous or "kinked," but no pressure difference is noted across the involved area, the patient is often labeled as having a "pseudocoarctation." In such cases, there is no posterior obstructive shelf. Proximal and distal pulses as well as blood pressures are equal. Occasionally, "pseudocoarctation" is found in connective tissue disorders. Certain individuals with "pseudocoarctation" have developed aortic aneurysms.[37] Therefore, these patients deserve periodic evaluation. However, unless aortic aneurysm is found, surgery is not indicated.

Summary

Coarctation of the aorta is an important cause of hypertension in the young, yet the mechanisms involved in producing the hypertension are not fully elucidated. Fortunately, the diagnosis of aortic coarctation usually is readily apparent in the child because of proximal systolic hypertension with lower pressures in the lower extremities. Coarctation must also be considered in infants with early cardiac decompensation. In most instances, the clinical diagnosis can be confirmed by echocardiography. However, in complex cases and in those suspected of having poor collateral circulation, aortography and/or cardiac catheterization may be necessary.

The usual approach to treatment of coarctation has been surgical resection or aortoplasty after 1 year of age. Balloon-dilation aortoplasty has now been shown to be effective and safe in reducing aortic narrowing even in infants and especially in those with residual or recurrent coarctation. Current results are encouraging but long-term data are awaited to decide on the procedure of choice.

A number of postoperative complications are known, including the postcoarctation syndrome, late postoperative hypertension, and paraplegia. While intriguing pathophysiologic questions are raised by such findings, it is clear that mechanical, aortic impedance, and humoral factors are involved. Thus treatment of postoperative problems usually involves sympatholytic or renin-angiotensin-blocker agents. For hypertension which does not resolve after operation, balloon aortoplasty may be required.

Despite the fact that coarctation of the aorta has been treated and various modes of repair investigated since 1945, general agreement on therapy does not exist. Future developments promise exciting treatment regimens as well as important physiologic information. Coarctation of the aorta remains far from a mundane condition.

References

1. Leuman EP: Blood pressure and hypertension in childhood and adolescence. In: Frick P, von Harnack GA, Martini GA, Prader A, Schven R, Wolff HP, eds. *Advances in Internal Medicine and Pediatrics*. Berlin: Springer-Verlag; 1979:111-183.
2. Lang P, Jonas RA, Norwood WI, Mayer JE, Castaneda AR. Palliation for aortic atresia: hypoplastic left heart syndrome: an update . *Circulation* 72(suppl III):260, 1985. Abstract.
3. Rudolph AM, Heymann MA, Spitznas U. Hemodynamic consideration in the development of narrowing of the aorta. *Am J Cardiol* 30:514-25, 1972.
4. Scott HW, Bahnson HT. Evidence for a renal factor in the hypertension of experimental coarctation of the aorta. *Surgery* 30:206-217, 1951.
5. Goldblatt H, Kahn JR, Hanzal RF. Studies on experimental hypertension: the effect on blood pressure of constriction of the abdominal aorta above and below the site of origin of both main renal arteries. *J Exper Med* 69:649-674, 1939.
6. Parker FB Jr, Farrell B, Streeten DHP, Blackman MS, Sondheimer HM, Anderson GH Jr. Hypertensive mechanisms in coarctation of the aorta. Further studies of the renin-angiotensin system. *J Thoracic Cardiovasc Surg* 80:568-573, 1980.
7. Thoele DG, Muster AJ, Paul MH. Recognition of coarctation of the aorta: a continuing challenge for the primary care physician. *Am J Dis Child* 141:1201-1204, 1987.
8. Shone JD, Selders RD, Anderson RC, Adams P, Lillehei CW, Edwards JE. The developmental complex of "parachute mitral valve," supravalvar ring of the left atrium, subaortic stenosis, and coarctation of the aorta. *Am J Cardiol* 11:714-725, 1963.
9. Gersony WM. Coarctation of the aorta. In: Adams FA, Emmanouillides GC, Riemenschneider TA, eds. *Moss' Heart Disease in Infants, Children, and Adolescents, 4th ed*. Baltimore: Williams & Wilkins Co; 1989:243-255.
10. Rowe RD, Freedom RM, Mehrizi A, Bloom KR. Syndrome of coarctation of the aorta. In: Rowe RD, Freedom RM, Mehrizi A, Bloom KR, eds. *The Neonate With Congenital Heart Disease*. Philadelphia: WB Saunders; 1981:166-192.
11. Becker AE, Becker MJ, Edwards JE. Anomalies associated with coarctation of the aorta: particular reference to infancy.*Circulation* 41:1067-1075, 1970.
12. Smallhorn JF, Huhta JC, Adams PA, Anderson RH, Wilkinson JL, Macartney FJ. Cross-sectional echocardiographic assessment of coarctation in the sick neonate and infant. *Br Heart J* 50:349-361, 1983.
13. McNamara DG. Coarctation of the aorta: difficulties in clinical recognition. *Heart Dis Stroke* 1:202-206, 1992.
14. Heymann MA, Berman W Jr, Whitman V. Dilatation of the ductus arteriosus by prostaglandin E-1 in aortic arch abnormalities. *Circulation* 59:169-173, 1979.

15. Lock JE, Bass, JL, Amplatz K, Fuhrman BP, Castaneda-Zuniga W. Balloon dilation angioplasty of aortic coarctation in infants and children. *Circulation* 68:109-116, 1983.

16. Rao PS. Balloon angioplasty of aortic coarctation. *Am J Cardiol* 71:256-257, 1993. Readers' Comments.

17. Rao PS, Wilson AD, Brazy J. Transumbilical balloon coarctation angioplasty in neonates with critical aortic coarctation. *Am Heart J* 124: 1622-1624, 1992.

18. Marvin WJ, Mahoney LT, Rose EF. Pathologic sequelae of balloon dilation angioplasty for unoperated coarctation of the aorta in children. *J Am Coll Cardiol* 7:117A, 1986. Abstract.

19. Lababidi ZA, Daskalopoulos DA, Stoeckle H. Transluminal balloon coarctation angioplasty: experience with 27 patients. *Am J Cardiol* 54:1288-91, 1984.

20. Beekman RH, Rocchini AP, Dick M, Snider R, Crowley DC, Serwer GA, Spicer RL, Rosenthal A. Percutaneous balloon angioplasty for native coarctation of the aorta. *J Am Coll Cardiol* 10:1078- 84, 1987.

21. Tynan M, Finley JP, Fontes V, Hess J, Kan J. Balloon angioplasty for the treatment of native coarctation: results of valvuloplasty and angioplasty of congenital anomalies registry. Am J Cardiol 65:790-792, 1990.

22. Crafoord C, Nylin G. Congenital coarctation of the aorta and its surgical treatment. *J Thorac Surg* 14:347-361, 1945.

23. Gross RE, Hufnagel CA. Coarctation of the aorta: experimental studies regarding its surgical correction. *N Engl J Med* 233:287-293, 1945.

24. Waldhausen JA, Nahrwold DL. Repair of coarctation of the aorta with a subclavian flap. *J Thorac Cardiovasc Surg* 51:532-533, 1966.

25. Clarkson PM, Brandt PWT, Barratt-Boyes BG, Rutherford JD, Kerr AR, Neutze JM. Prosthetic repair of coarctation of the aorta with particular reference to dacron onlay patch grafts and late aneurysm formation. *Am J Cardiol* 56:342-346, 1985.

26. Hesslein PS, McNamara DG, Morris MJH, Hallman GL, Cooley DA. Comparison of resection versus patch aortoplasty for repair of coarctation in infants and children. *Circulation* 64:164-168, 1981.

27. Smith RT Jr, Sade RM, Riopel DA, Taylor AB, Crawford FA Jr, Hohn AR. Stress testing for comparison of synthetic patch aortoplasty with resection and end-to-end anastomosis for repair of coarctation in childhood. *J Am Coll Cardiol* 4:765-770, 1984.

28. Rocchini AP, Rosenthal A, Barger AC, Castaneda AR, Nadas AS. Pathogenesis of paradoxical hypertension after coarctation resection. *Circulation* 54:382-387, 1976.

29. Fox, S, Pierce WS, Waldhausen JA. Pathogenesis of paradoxical hypertension after coarctation repair. *Ann Thorac Surg* 29:135-141, 1980.

30. Sehested J, Baandrup U, Mikkelsen E. Different reactivity and structure of the prestenotic and poststenotic aorta in human coarctation: implications for baroreceptor function. *Circulation* 65:1060-1065, 1982.

31. Gidding SS, Rocchini AP, Beekman R, Szpunar CA, Moorehead C, Behrendt D, Rosenthal A. Therapeutic effect of propranolol on paradoxical hypertension after repair of coarctation of the aorta. *N Engl J Med* 312:1224-1228, 1985.

32. Sealy WC. Coarctation of the aorta and hypertension. *Ann Thorac Surg* 3(1):15-28, 1967.

33. Brewer LA III, Fosburg RG, Mulder GA, Verska JJ. Spinal cord complications following surgery for coarctation of the aorta. *J Thorac Cardiovasc Surg* 64:368-381, 1972.

34. Freed MD, Rocchini AP, Rosenthal A, Nadas AS, Castaneda AR. Exercise-induced hypertension after surgical repair of coarctation of the aorta. *Am J Cardiol* 43:253-258, 1979.

35. Beekman RH, Katz BP, Moorehead-Steffens C, Rocchini AP. Altered baroreceptor function in children with systolic hypertension after coarctation repair. *Am J Cardiol* 52:112-117, 1983.

36. Scott HW Jr, Dean RH, Boerth R, Sawyers JL, Meacham P, Fisher RD. Coarctation of the abdominal aorta pathophysiologic and therapeutic considerations. *Ann Surg* 189:746-757, 1979.

37. Dungen WT, Char F, Gerald BE, Campberg SG. Pseudocoarctation of the aorta in childhood. *Am J Dis Child* 119:401-406, 1970.

Chapter 6

Renal Hypertension

Introduction

Considering that renal physiology is intimately tied to blood pressure regulation, it is hardly a surprise that renal disorders are by far the most common causes of secondary hypertension in both child- and adulthood.[1] In fact, early workers ascribed nearly all hypertension to renal disease. General agreement now holds that between 70% and 80% of secondary hypertension is renal in origin. Hypertension of renal origin is commonly severe and sustained. It may be acute or chronic. The seat of the disease may be in the renal vasculature or in the parenchyma (Table 1). Parenchymal disorders may occur at three sites: the glomeruli (e.g., glomerulonephritis); the tubules (e.g., polycystic diseases); and the interstitium (e.g., pyelonephritis). When renal disease causes blood pressure elevation, a vicious cycle is established: the high blood pressure causes more renal damage, in turn causing further pressure elevation. Thus, the goal becomes one of early disease detection.

Then, when possible, treatment of the original disorder is undertaken. At the very least, the hypertension should be controlled to interrupt the cycle thereby preserving remaining renal function.

At the onset, certain pathophysiologic concepts involving end-stage renal disease and transplant deserve mention prior to consideration of specific diagnostic measures and diseases with their treatment. End-stage renal disease with chronic renal failure may necessitate dialysis, then transplantation. A few of those on dialysis with hypertension may continue to have uncontrollable pressure

Table 1.
Renal Disorders Causing Hypertension

Renal Parenchymae	Renovascular
Acute	renal artery thrombosis
glomerulonephritis	sickle cell crisis
pyelonephritis	vasculitis
hemolytic uremic syndrome	
renal trauma	
ureteral obstruction	
Chronic	
glomerulonephritis	fibromuscular dysplasia
pyelonephritis	renal artery aneurysm
reflux nephropathy	arteriovenous fistula
obstructive uropathy	vasculitis
polycystic diseases	
renal dysplasia	
hemolytic uremic syndrome	
renal tumors	

despite maximum medication.[2] Rarely these patients will require bilateral nephrectomy while awaiting transplant. The result of bilateral nephrectomy is dependency on fluid volume for blood pressure regulation. The absence of renal vasodepressor substances such as renal prostaglandin or kallikrein and extrarenal renin appears not to have much of a role in systemic pressure control in such patients. Patients hypertensive prior to transplant are prone to hypertension following transplant. Hypertension may lead to parenchymal damage in the transplanted kidney and increases the likelihood of early atherosclerotic renovascular disease.[3] Thus, prevention and control of hypertension are dominant issues in both those with transplanted and in those with diseased native kidneys.

Investigation for Renal Forms of Hypertension

With current emphasis on recording blood pressures in children, renal hypertension may first be suspected on the basis of incidental pressure measurements. Some may initially present withweight loss and fatigue, edema, headaches, abnormal urine findings, or even seizures. In the course of their evaluation, the blood pressure will be found to be quite high (i.e., consistently over the 99th percentile). With such elevation of blood pressure, the first etiologic consideration should be renal disease. Initial workup by history and physical should include blood pressures in at least three limbs (both arms and one lower limb) and careful fundoscopic study. Basic laboratory studies consist of urinalysis and culture, blood count and chemistry, as well as an echocardiogram (Table 2).

Renal ultrasound and measurement of plasma renin may be in order as determined by the basic workup. Assessment of end-organ involvement by chest x-ray and excretory function by urography may then be indicated. Depending on the findings of the initial workup, further studies can be obtained in a focused fashion. It is important to maintain patient comfort as well as minimize financial expenditures by avoiding unneeded tests.

Table 2.
Laboratory Investigation for Hypertension of Renal Origin[63]

Basic Screening tests (for office evaluation of hypertension)

Urinalysis and culture
Complete blood count
Serum creatinine, urea, electrolytes, uric acid, calcium, and phosphorus
Echocardiogram

Additional tests (also available on ambulatory basis)

Abdominal (renal) ultrasound
Chest x-ray
Excretory urogram
Plasma renin activity
Urine sodium and chloride

Other Useful Tests (usually performed at a medical center)

DMSA/DTPA renal scans
Glomerular filtration rate
Voiding cystourethrogram
CT/MR scan of kidneys
Renal angiography or digital subtraction angiography
Renin sampling from renal veins and vena cava
ACE inhibitor test
Renal biopsy

DMSA = ^{99m} TC = dimercaptosuccinic acid; DTPA = ^{99m} TC = diethylenetriamine = penta = acetic acid; CT = computer tomography; MR = magnetic resonance; ACE = angiotensin = converting enzyme.

Renal Imaging

Renal imaging has undergone a revolution in the past decade. The intravenous pyelogram (IVP) has largely been replaced by moresophisticated scans.[4] The complications of injecting a large solute load of contrast media to poorly functioning kidneys can now be avoided. Scans currently employed allow visualization of renal architecture even when renal function is poor. On the other hand, the voiding cystourethrogram remains a useful diagnostic modality readily identifying obstructive uropathy and vesicoureteral reflux.

Renal ultrasound can provide satisfactory images of abdominal masses by differentiating solid from cystic lesions. Dilation of collecting systems, calculi, and gross scarring also can be seen. However, renal polar lesions may be missed and the technique does not allow determination of renal function information.[5]

Once pathology has been uncovered, detailed information may be obtained by either computerized tomographic (CT) or magnetic resonance (MR) scans. The latter is useful in the evaluation of suspected renovascular hypertension. However, renal arteriography with or without digital subtraction contrast enhancement is advocated for the most detailed arterial anatomical information, particularly in adolescents and those for whom surgery or catheter dilatation is planned.

When necessary, radionuclide imaging may provide additional information to the workup. ^{99m}Tc-dimercaptosuccinic acid (DMSA) scintigraphic perfusion scans are particularly helpful in detecting areas of pyelonephritic scarring[6] and ischemic areas of the kidney.[5] ^{99m}Tc-diethylenetriamine-penta-acetic acid) (DTPA) scans are useful for information of renal perfusion and glomerular filtration rate, as well as in demonstrating obstructive uropathy.[7]

With the array of advanced imaging technologies available, the decision of which procedure to use first requires an organized approach.[8] Following the basic initial evaluation outlined in Table 2, renal ultrasound is recommended. Depending on the findings, other tests can then be planned.

Plasma Renin Activity

Plasma-renin activity (PRA) assays, while not performed in all laboratories, still find use in the initial workup of hypertension in pediatrics. In contrast to adults, elevated peripheral PRA levels may be found in children with reflux uropathy before hypertension is clinically evident. Conversely, the renin-dependent hypertension of renal disease is unlikely with low or normal peripheral PRA. Measurements of PRA are expressed in nanograms per milliliter per hour (ng/mL per hour) angiotensin I generated when incubated with angiotensinogen. They vary with age (Fig. 1). Normal peripheral PRA values are based on samples drawn after an overnight fast, preferably in a supine posture. It is preferable that the individual undergoing the test be free of medication for at least a week and on a regular diet. Furosemide and radiographic contrast agents increase renin production but prostaglandin synthetase and angiotensin-converting enzyme (ACE) inhibitors reduce PRA. From a practical standpoint, a therapeutic trial with an ACE inhibitor such as captopril can provide information concerning the involvement of the renin-angiotensin (RA) system in hypertension. Reduction in blood pressure with captopril treatment is presumptive evidence of RA system involvement.

If a peripheral PRA value is found to be elevated, direct renal vein sampling may be indicated. If asymmetric renin release is present, it will be demonstrated by such sampling. In turn, surgical

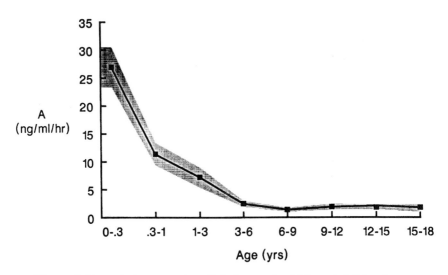

Figure 1: Normal plasma renin activity by age in children. Adult levels are reached at about 9 to 12 years of age.[9,64] The heavy line represents the mean and the shaded area ± 2 standard deviation.

success may be predicted from the values determined. A ratio of 1.5 or more between PRA in the right and left main renal veins indicates asymmetric renin release and has predicted successful surgical treatment of unilateral disease.[9] This ratio is also applicable for prediction of outcome in renal segmental disease when segmental vein renin samples are obtained.

Specific Renal Parenchymal Disorders Causing Hypertension

A useful rule is that practically all disorders of the kidney can cause hypertension especially if chronic renal failure ensues. Major groups of renal diseases and their relative frequency as a cause for hypertension are presented in Table 3. The three major causes of renal hypertension are renal scarring, glomerular diseases, and renovascular disease. Diseases that result in scarred kidneys account for the largest number of hypertensive patients. This is a heterogeneous group of conditions that results in coarse renal scarring and small kidneys. Chronic pyelonephritis and reflux nephropathy are the major causes of scarring.

Renal Scarring

This heterogenous group includes several disorders which result in progressive scarring of renal parenchymal. The process may be

Table 3.
Frequency of Various Causes of Sustained
Renal Hypertension [1,28]

Causes	Percent
Renal scarring (including obstructive uropathy)	42
Chronic glomerular disease*	29
Renovascular	15
Hemolytic uremic syndrome	6
Polycystic disease	4
Renal tumors	3
Trauma	1

*Acute glomerulonephritis not included because of its usual transient nature.

either uni- or bilateral and occurs over a number of years. The group comprises more than 40% of all causes of renal-induced hypertension (Table 3). Whether the original process is chronic pyelonephritis or reflux uropathy, the end result is similar with hypertension developing in about 10% of cases.[10] The hypertension is likely to be sudden in onset and rather high or even malignant in nature. Although not universally accepted, the pressure elevation appears related to RA-system hyperactivity.[11] The normal physiologic fall in PRA level with age may fail to occur as a result of renal inflammation and scarring.[12] Late exacerbation of the parenchymal disorder may further elevate PRA levels, leading to manifest hypertension. This chain of events points out the need for aggressive treatment of childhood urinary tract infections and vesicoureteral reflux. Renal scarring is rarely found in the first 5 years of life. Consequently, there is opportunity for early diagnosis and treatment to prevent serious complications and hypertension.

Pyelonephritis

As a major cause of renal scarring, pyelonephritis is an acute or chronic disease of the interstitium which may cause hypertension mostly in the chronic phase of the illness. The usual situation occurs as a result of repeated infections from vesicoureteral reflux.[13] Bacteriuria is frequently present and intrarenal reflux may be demonstrated by a voiding cystourethrogram. Further imaging studies can be used to demonstrate whether there is significant scarring. At this point, preventive measures should be undertaken to maintain sterile urine. With growth, over time, the reflux may resolve. Those with marked reflux should have early surgical intervention.

Most individuals with chronic pyelonephritis will remain normotensive. However, once hypertension is established, it is likely to be volume dependent[14] and often associated with elevated PRA.[12] Restriction of fluids and sodium is a mainstay in the treatment of this hypertension along with judicious use of diuretics. Daily furosemide has found favor in such cases. Antihypertensive drugs may be needed and are safe to use with appropriate adjustment for degree of renal impairment. Angiotensin-converting enzyme inhibitors such as captopril (Table 4) may be especially efficacious because of involvement of the RA system. Even at a late stage in the disease, if marked reflux is still present, surgical repair may be worthwhile

Table 4.
Medications Commonly Used in the Treatment of Renal Hypertension

Medication	Dose	Route	Side Effects	Comment
β: blockers				
Propranolol	0.5–1 mg/kg per dose	Oral q 6h–8h	Avoid with CHF* +bronchospasm	Affects diabetic management + lipids (lower HDL)
	0.1–0.2 mg/kg per dose	I.V.	Bronchospasm	same
Labetalol	2 mg/kg per dose	Oral q12h	Orthostatic hypotension esp. with I.V. doses	same also causes fatigue, nasal congestion, paresthesia (dose related)
	0.2–1 mg/kg per dose MAX 20 mg	I.V. push		
	0.25–1.5 mg/kg per h MAX 3 mg/kg per h	I.V. con't infusion		
Atenolol	1–2 mg/kg per dose	Oral qd	Bradycardia Dizziness	? less side effects Single dose Rx
ACE inhibitors				
Captopril	< 2 mo of age per dose 0.05–0.25 mg/kg	Oral q12h	Hyperkalemia	Low doses avoid renal failure/hypotension
	> 2 mo of age per dose 0.5–6 mg/kg	Oral q8h	Same WBC decreased	Use < 2 mo doses with renal insufficiency
Enalapril	0.2–1 mg/kg per dose[34]	Oral qd	Proteinuria	Same concerns, single dose Rx

Table 4.
Medications Commonly Used in the Treatment of Renal Hypertension (*Cont.*)

Calcium-channel blocker				
Nifedipine *Norvasc*	0.25–0.5 mg/kg per dose	Oral q6h	Dizziness, headache	Many other including GI, hematol, vision, joints
Other vasodilators				
Hydralazine	0.75–7 mg/kg per day	Oral q8h	Reflex tachycardia, abd Sx, headache	Palpitations main Sx-usually well tolerated
	1.7–3.5 mg/kg per day	I.M./I.V. q4–6h	Periph neuritis Weakness	SLE (rare)
Nitroprusside	0.5–10 mcg/kg per min	I.V.	Hypotension Thiocyanate toxicity (with higher doses)	Titrate (use in ICU only)
Diuretics				
Hydrochlorothiazide	1 mg/kg per dose	Oral q12h	K+deplete incr trig + cholesterol	Not effective with GFR decreased
Furosemide	1–2 mg/kg per dose	Oral/I.M. I.V. q6–12h	'lyte depletion dehydration, alkalosis	For neonates dose I.M./I.V. only q12h
Metolazone	0.2–.4 mg/kg per day	Oral qd	fluid/'lyte depletion, abd Sx	Strong diuretic hypotension

MAX = maximum; CHF = congestive heart failure; HDC = high-density lipoprotein; WBC = white blood cell; Sx = symptoms; GI = gastrointestinal; 'lyte = electrolytes; SLE = systemic lupus erythematosis; GFR = glomerular filtration rate.

to salvage remaining renal parenchyma. Ultimately, dialysis and transplantation may be necessary.

Segmental Hypoplasia (Ask-Upmark Kidney)

There remains some doubt as to whether demarcated segmental cortical and medullary hypoplasia is the result of a developmental vascular occlusion or the outcome of renal reflux. Support for the reflux etiology may be the fact that the disorder is at least twice as common in females and reflux can be demonstrated in many with the disease. The disorder is usually progressive. Some of these lesions may appear as a polar pyelonephritic scar. On close examination, a disarray of renal architecture with few glomeruli may be seen. Infection has been noted in over half of the reported cases.[15] Plasma-renin activity levels are variable, but over three fourths are hypertensive. Surgical relief of reflux seldom leads to control of the hypertension. While segmental renal resection is useful with a single lesion, nephrectomy may be necessary with widespread unilateral disease. Those with bilateral disease may require bilateral nephrectomy and transplantation. Diuretics and ACE inhibitors are helpful in the initial treatment of the hypertension along with infection control.

Reflux Uropathy

Persisting renal reflux over time can, even in the absence of infection, result in renal parenchymal scarring.[16] Mention has been made that urinary reflux into the kidney is a cause for concern.[13] Unless there is improvement or disappearance of the reflux known to occur with age, ultimately the reflux causes parenchymal destruction. Hypertension may develop in some of the latter afflicted individuals. Most often, however, concomitant infection plays a role in the parenchymal destruction. Basic workup and voiding cystourethrography lead to the diagnosis. Once renal reflux is discovered, regardless of the nature of the disorder, it is imperative to maintain sterile urine. If follow-up studies show increased renal tissue destruction, surgical intervention will be needed.

Hydronephrosis–Obstructive Uropathy

Obstruction to urine flow at the ureteropelvic junction is known to cause hypertension in young children. Distension of the small intrarenal pelvis found in the young may lead to parenchymal ischemia. This, in turn, results in elevated renin levels and hypertension. Accordingly, this process may affect infants more than older children.[17] Surgical removal of the obstruction or the obstructed kidney relieves the hypertension. High renin hypertension may also follow trauma to a hydronephrotic kidney. An acute elevation in pressures follows the injury and may require vigorous medical then surgical treatment.

Glomerular Diseases

Acute Glomerulonephritis

A spectrum of disorders exists between classical acute glomerulonephritis and classical nephrotic syndrome. In nephritis, primarily a disease of the glomerular endothelium, there is hematuria, azotemia, dependent edema, and hypertension. In contrast, nephrosis is mainly a disorder of glomerular basement membrane, with gross edema and proteinuria and hypoalbuminemia, but no hypertension. Many intermediate forms exist and, in the acute disorder, the presence of hypertension depends on the degree of glomerulovascular involvement. It is the acute postinfectious nephritis, often due to streptococcal infection, that can trigger sudden blood pressure elevation severe enough to result in encephalopathy and a hypertensive emergency.

Some degree of blood pressure elevation in acute nephritis occurs in about 90% of cases. Glomerulonephritis is the most common cause of acute hypertension in childhood. The hypertension is volume related and biphasic in nature. Although the initial phase lasts less than a week, the degree of hypertension is often severe and may be malignant. Cardiac failure, retinopathy, and/or encephalopathy may develop rapidly in about 5% of patients.[18] These hypertensive emergencies require aggressive treatment, usually in an intensive care setting. Pressure control can be accomplished rapidly by titrating an infusion of nitroprusside beginning with 0.5 µg/kg per minute. A maximum of 10 µg/kg per minute can be given. Thiocyanate poisoning can be avoided by limiting infusions to a few days. Once the pressure is controlled, other antihypertensives such as nifedipine may be substituted and volume controlled by diuretics such as furosemide.

The second phase of blood pressure elevation in acute nephritis follows a short return to a more normal pressure. This phase is characterized by a mild but more persistent hypertension which lasts several weeks. Pressure elevation lasting more than a month suggests progression to chronic nephritis. Second-phase hypertension treatment again involves restricted fluid and electrolyte intake, use of diuretics, and antihypertensive medication, and rarely dialysis.

Nephrotic Syndrome

About three fourths of children who are grossly edematous because of albuminuria have classic minimal change disease or lipoid nephrosis. They generally are not hypertensive in contrast to adults with similar disease. However, as many as 10% of children with minimal change disease will have some elevation of blood pressure. In some, it will be as a result of steroid therapy. In others, it will be as a result of a degree of nephritic involvement. On the other hand, 20% of those who have the nephrotic syndrome as a result of other disorders, such as focal glomerulosclerosis, or membranous glomerulonephritis have hypertension.[19] Patients with the nephrotic syndrome who are found to have hypertension due to a nephritic component of their illness will have hematuria and reduced glomerular filtration. Their hypertension, like those with nephritis, is dependent on intravascular volume. General nephrosis treatment schemes must be modified for treatment of the hypertension. Measures outlined for nephritis may be applicable. Nephrotic syndrome-steroid therapy especially needs close monitoring. Alternate day treatment may be beneficial.

Chronic Glomerulonephritis

In cases where nephritis is rapidly progressive or is found to be a chronic process such as membranous or membranoproliferative glomerulonephritis, hypertension is common. Indeed renal hypertension may be attributed to chronic glomerulonephritis inmore than one fourth of patients (Table 3). The prevalence of hypertension varies with the type of glomerular disease. When the pathologic process reduces renal function to the point that serum creatinine rises above 1.5 mg/dL, hypertension usually develops.[20] Both volume and vasoconstriction are significant factors in blood pressure regulation in chronic glomerulonephritis with hypertension.[21] In addition, neurogenic factors, such as β-adrenergic stimulation which cause increased cardiac output and increased peripheral resistance, may contribute to the problem. It also must be recalled that the hypertension itself can contribute to decreased renal function leading to end-stage renal disease. With severe chronic renal failure, about 80% of patients will have hypertension.[22]

Regardless of the pathologic variety of chronic nephritis, once hypertension is recognized it must be treated aggressively. As in other chronic renal parenchymal disorders, it is likely that measures directed both at volume and vascular factors will be needed. Some limitation of salt intake may be useful. However, too little as well as too much salt can be detrimental. Careful monitoring of electrolyte balance is necessary. From a practical standpoint, effective volume control is best achieved using diuretics. Since these patients usually have some degree of renal insufficiency, diuretic dosage must be titrated to high levels. Furosemide, usually given in doses of 1 to 2 mg/kg (Table 4) once or twice daily, may have to be increased to 6 mg/kg per day. Care must be taken with other diuretics like spironolactone and triamterene, for they may cause hyperkalemia. Intermittent doses of metolazone 0.2 to 0.4 mg/kg per day may be a help in those patients whose conditions are refractory to furosemide and provide 24 hours of diuretic effect. Ultimately, dialysis may be needed. Both ACE inhibitors (i.e., captopril) and calcium-channel blockers (i.e., nifedipine) have found favor in treatment of the vascular component of the hypertension. Attention must be paid so that renal perfusion pressure is maintained.

Hemolytic Uremic Syndrome

Similar to glomerulonephritis, the hypertension associated with the hemolytic uremic syndrome (HUS) may occur in both the acute and chronic phases. The acute phase is often heralded by a viral syndrome or gastroenteritis. Characterized by glomerular fibrin deposition, there is a sudden decline in renal function leading to oligouria and anuria with elevated creatinine.[23]

There is associated microangiopathic hemolytic anemia, low platelets, and evidence of intravascular coagulopathy. Hypertension has been found in as many as half of the cases and is particularly frequent with severe disease.[19] It is apparently related to glomerular ischemia leading to increased renin production. Volume expansion resulting from the decline in filtration rate with water and salt retention often complicates the problem. Malignant hypertension may supervene and requires vigorous treatment. Fluid restriction, diuretics and, not uncommonly, dialysis are needed. Antihypertensive medications such as captopril or nifedipine may rapidly affect relief.[24,25] In a hypertensive crisis, intravenous nitroprusside is advocated. With current medical management regimens, emergency nephrectomy, formerly needed in accelerated malignant hypertension, can usually be avoided.

Between 5% and 20% of those with HUS will have hypertension beyond the acute phase.[26] Those with anuriaduring the acute phase and continued proteinuria and/or low creatinine clearance are likely to be afflicted. Increased risk for chronic renal disease in the HUS may be indicated if the ratio of urine protein to urine creatinine fails to become normal (i.e., = < 21 mg/mmol).[27] The hypertension in chronic renal disease from the HUS is similar in manifestation to chronic glomerulonephritis and is so treated.[28]

Cystic Kidney Diseases

Comprising a variety of renal parenchymal disorders, cystic kidney diseases are generally congenital but often escape detection until infancy, childhood, or even adulthood. A flank mass or symptoms such as hypertension may lead to the diagnosis. While the hypertension is classified as renin dependent, its cause is not known and usually not related to renal function. It is common for renal failure to supervene at some time in the course of most of the diseases in the group.

Infantile Polycystic Disease of the Kidney and Liver (IPKD)

Infantile polycystic disease of the kidney and liver is an autosomal-recessive disease manifesting itself in a variety of ways and ages. It is usually diagnosed when a flank mass or masses are found in early life. In other instances, the disease may not be found until childhood. Renal ultrasound and DMSA scans (Table 2) may be helpful in making the diagnosis. The renal enlargement is due to numerous elongated collecting duct cysts. The ducts apparently are functional but displace glomeruli.[29] The number of remaining functioning glomeruli determine survival in childhood. Newborns with the disorder may have pulmonary hypoplasia. Such babies present in respiratory distress. Pulmonary disorders are a major cause of death in IPKD. Periportal cysts may also be associated with IPKD. The result is liver disease with hepatic fibrosis.[30]

Half or more of those with IPKD develop hypertension, especially if they survive infancy.[31] The pressure elevation does not seem to influence survival, which is more dependent on the progression of renal dysfunction. Dialysis and transplant may berequired, sometimes at a relatively early age. However, hypertension may be severe in infants, leading to heart failure. Treatment of hypertension in these young patients with IPKD is difficult and may require more than one drug.[19] A combination of nifedipine or captopril and a diuretic (Table 4) may be effective. While the hypertension does not abate with age it usually becomes less difficult to control.

Adult-Type Polycystic Kidney Disease (APKD)

Characterized by an enlarged kidney in an otherwise asymptomatic infant or child, APKD is an autosomal-dominant disease. It is seldom found in the young and is most commonly diagnosed in adults.[32] While the palpable renal mass is a prominent feature, there may be hematuria and hypertension. Intracranial aneurysms have been reported.[33] Often, more than one family member is involved. Renal ultrasound is helpful in detecting APKD in asymptomatic relatives.[34] Adult-type polycystic kidney disease must be differentiated fromthe sporadic disorder of embryogenesis: multicystic dysplastic kidney. Hypertension is not found with the latter problem. In APKD, the hypertension seems to be both volume and renin dependent.[35] Hypertension usually is not a problem in childhood APKD for, when present, it is readily controlled with medication especially diuretics.

Other Renal Cystic Disorders

Other disorders in which renal cysts are found are rare. They include tuberous sclerosis with angiomyolipomas and cystic changes; Goldenhar's, Ehlers-Danlos and trisomy syndromes, and medullary cystic disease. Hypertension is thought to be frequent with them.[19]

Renal Tumors

A small number of cases of childhood renal hypertension are caused by tumors. They must be differentiated from renal cystic diseases. Of these, Wilms' tumor is most common. About half the cases of Wilms' tumor have hypertension. While not contributing to mortality, the elevation in pressure may increase morbidity.[19] Renal vascular compression by the tumor and elevated renin content of tumor tissue are postulated to cause the hypertension. While surgical resection resolves the hypertension, β-blockade with propranolol may provide initial relief.

Hamartoma, sympathoblastoma, and the juxtaglomerular cell-renin- secreting tumor, hemangiopericytoma, as well as renal neuroblastoma have all been identified as renal tumors with hypertension. High renin levels which, on further workup, can be localized to a segmental vein, may lead to the diagnosis of the extraordinarily rare hemangiopericytoma.[28]

Renal Trauma

Trauma to the kidney may injure the parenchyma or bloodvessels either directly or by compression. Hypertension was a sequela in 21% of a published series of 622 patients with renal trauma.[36] Fortunately, it was short-lived in the survivors. Hypertension in renal trauma is renin mediated and may be responsive to ACE inhibitors. Most injuries heal without residua although, when a subcapsular hematoma follows blunt trauma, the hypertension may be persistent. Removal of the hematoma will cure the hypertension. Renal artery thrombosis may also follow injury and lead to hypertension. If discovered early, thrombectomy with or without autotransplantation, may salvage the kidney and relieve the hypertension. However, in young infants, medical management generally preserves renal function and late resolution ensues.

Renovascular Hypertension

As many as one in 10 young patients found to have severe sustained hypertension will have a renovascular disorder.[37] While relatively uncommon (< 1/10,000 young people), especially among blacks, renovascular disease represents a potentially curable form of hypertension. Thus, it should be considered in workup of sustained significant hypertension. Unlike older patients who are likely to suffer from atherosclerosis, in children renovascular disease most often is caused by renal artery stenosis from fibromuscular dysplasia. Other causes like neurofibromatosis, arteritis, renal artery thromboembolism, and extrinsic compression (Table 5) are very rare. Renovascular hypertension in neonates is most commonly iatrogenic as a result of umbilical arterial cannulation damage (see Chapter 8).[38]

Fibromuscular Dysplasia

Since first described in children in 1938,[39] fibromuscular dysplasia has been reported in all age groups including infants.[40] No one cause for the disease is known although humoral, mechanical, genetic, and ischemic factors have been implicated. The pathologic process is a circumferential intimal or muscular accumulation of loose fibrous matrix tissue which is often eccentric. Inflammation is absent. There may be duplications of the internal elastic lamellae.

Table 5.
Causes of Renovascular Hypertension

Disorder	Pathology
Renal artery stenosis	fibrous, fibromuscular dysplasia (intimal, medial)
Neurofibromatosis	vascular
Arteritis	polyarteritis nodosa Takayasu's syndrome, congen. rubella phacomatosis, hypercalcemia infectious tumor, other tumor
Emboli Thrombosis Renal artery aneurysm Arteriovenous malformation Trauma Congenital stenosis Fistulae Extrinsic compression	tumors, hemorrhage, iatrogenic
Atherosclerosis	hyperlipidemia progeria

The matrix tissue may be found in the intima, media, and/or adventitial vascular layers. It replaces elastic and displaces muscular cells in the media.[41] Five subclassifications have been proposed: intimal fibroplasia, medial fibroplasia, perimedial fibroplasia (the type most often seen in childhood), medial hyperplasia, and periarterial fibroplasia.[42] Those with forms of medial involvement are usually grouped as fibromuscular dysplasia. Medial dissection, aneurysm, and arteriovenous fistula may complicate the disease process. In addition to the renal arteries, fibromuscular dysplasia can affect carotid, axillary, iliac, and even proximal coronary arteries.

Fibromuscular dysplasia accounts for three fourths of renovascular hypertension in children. The process may involve the main renal artery, segmental branches, or both. Focal areas of thickening often alternate with areas of extreme thinning (Fig. 2). The latter may predispose to aneurysm formation. Angiographically, the lesions have

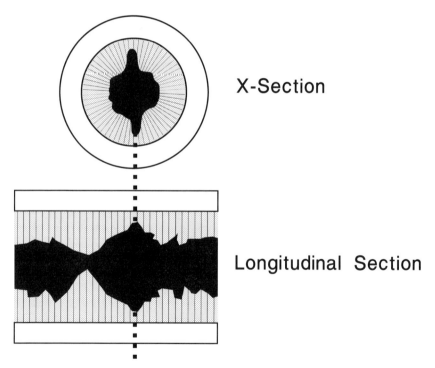

X-Section

Longitudinal Section

Figure 2: Diagram of longitudinal and cross-sectional histopathology of fibromuscular dysplasia. (Modified from Luscher et al[41]).

been characterized as having the appearance of "a string of beads."[43] The disorder is usually unilateral, more often on the right. About one fourth of cases have bilateral involvement. In most instances, fibromuscular dysplasia remains a stable condition. However, in about a third of those involved, the disease is progressive although complete vascular occlusion has not been reported.[41] Generally, renal function is not compromised with renal fibromuscular dysplasia and many individuals with the disorder are normotensive.

Neurofibromatosis

As a hereditary dysplasia of meso- and ectoderm resulting from a neural crest abnormality, many children with the disorder have some form of vascular dysplasia. Often, this is found in the proximal renal artery. The dysplastic process usually involves the intima with a nodular arrangement of cells of neural origin between the intima and medial vascular layers.[44] The disease may be mistaken for fibromuscular dysplasia but the history, proximal renal arterial involvement, and presence of lesions in the skin and bones usually provides for a distinct diagnosis.

Pathophysiology

The renin-angiotensin system has been demonstrated to be involved in the hypertension of renovascular disease. Because individual renal artery stenoses develop at variable rates, plasma renin (and volume) changes are found in both uni- and bilateral disease. Plasma-renin activity levels are normal or high. Low levels are not found. As in animal models, when PRA levels are normal, plasma volume is high. That is, the PRA level has been normalized through the mechanism of sodium retention and expansion of intravascular volume. Conversely, when PRA values are high, plasma volume isnormal.[45] Secondary hyperaldosteronism has been noted but is less common than in other high renin states.

Clinical Features

There are few specific findings to alert the examiner to renovascular hypertension. The disorder may be uncovered as the result of a casual blood pressure determination, particularly in syndromes like rubella, phacomatoses, and hypercalcemia of infancy. More often, vague symptoms lead to a blood pressure determination. This is the predominant way the hypertension of renovascular disease is discovered. As a rule, the degree of hypertension is quite high and may appear to have a sudden onset. However, close questioning will often suggest exacerbation of a chronic process. Infants with the disorder do not thrive and may present with seizures or heart failure. Older children may complain of fatigue or headache. Rarely, patients may present in pulmonary edema.

The presence of an abdominal bruit, found in about 40% ofcases, is about the only definite feature leading to the diagnosis. The murmur is usually high pitched and located over the flank or over the abdominal aorta. It may be heard posteriorly in the subcostal region. Other nonspecific findings include those of a hyperdynamic circulation with active precordium and strong pulses. Carotid and/or femoral arterial bruits are also reported. Retinoscopic examination may demonstrate severity of the disease. Hemorrhages or exudates may be seen in the fundi with severe disease.

Diagnosis

The finding of persistent, task force defined,[40] significant or severe hypertension, necessitates evaluation by a careful history and physical examination with search for abdominal bruits and femoral artery pulses.[46] Then a basic hypertension laboratory screening workup (Table 2) is carried out. If renal parenchymal disease and coarctation of the aorta can be ruled out, further testing for renovascular disease is in order, especially in those unresponsive to three-drug therapy or with increasing blood pressure.[47] It should be noted that, in those with renovascular disease, screening tests may show proteinuria and casts in the urine. These are the result of a major degree of renal arterial obstruction leading to ischemic injury. Release of the obstruction may restore renal function with resolution of the proteinuria. A slight reduction in serum potassium is found in a minority of patients as a result of hyperaldosteronism. However, blood urea nitrogen and creatinine are normal unless renal function has been compromised by ischemia.

Since renovascular hypertension depends on a hyperactive renin-angiotensin system, peripheral PRA levels may furnish useful albeit nonspecific information. As noted, values may be normal or high. Low PRA values rule out renovascular-induced hypertension. Currently the captopril test is regarded as a more sensitive office screening test in adults.[48] A peripheral venous sample for PRA analysis is drawn. Then a single oral dose (Table 4) of captopril is given and PRA is sampled again. The result is suggestive of renovascular disease if three criteria are met: 1) stimulated PRA of greater than to 12 ng/mL per hour; 2) absolute increase of PRA greater than 10 ng/mL per hour; and 3) 150% increase in PRA (400% increase if baseline PRA is less than 3 ng/mL per hour). Pediatric experience with the captopril test is limited[49] but a recent report found the test useful in 23 children and/or adolescents.[50] Such PRA tests do not lateralize the side of renal involvement or detect whether bilateral disease is present. Although requiring invasive testing, renal vein renin sampling, described at the beginning of the chapter, may lateralize the disease and be helpful in predicating surgical outcome. When renal vein sampling is done it is usually in conjunction with renal arteriography.

Other tests used in the evaluation of renovascular disease include the previously described renal isotope scans and digital subtraction angiography. Both modalities furnish gross information but little detail. Scans after captopril administration may be more specific and furnish predictive interventional information.[51] The technique of duplex echo- Doppler imaging can detect renal artery stenosis. However, the degree of narrowing may be uncertain and only proximal vessels can be sampled. With this test peak renal artery flow, velocity can be measured and compared to the aorta. A ratio of more than 3.5 predicts renal artery stenosis of greater than 60% with specificity and sensitivity in the 90% range.[48] Split renal function studies, while accurate, require cystoscopy and bilateral ureteral catheterization and are little used.

Thus, there does not exist one single test which can diagnose and predict outcome in renovascular disease. Accordingly, schemes have been developed to promote diagnosis and treatment of these relatively uncommon disorders.[52] One such scheme is presented in Figure 3. When severe, persistent hypertension is present and initial screening test unrevealing, use of the scheme may lead to the diagnosis without excessive testing. It should be noted that invasive testing by renal vessel catheterization and angiography is often combined with treatment by balloon renal artery angioplasty, size permitting.

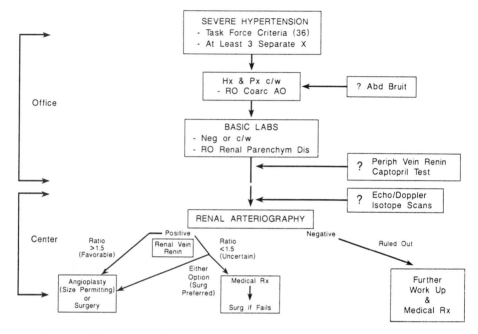

Figure 3: Diagnostic and management scheme for renovascular hypertension. Both the initial office-based measures and the further center-based procedures needed to diagnose the disorder are indicated.

Treatment

There are three treatment modalities available for hypertension with demonstrated renovascular disease: 1) use of antihypertensive medications; 2) balloon angioplasty; and 3) surgery, either reconstruction or resection. Since renovascular hypertension is potentially curable, the goal should be elimination of obstructing lesions once they are found. Medical management (Table 4) may be required before and after such efforts but should not be the sole therapy. In this renin-angiotensin- mediated disease it is logical to use β-blockers or angiotensin-converting enzyme (ACE) inhibitors as initial treatment.

Among β-blockers, atenolol has found favor over propranolol. Despite the wide experience with propranolol, the reduced number of side effects with atenolol and the single daily dose make it advantageous to use (Table 4). However, all β-blockers may increase heart failure and must be used with caution in that condition. They should be used only when it is felt the heart failure will respond to control of the hypertension by β-blockade.

ACE inhibitors like captopril also have few side effects and are particularly useful in high renin situations. Care must be taken to monitor for first-dose hypotension. After the initial pressure-fall response, recurrence of hypertension may be seen. Accordingly, the dose may require titration. More recently, enalapril has found favor, again because only a single daily dose is required.

A word of caution is needed here. Angiotensin-converting enzyme inhibitors, especially if used with diuretics, may cause a serious decrease in renal blood flow in those who have severe bilateral artery stenosis.[53] For the same reason, ACE inhibitors should not be used in those with a single kidney and a stenosed renal artery. The resulting renal ischemia may lead to renal failure and/or severe hypotension. Fortunately, return of function follows withdrawal of medication.

Preservation of renal function and elimination or control of hypertension are the achievable aims of catheter interventional and/or surgical therapy. Prolonged medical management has no place in childhood renovascular disease.[54] The first choice is renal artery balloon-catheter angioplasty (Fig. 4). Initially reported as successful in 1978,[55] the usefulness of balloon renal arterioplasty is dependent on size and the location of the renal arterial lesions (i.e., catheter accessibility).[56] In the very young, and in those with branch renal artery stenoses, balloon-catheter angioplasty may not be feasible. If the lesions of fibromuscular dysplasia can be reached by catheter, the immediate success rate is high. Arterial patency has been published to be as much as 100% with long-term patency of 87%.[57] Ten percent of the same group had recurrences, but 39% were cured of their hypertension as judged by diastolic pressure below 90 mm/Hg off medication. Almost 59% improved to the point of satisfactory blood pressure control with medication. There were 2% failures. Renal function improved in 86%. Similar results were noted in a summary of the literature by Pickering with over 90% of cases having successful arterial dilation.[52]

Complications of renal artery angioplasty are similar to all angioplasty procedures and occur in 5% to 10% of cases.[58] They vary from renal artery injury and dissection to injury of the insertion site and artery. Most use the femoral artery with pulse loss or, rarely, limb loss as potential untoward events. Many children with reno-

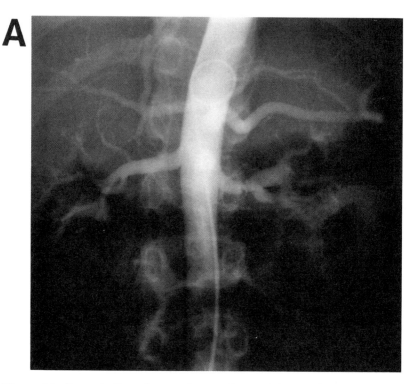

Figure 4A: Reproduction of an aortogram from a 12-year-old child showing stenosis of the left renal artrey prior to its branching.

vascular hypertension will have lesions not accessible to the balloon catheter. They will require some form of renal surgery. Once the need for operation is recognized, it should be done as soon as feasible. Waiting for growth can lead to renal deterioration. Nephrectomy, once the mainstay of treatment, is reserved for the atrophic or infarcted kidney or the kidney with multiple small vessel involvement.[49] Current surgical technology offers a variety of reconstructive methods to overcome renal arterial obstruction (Table 6). Using modern techniques, Martinez and coworkers reported results from 56 patients under 21 years of age.[59] In the 28 patients operated on after 1977, hypertension was cured in 96%. Aortorenal bypass using the hypogastric artery in small children or the saphenous vein in older children is the usual method of renal revascularization (Fig. 5). The saphenous graft, however, has been noted to have aneurysmal

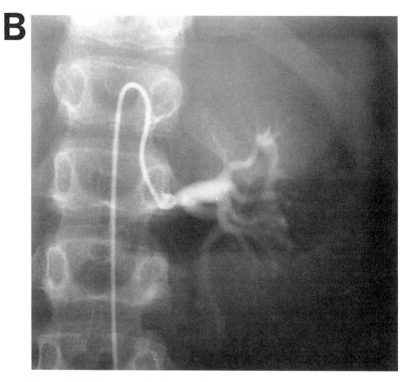

Figure 4B: Balloon angioplasty catheter in place dilating the stenosis.

expansion on occasion. End of graft-to-end of renal artery is the preferred anastomosis. In a few cases with a long renal artery and proximal stenosis, the distal renal artery can be reanastomosed to the aorta or the kidney autotransplanted into the iliac fossa.

Reinforced saphenous vein grafts in one series of 29 grafts in 17 cases (mean age 10.2 years) appeared to avoid the saphenous graft aneurysm problem.[60] One early and one late graft occlusion were noted. Three grafts required percutaneous transluminal angioplasty for late stenoses. There were no deaths. Thirteen of 17 were normotensive after a mean follow-up of 6 years. The rest were considered improved with the hypertension controlled on lower dose medication.

When extensive renal artery branch stenosis exists, the kidney can be removed for extracorporeal microvascular reconstruction with the aid of hypothermic ischemia. Then the repaired kidney is autotransplanted into the iliac fossa. With this technique, Novick

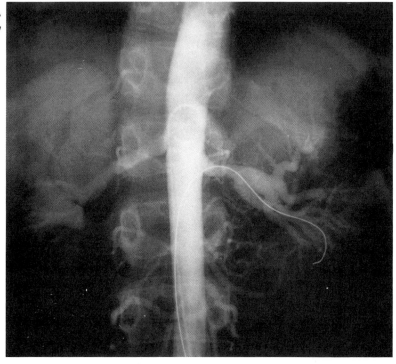

Figure 4C: Postangioplasty with guide wire in place. Considerable increase in lumen size at the previously stenotic area can be seen. (Reproductions courtesy of Phillip Stanley, MD, Dept. of Radiology, CHLA).

Table 6.
Techniques for Reconstructing Renal Artery Stenosis in Children

Bypass Anastomosis
    Autogenous hypogastric artery
    Autogenous saphenous vein +/– reinforcement
Reanastomosis
Reimplantation (autotransplantation)
Ex vivo microrepair (with ischemic hypothermia)

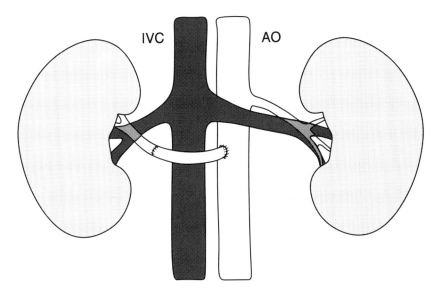

Figure 5: The technique of aortorenal bypass graft. An arterial graft is preferred when direct resection and reanastomosis cannot be done. The end of the graft is anastomosed to the side of the aorta and then end-to-end with the renal artery (based on Novick[54]).

restored renal circulation to normotensive levels in all 54 patients so operated, although nine still required medications.[54] Sixteen of the patients were 21 or less years in age and all had excellent return of renal function and blood pressure to normal. From these data, it can be seen that surgical relief of renovascular obstruction is usually safe and effective. However, nephrectomy may be required in the few children where uncorrectable renal disease is present.[61]

A few hypertensive patients with renovascular disease will beunsuitable for either angioplasty or surgery. For these individuals, a recent report found partial or total renal ablation by injecting ethanol through a catheter placed in the renal artery to be efficacious.[62] All 15 cases so injected improved and five were cured of their hypertension on 2-year follow-up.

Summary

Chronic renal parenchymal disorders are responsible for over 70% of severe sustained hypertension in childhood. Glomerular and interstitial diseases are the predominant causes, but tubular cystic diseases also result in hypertension. These diseases are usually renin mediated. Volume also may play a role. Acute parenchymal disease such as acute glomerulonephritis and pyelonephritis are likewise often associated with severe hypertension, albeit of shorter duration. They must be managed aggressively to avoid complications such as heart failure and seizures. Similarly, children who have chronic glomerular diseases or obstructive uropathies, with or without infection, require control of their hypertension before it leads to further renal parenchymal damage and more hypertension. Calcium-channel blockers, ACE inhibitors, β-blockers, and diuretics (Table 4) may be useful; sometimes in combinations. Where possible, the cause should be removed as soon as feasible, i.e., the surgical elimination of a progressive urologic obstruction.

Renovascular diseases are a potentially curable group of renal disorders which comprise another 7% of childhood hypertension. Renovascular diseases are also renin mediated and renin assays may be helpful in diagnosis and predicting outcome. Fibrous dysplasia of the renal arteries is by far the most common pathologic process. A simple algorithm for diagnosis and management has been proposed (Fig. 3). Use of the scheme should minimize testing. Percutaneous transluminal angioplasty (PTA) is the treatment of choice if size permits, but surgical removal of the obstruction(s) may be successful when PTA is not possible or a failure.

References

1. Dillon MJ. Hypertension. In: Postlethwaite RJ. *Clinical Paediatric Nephrology*. Bristol: Wright; 1986.
2. Lee JB. Antihypertensive activity of the kidney: the renomedullary prostaglandins. *N Engl J Med* 277:1073-1079, 1967.
3. Lindner A, Charra B, Sherrard DJ, Scribner BH. Accelerated atherosclerosis in prolonged maintenance hemodialysis. *N EnglJ Med* 290:697, 1974.
4. Rosen PR, Treves S, Ingelfinger, J. Hypertension in children. Increased efficacy of technetium Tc[99m] succimer in screening for renal disease. *Am J Dis Child* 139:173-177, 1985.
5. Stringer DA, de Bruyn R, Dillon MJ, Gordon I. Comparison of aortography, renal vein renin sampling, radionuclide scans,ultrasound, and the IVU in the investigation of childhood renovascular hypertension. *Br J Radiol* 57:111-121, 1984.
6. Dillon MJ, Gordon I, Shah V. [99m Tc]DMSA scanning and segmental renal vein renin estimations in children with renal scarring. In:

Hodson CJ, Heptinstall RH, and Winberg J, eds. *Contributions to Nephrology 39. Reflux Nephrology Update: 1983.* Basle: Karger; 1984.

7. Fine EJ, Scharf SC, Blavfox MD. The role of nuclear medicinein evaluating the hypertensive patient. *Nucl Med Ann* 23-79, 1984.

8. Diament MJ, Stanley P, Boechat MI, Kangarloo H, Gilsanz V, Lieberman ER. Pediatric hypertension: an approach to imaging. *Pediatr Radiol* 16: 461-467, 1986.

9. Stalker HP, Holland NH, Kotchen JM. Plasma renin activity in healthy children. *J Pediatr* 89:256-258, 1976.

10. Wallace DMA, Rothwell DL, Williams DI. The long-term follow- up of surgically treated vesicoureteric reflux. *Br J Urol* 50:479-484, 1978.

11. Pfau A, Rosenmann E. Unilateral chroric pyelonephritis and hypertension: coincidental or causal relationship? *Am J Med* 65:499-506, 1978.

12. Savage JM, Dillon MJ, Shah V, Barratt TM, Williams DI. Renin and blood pressure in children with renal scarring and vesicoureteric reflux. *Lancet* 2:441-444, 1978.

13. Bailey RR. An overview of reflux nephropathy. In: Hodson J, Smith PK, eds. *Reflux Nephropathy.* New York: Mason Pub; 1979.

14. Frohlich ED, Tarazi RC, Dustin HP. Hemodynamic and functional mechanisms in two renal hypertensions: arterial and pyelonephritis. *Am J Med Sci* 261:189-195, 1971.

15. Arant BS Jr, Sotelo-Avila C, Bernstein J. Segmental "hypoplasia" of the kidney (Ask-Upmark). *J Pediatr* 95:931- 939, 1979.

16. Braren V, West JC Jr, Boerth RC, Harmon CMcW. Management of children with hypertension from reflux or obstructive nephropathy. *Urology* 32:228-233, 1988.

17. Munoz AI, Pascual Y, Baralt JF, Melendez MT. Arterial hypertension in infants with hydronephrosis. *Am J Dis Child* 131:38-40, 1977.

18. Travis LB. Acute post-infectious glomerulonephritis. In: Edelmann CM. *Pediatric Kidney Disease.* Boston: Little Brown; 1978.

19. Ingelfinger JR. *Pediatric Hypertension.* Philadelphia: WB Saunders Co, 1982.

20. Kincaid-Smith P, Whitworth JA. Pathogenesis of hypertension in chronic renal disease. *Semin Nephrol* 8:155-162, 1988.

21. Smith MC, Dunn MJ. Hypertension in renal parenchymal disease. In: Laragh JH, Brenner BM. *Hypertension: Pathophysiology, Diagnosis, and Management.* New York: Raven Press; 1990.

22. Danielson H, Kornerup HJ, Olsen S, Posborg V. Arterialhypertension in chronic glomerulonephritis: an analysis of 310 cases. *Clin Nephrol* 19:284-287, 1983.

23. Bergstein JM, Riley M, Bang NU. Role of plasminogen-activator inhibitor type 1 in the pathogenesis and outcome of the hemolytic uremic syndrome. *N Engl J Med* 327:755-759, 1992.

24. Monnens L, Drayer J, deJong M. Malignant hypertension in a child with hemolytic uremic syndrome treated with captopril. *Acta Paediatr Scand* 70:583-585, 1983.

25. Lieberman E. Hypertension in childhood and adolescence. In: Kaplan NM: *Clinical Hypertension, 5th ed.* Baltimore: Williams & Wilkins; 1990.

26. Siegler RL, Milligan MK, Burningham TH, Christofferson RD, Chang S-Y, Jorde LB. Long-term outcome and prognostic indicators in the hemolytic-uremic syndrome. *J Pediatr* 118:195-200, 1991.
27. Milford DV, White RHR, Taylor CM. Prognostic significance of proteinuria one year after onset of diarrhea-associated hemolytic uremic syndrome. *J Pediatr* 118:191-194, 1991.
28. Broyer M, Bacre J-L, Royer P. Renal forms of hypertension in children: report on 238 cases. In: Giovannelli G, New MI, Gorini S. *Hypertension in Children and Adolescents.* New York: Raven Press; 1981.
29. Blyth H, Ockenden BG. Polycystic disease of kidneys and liver presenting in childhood. *J Med Genet* 8:257-284, 1971.
30. Lieberman E, Salinas-Madrigal L, Gwinn JL, Brennan LP, Fine RN, Landing BH. Infantile polycystic disease of the kidneys and liver: clinical, pathological and radiological correlations and comparison with congenital hepatic fibrosis. *Medicine* 50:277-318, 1971.
31. Lewy PR, Holland NH. Renal parenchymal diseases and hypertension. In: Kotchen TA, Kotchen JM, eds. *Clinical Approaches to High Blood Pressure in the Young.* Boston: John Wright PSG Inc; 1983.
32. Stickler GB, Kelalis PP. Polycystic kidney disease: recognition of the "adult form" (autosomal dominant) in infancy. *Mayo Clin Proc* 50:547-548, 1975.
33. Chapman AB, Rubinstein D, Hughes R, Stears JC, Earnest MP, Johnson AM, Gabow P, Kaehny WD. Intracranial aneurysms in autosomal dominant polycystic kidney disease. *N Engl J Med* 327:916-920, 1992.
34. Lufkin EG, Alfrey AC, Trucksess ME, Holmes JH. Polycystic kidney disease: earlier diagnosis using ultrasound. *Urology* 4:5-12, 1974.
35. Chapman AB, Johnson A, Gabow PA, Schrier RW. The renin-angiotensin-aldosterone system and autosomal dominant polycystic kidney disease. *N Engl J Med* 323:1091-1096, 1990.
36. Monstrey SJ, Beerthuizen GI, vander Werken C, Debruyne FM, Goris RJ. Renal trauma and hypertension. *J Trauma* 29:65-70, 1989.
37. Hanna JD, Chan JC, Gill JR Jr. Hypertension and the kidney. *J Pediatr* 118:327-340, 1991.
38. Adelman RD. Neonatal hypertension. In: Loggie JMH, Horan MJ, Gruskin AB, Hohn AR, Dunbar JD, Havlik RJ. *NHLBI Workshop on Juvenile Hypertension.* New York: Biomedical Information Corp, 1984.
39. Leadbetter WF, Burkland CE. Hypertension in unilateral renal disease. *J Urol* 39:611-626, 1938.
40. Task Force on Blood Pressure Control in Children. Report of the second task force on blood pressure control in children, 1987. *Pediatrics* 79:1-25, 1987.
41. Luscher TF, Lie JT, Stanson AW, Houser OW, Hollier LH, Sheps SG. Arterial fibromuscular dysplasia. *Mayo Clin Proc* 62:931-952, 1987.
42. Harrison EG Jr, McCormack LJ. Pathologic classification of renal arterial disease in renovascular hypertension. *Mayo Clin Proc* 46:161-167, 1971.
43. McCormack LJ, Dustan HP, Meaney TF. Selected pathology of the renal artery. *Semin Roentgenol* 2:126, 1967.

44. Blackburn WR. Vascular pathology in hypertensive children. In: Loggie JMH, Horan MJ, Gruskin AB, Hohn AR, Dunbar JD, HavlikRJ. *NHLBI Workshop on Juvenile Hypertension.* New York: Biomedical Information Corp, 1984.
45. Bianchi G, Campolo L, Vegeto A, Piazza U. The value of plasma renin concentration per se, and in relation to plasma and extracellular fluid volume in diagnosis and prognosis of human renovascular hypertension. *Clin Sci* 39:559-578, 1970.
46. Hiner LB, Falkner B. Renovascular hypertension in children. *Pediatr Clin North Am* 40:123-140, 1993.
47. Aristizabal D, Frohlich ED. Review. Hypertension due to renal arterial disease. *Heart Dis Stroke* 1:227-234, 1992.
48. Pickering TG. Diagnosis and evaluation of renovascular hypertension: indications for therapy. *Circulation* 83(suppl I):I-147-I-154, 1991.
49. Feld LG, Springate JE. Hypertension in children. *Curr Probl Pediatr* 18:317-373, 1988.
50. Daman-Williams CE, Shah V, Uchiyama M, Dillon MJ. The captopril test: an aid to investigation of hypertension. *Arch Dis Child* 64:229-234, 1989.
51. Davidson RA, Wilcox CS. Newer tests for the diagnosis of renovascular disease. *JAMA* 268:3353-3358, 1992.
52. Pickering TG. Renovascular hypertension: medical evaluation and non-surgical treatment. In: Laragh JH, Brenner BM. *Hypertension: Pathophysiology, Diagnosis, and Management.* New York: Raven Press; 1990.
53. Postma CT, Hoefnagels WH, Barentsz JO, DeBoo T, Thien T. Occlusion of unilateral stenosed renal arteries: relation to medical treatment. *J Hum Hypertens* 3:185-190, 1989.
54. Novick, AC. Management of renovascular disease: a surgical perspective. *Circulation* 83(suppl I):I-167-I-171, 1991.
55. Gruntzig A, Kuhlmann U, Vetter W. Treatment of renovascular hypertension with percutaneous transluminal dilation of a renal artery stenosis. *Lancet* 1:801-802, 1978.
56. Norling LL, Chevalier RL, Gomez RA, Tegtmeyer CJ. Use ofinterventional radiology for hypertension due to renal arterystenosis in children. *Child Nephrol Urol* 12:162-166, 1992.
57. Tegtmeyer CJ, Bayne Selby J, Hartwell GD, Ayers C, Tegtmeyer V. Results and complications of angioplasty in fibromuscular disease. *Circulation* 83(suppl I):I-155-I-161, 1991.
58. Hayes J, Risius B, Novick AC, Geisinger M, Zelch M, Gifford RW Jr, Vidt DG, Olin JW. Experience with percutaneous transluminal angioplasty for renal artery stenosis at the Cleveland clinic. *J Urol* 139:488-492, 1988.
59. Martinez A, Novick AC, Cunningham R, Goormastic M. Improved results of vascular reconstruction in pediatric and young adult patients with renovascular hypertension. *J Urol* 144:717-720, 1990.
60. Berkowitz HD, O'Neill JA Jr. Renovascular hypertension in children. Surgical repair with special reference to the use of reinforced vein grafts. *J Vasc Surg* 9:46-55, 1989.

61. Deal JE, Snell MF, Barratt TM, Dillon MJ. Renovascular disease in childhood. *J Pediatr* 121:378-384, 1992.
62. Iaccarino V, Russo D, Niola R, Muto R, Testa A, Andreucci VE, Porta E. Total or partial percutaneous renal ablation in the treatment of renovascular hypertension: radiological and clinical aspects. *Br J Radiol* 62:593-598, 1989.
63. Second international symposium on hypertension in children and adolescents: recommendations for the management of hypertension in children and adolescents. *Pediatr Nephrol* 1:56-58, 1987.
64. Sassard J, Sann L, Vincent M, Francois R, Cier JF. Plasmarenin activity in normal subjects from infancy to puberty. *J Clin Endocrinol Metab* 40:524-525, 1975.

Chapter 7

Hypertension Caused by Endocrine Disorders

Introduction

Over the years, endocrinopathies have intrigued physicians and medical scientists as they unraveled the intricacies of hormonal function. As a group, endocrine disorders are relatively infrequent causes of hypertension. They are mainly adrenal in origin[1] and account for perhaps 2% of all causes of pediatric hypertension.[2] Nevertheless, when glandular dysfunction does cause hypertension, it may be severe. For example, adrenal disorders may result in significant elevation of blood pressure, whether it be paroxysmal with some pheochromocytomas or sustained with Cushing's syndrome. Other rare adrenal endocrine-secreting tumors like Conn's syndrome are also known to cause hypertension in young patients.

Some children with diabetes mellitus may be found to be hypertensive and a few with parathyroid and thyroid disorders can be similarly afflicted. From this view of endocrine-induced hypertension, it is apparent that these disorders require some consideration when hypertension of uncertain etiology is discovered (Table 1).

Adrenal Cortical Conditions

Adrenal cortical physiology is well understood. As adrenal cortical cells migrate centrally from the subcapsular region, their hormonal production changes. In the outermost adrenal zone, the zona glomerulosa, mineralocorticoids (primarily aldosterone) are

159

Table 1.
Endocrinopathies Leading to Hypertension

Adrenal Cortical Conditions

Mineralocorticoid hypertension
    Secondary hyperaldosteronism
    Conn's syndrome
    Adrenal hyperplasia

Other Mineralocorticoid disorders
    Syndrome of apparent mineralocorticoid
      excess
    Glucocorticoid suppressible hyperaldosteronism
    Doc excess
    Licorice ingestion

Glucocorticoid hypertension
    Cushing's syndrome
      ACTH dependent: pituitary adenoma,
        lung cancer; carcinoids
      ACTH independent: adrenal adenoma/carcinoma

Adrenal Medullary-type Conditions

Pheochromocytoma tumors
    Benign
    Malignant
    Extra-adrenal catechol-secreting tumors
Neuroblastoma
Ganglioneuroblastoma
Renal tumors (incl. Wilms')

Other Endocrinopathies

Hyperthyroid and parathyroid conditions
Diabetes mellitus
Syndrome of IADH secretion
Estrogen Rx of Turner's Syndrome
Estrogen contraceptive therapy

ACTH = adrenocorticotrophic hormone; DOC = deoxycorticosterone; IADH = inappropriate antidiurectic hormone.

produced. The intermediate zone, the fasciculata, secretes glucocorticoids as well as some mineralocorticoids. The inner zona reticularis provides androgens and estrogens. Complex steroidal genesis takes cholesterol through a series of hydroxylations and oxidation to produce the end-product, biologically active steroids (Fig. 1).

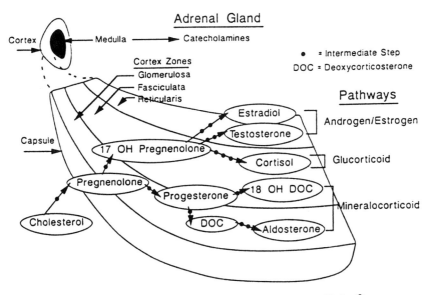

Figure 1: Adrenal steroidal genesis. (Modified from Biglieri[3]).

Alterations in enzymatic activity at any level, whether genetically determined or induced by another disease process, can result in hormonal hypersecretion with resultant syndrome consequences,[3] which include hypertension.

Mineralocorticoid Disorders

Primary Aldosteronism

Clinically, this disorder is characterized by hypertension, often severe, and unprovoked hypokalemia. It is the result of inappropriate hypersecretion of mineralocorticoids. However, primary aldosteronism is a rare cause of hypertension, especially in childhood. Its general incidence has been put at less than one per million people per year.[4] In contrast, secondary hyperaldosteronism is relatively common and usually the result of renin excess. Conditions with volume depletion, edema, renovascular obstruction, elevated estrogen levels, and excess of catechols, potassium, or adrenocorticotrophic hormone (ACTH) all lead to increased aldosterone secretion on the basis of increased renin production.

Primary aldosteronism is marked by low renin hypertension. The elevation of blood pressure is mainly the result of increased sodium reabsorption from the distal nephron brought about by the elevated level of circulating aldosterone. Plasma and extracellular volume expansion ensue and suppress renin secretion. Increased peripheral resistance may occur as a direct central nervous system effect of aldosterone[5] or from an enhanced renal vasopressin effect. The mineralocorticoid excess also leads to hypokalemia and alkalosis through increased hydrogen ion excretion in exchange for sodium. Because of increased renal perfusion pressure and an increase in atrial natriuretic factor[6] there is "escape" of the sodium retention but the excess potassium excretion does not remit. The potassium depletion may lead to increased fasting glucose levels through its effect on insulin secretion.

The insidious symptoms of primary aldosteronism include muscular weakness, paresthesias, constipation, growth delay, and downy hair growth. Polyuria, nocturia, and enuresis may occur as a result of hypokalemia-induced diabetes insipidus.[7] More likely, however, primary aldosteronism will be found in the course of a workup for blood pressure elevation in an asymptomatic individual. Initial or screening tests will reveal hypokalemia without obvious cause along with high 24-hour levels of urinary potassium.[8] In some patients, the hypokalemia may not be clinically evident, for they will have borderline low- normal serum potassium values. If such patients are given a higher sodium intake the hypokalemia will become obvious. Electrocardiographic signs of hypokalemia may be found such as prolonged ST segment, T-wave inversion, and the presence of prominent U waves.

The diagnosis of hyperaldosteronism is made by obtaining elevated levels of plasma aldosterone (PA). In primary aldosteronism, PA levels will not only be high but also autonomous. That is, aldosterone secretion is independent of the usual regulatory mechanisms. Several PA determinations should be done and compared to normal levels for age. As a rule, PA levels are usually below 10 ng/dL. Multiple sampling is important, for PA levels may vary widely with age. There is also diurnal variation. The autonomous nature of the hyperaldosteronism can be verified by failure of PA secretion suppression by saline infusion[9] or a captopril dose[6] if necessary. With primary hyperaldosteronism, plasma renin activity (PRA) levels are characteristically low. These levels vary by laboratory and sampling conditions. Generally, to be considered low the PRA should be in the range of 0.1 ng/mL per hour. A diagnostic protocol is presented in Figure 2[10] and can be used to screen and confirm the diagnosis of primary aldosteronism.

Two major pathologic forms of primary aldosteronism exist: bilateral adrenal hyperplasia and unilateral adrenal adenoma (Conn's syndrome).[11] Hyperplasia is the main variant affecting children. Adenomas are more common in females and more often left-sided. Biochemical abnormalities tend to be more severe with adenomas. Once the diagnosis of primary aldosteronism seems likely, it is necessary to discover whether it is from an adenoma or from hyperplasia. The distinction between adenoma and hyperplasia may be difficult but it is important because of therapeutic implications. Adenoma requires surgery but hyperplasia is treated medically.

A variety of diagnostic measures are available to separate hyperaldosteronism due to bilateral adrenal hyperplasia from the usually unilateral adrenal adenoma. Patients with adrenal adenoma may have a paradoxical fall in aldosterone level upon standing,[8] whereas those with hyperplasia generally have an increase of over one third the baseline value.[10] Selective adrenal vein catheterization for hormonal

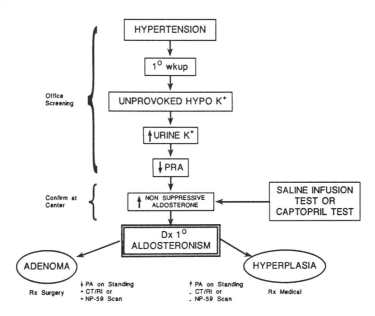

Figure 2: Diagnostic protocol for the detection of primary aldosteronism. (Modified from Kaplan[10]).

assay has been described as accurate in adults to detect adenomas which are usually unilateral.[12] In most children the vessels are small, making this approach very difficult. For the most part, adenomas as small as 7 mm in diameter can be separated from hyperplasia by high resolution computerized tomography or magnetic resonance imaging techniques. For smaller lesions, sophisticated radionuclide imaging may be helpful. The patient is given dexamethasone for about a week prior to isotope scanning with 131-I-normethylcholesterol (NP-59 scan). Images become positive in about 4 days and may be enhanced by digital subtraction techniques.[13]

Once the lesion is located, excision of the adenoma via lumbar or transabdominal route is recommended. Preoperative preparation with medical treatment for several weeks will speed recovery after surgery. Spironolactone is especially useful in this regard as it blocks the effect of aldosterone by competitive antagonism. High doses are required (125 to 325 mg/m^2 per day in divided doses). Postoperative aldosterone deficiency generally is short- lived and responds to the administration of electrolytes. However, hypertension may persist for a while longer and may require treatment with a diuretic. Cure rates for children approach 100%.[14]

Medical management is advocated for those with adrenal hyperplasia. Spironolactone, usually with a thiazide diuretic, will provide control of the hormonal excess. Aspirin should be avoided because of antagonism to spironolactone. The rare case of spironolactone intolerance may respond to a low sodium diet and the use of Triamterene.[15] If blood pressure control is not obtained with thiazides, captopril may provide relief and has the additional advantage of having a potassium-sparing effect. However, care must be taken to avoid hyperkalemia if large doses of spironolactone are used concomitantly.

Other Mineralocorticoid Disorders

Lesser and therefore very rare forms of mineralocorticoid excess include the syndrome of apparent mineralocorticoid excess, licorice ingestion, glucocorticoid-suppresible hyperaldosteronism,[8,16] deoxycorticosterone (DOC) excess, and adrenal carcinoma. These conditions may mimic primary aldosteronism in that they have hypokalemia and hyperkaluria with alkalosis. However, aldosterone levels are low.

In addition to the low renin hypertension and hypokalemia, there is responsiveness to spironolactone in the syndrome of apparent mineralocorticoid excess along with a general reduction in steroid secretion. A genetic defect of 11-β-hydroxysteroid dehydrogenase (11-β-OHSD) with prolonged half life of cortisol results in normal cortisol levels despite decreased secretion. There is also an abnormal affinity for cortisol by the mineralocorticoid receptors with cortisol acting as a mineralocorticoid.[17]

In licorice ingestion, renal blockage of the same enzymatic(11-β-OHSD) conversion of cortisol (again active as a mineralocorticoid) to cortisone (inactive) by the glycyrrhetinic acid of licorice is responsible for excess mineralocorticoid activity. Relatively small amounts of licorice over little more than a week may lead to the syndrome.[18] Removal of the licorice leads to recovery of the 11-β-hydroxysteroid in about 2 weeks but the renin-aldosterone axis may not recover for several months.[19]

Administration of dexamethasone or another glucocorticoid for about a week will completely resolve symptoms and hypertension in glucocorticoid-suppressible hyperaldosteronism.[20]

Glucocorticoid Disorders

Cushing's Syndrome

Hypertension from endogenous glucocorticoid excess is due to another rare set of adrenal hormonal disorders. Cushing's syndrome involving cortisol excess is the most common of these. Over half the children and three fourths of adults with the syndrome have hypertension.[21] This contributes to the high mortality found in the disorder. Exogenous glucocorticoid excess is a far more common cause of the syndrome. Fortunately, hypertension is less frequent in Cushing's syndrome resulting from steroid therapy, especially if alternate day dosage is used. The mineralocorticoid activity in the therapeutic steroids is generally low. Accordingly, the incidence of hypertension is greatly reduced. Thus, most children being treated with steroids will have normal blood pressures.

Both adrenocorticotrophic hormone (ACTH)-dependent and independent mechanisms can cause the excess endogenous adrenal cortisol secretion leading to Cushing's syndrome. The former includes pituitary tumors with hypersecretion of ACTH. That disorder is actually the disease first described by Cushing.[22] It accounts for about 70% of the syndrome cases. Other ACTH-dependent Cushing disorders are caused by tumors secreting the hormone, such as lung cancers and carcinoids of the thorax or abdomen. In addition, lesions with excess production of corticotropin-releasing hormone (CRH) may result in the syndrome.[23] They are rare in children but account for approximately 12% of the cases of Cushing's syndrome in adults.[24]

Adrenocorticotrophic hormone-independent disorders causing Cushing's syndrome are adrenal adenomas mainly, adrenal cortical carcinomas, and adrenal nodular dysplasias. These ACTH- independent disorders are more frequent causes for Cushing's syndrome in children than adults.[21] Sporadic cases have been reported as variants of ACTH-dependent and independent disorders.

The pathophysiology behind the hypertension in all Cushing's syndrome disorders is most likely the result of an interplay between the hormonal excesses which accompany them. Although the mineralocorticoid activity of cortisol is weak, the large amounts secreted in Cushing's syndrome lead to salt retention and fluid volume expansion.[25] Deoxycorticosterone and other mineralocorticoids including aldosterone are also secreted in greater than normal amounts thereby promoting further volume expansion.[26] In addition, both the renin-angiotensin system and the sympathetic nervous system activity are increased by cortisol excess. Other effects such as inhibition of vasodilator prostaglandin production[27] and hyperinsulinemia[28] may be involved as well.

From a clinical standpoint, most children are referred because of obesity,[21] perhaps with recent rapid weight gain. At that point, hypertension may be discovered. The typical obesity of Cushing's syndrome is progressive upper truncal and facial obesity. This is often manifested by the "buffalo hump" and "moon facies" appearance characteristic of the syndrome. Extremity wasting and osteoporosis from the catabolic effect of cortisol are other signs of the disorder. However, in infants, wasting may not be seen and obesity is generalized. Arrest or improvement in linear growth is a prominent finding in Cushing's syndrome in childhood.[28] Behavior changes including poor school performance and depression, may be the presenting complaint in older children.[24] Facial plethora, red striae on the proximal extremities and abdomen, acne, posterior truncal downy hair growth, virilization, and secondary amenorrhea in females, osteoporosis, and diabetes mellitus are other features of the syndrome.

When hypertension is found in the company of several of the above described features, Cushing's syndrome should be suspected. Confirmation of the diagnosis and localization of the lesion to the pituitary, ectopic ACTH-producing tumor or adrenal is a two- stage process. It requires both biochemical testing and imaging techniques. In the first stage, screening to verify the diagnosis may be accomplished by measuring urinary free cortisol (UFC). Over 100 μg UFC/day is strongly suggestive of the syndrome. The measurement of UFC to screen for Cushing's syndrome has largely replaced other urinary steroid measurements for this purpose.[24] An overnight dexamethasone suppression test may also be used for screening (Table 2).

If the UFC determination is equivocal, further confirmation of the diagnosis may be gained through the use of the low-dose dexamethasone suppression test. As outlined in Table 2, lack of cortisol suppression with the test confirms the diagnosis of the syndrome.[30] Unfortunately, the test requires hospitalization and is expensive. It is not necessary to use the low-dose dexamethasone suppression test if the UFC determination is diagnostic.

Table 2.
Biochemical Tests for Cushing's Syndrome

1. Screening tests
   a. 24-hour urine sample
      Cushing's syndrome RO with cortisol < 100μg/day (nl = <60μg/m^2)
   b. Overnight dexamethasone suppression test[31]
      1mg dexamethasone hs, plasma cortisol sample @ 8 AM (nl response = < 5 μg/dl cortisol)
2. Low-dose dexamethasone suppression
   a. baseline 24-h urine for cortisol (nl = < 60 μg/m^2/d)
   b. Dexamethasone 10 μg/kg (max 0.5 mg/dose) q6h for 2 d
   c. 24-hour urine sample:
      Non-Cushing's syndrome:
         suppresses urinary free cortisol to below 25 μg/d (< 50% baseline).
      Confirmation of Cushing's syndrome:
         no significant change from baseline
   d. Serum sample @ 8 AM:
      Non-Cushing's syndrome:
         serum cortisol level below 2.2 μg/dL
      Confirmation of Cushing's syndrome:
         serum cortisol level over 9.1 μg/dL[28]

Table 2.
Biochemical Tests for Cushing's Syndrome (*Cont.*)

3. High-dose dexamethasone suppression
  a. baseline 24-hour urine for free cortisol
  b. Dexamethasone 40 µg/kg (max 2 mg/dose) q6h for 2d:
  c. 24-hour urinary sample (nl response = urinary free
     cortisol < 10% baseline).
    1. ACTH-dependent Cushing's disease (pituitary)
       suppresses urinary free cortisol to 60% of
       baseline
    2. ACTH-dependent Cushing's syndrome (ectopic ACTH-producing tumor):
       no significant change from baseline urinary
       cortisol
    3. ACTH-independent Cushing's syndrome (adrenal tumor):
       no significant change from baseline urinary
       cortisol
4. Plasma ACTH levels ([30])
  a. Plasma from AM blood sample (nl = 20–100 pg/mL)
    1. Cushing's disease (pituitary)
       "normal" or high levels
    2. Cushing's syndrome (ectopic ACTH-producing tumor)
       very high levels
    3. Cushing's syndrome (adrenal tumors)
       undetectable
5. Plasma lipotropin (LPH) ([31])*
  a. Plasma from AM blood sample (radioimmunoassay)
    1. Cushing's disease = levels moderately elevated
    2. Cushing's syndrome (ectopic tumor) = very high levels
    3. Cushing's syndrome (adrenal) = very low levels

*As sensitive as ACTH levels but less overlap; ACTH = adrenocorticotrophic hormone.

Once Cushing's syndrome has been diagnosed, the next stage is to determine its cause. Additional biochemical testing is required to discover whether the disorder is ACTH dependent or independent. The high-dose dexamethasone suppression test is the standard test to identify ACTH-dependent pituitary Cushing's disease. As described in Table 2, suppression of UFC to below 60% of baseline confirms ACTH dependency. Lack of suppression indicates the presence of either an ectopic ACTH dependent, autogenous-secreting tumor or an ACTH-independent adrenal tumor.[31] Unfortunately, a few with ACTH-dependent lesions will not suppress cortosol production with dexamethasone while others with ACTH-independent disorders will have suppression. Plasma ACTH determinations,[32] also noted in Table 2, may be used to separate the pituitary from ectopic ACTH-secreting tumors. Pituitary tumors have normal ACTH levels whereas ectopic ACTH- secreting tumors have very high levels. Adrenal tumors have low levels of plasma ACTH. Use of plasma lipotropin levels may be more satisfactory as there is less overlap of plasma level between the three types of tumors.[33]

The failure to distinguish an ACTH-dependent pituitary tumor from an ectopic ACTH-producing tumor consistently has led to the development of other tests like the corticotropin-releasing hormone (CRH) stimulation test.[34] The test is simple but expensive. It can, however, be performed on an ambulatory basis. With the CRH test, a cortisol increase greater than 50% or ACTH rise over 100% essentially excludes an ectopic ACTH tumor.

Upon classifying the cause of Cushing's syndrome biochemically, the actual tumor site is sought by imaging techniques. For ACTH-dependent disorders, CT scans of the chest and abdomen have been the standard for locating the rare ectopic ACTH-producing tumor. On the other hand, pituitary CT scans in Cushing's disease are commonly unrevealing. Indeed, a positive scan may carry an unfavorable prognosis. Nearly all those without scan abnormalities in one report had surgical remission whereas only two thirds with positive scans responded favorably to surgery.[24] Most recently, high-resolution MR-imaging techniques have been shown to demonstrate over 70% of pituitary tumors along with lateralizing information.[35] Abdominal MR and CT scans as well as the NP-59 isotope scan are useful in locating adrenal tumors in those with ACTH-independent Cushing's syndrome.[36] The expensive, time consuming NP-59 scan should be reserved for difficult adrenal Cushing syndrome diagnoses such as small tumors or adrenal nodular dysplasias.[37] Most adrenal tumors are large enough to be seen with MR or CT imaging.

Rarely, in spite of exhaustive biochemical testing, the distinction of pituitary from ectopic ACTH-producing tumor remains in doubt. Similarly and not uncommonly, imaging techniques fail to demonstrate a biochemically verified pituitary tumor. In such situations, the use of petrosal sinus sampling for ACTH measurement may provide definitive surgically useful information.[38] Using this technique, both the right and the left inferior petrosal sinuses are catheterized. A blood sample is obtained for ACTH analysis from each sinus and compared with a peripheral venous ACTH analysis. The basal petrosal sinus to peripheral vein sample ratio should be less than 2:1. Petrosal sinus sampling is the most accurate and reliable method for separating pituitary from ectopic ACTH-secreting tumors. Lateralization can be accomplished by comparing the samples from the left and right sinuses.[39] Unfortunately, the technology is not widely available for the young and other pitfalls have been outlined.[40]

Initial management of Cushing's syndrome is directed at control of the associated hypertension. A combination of lasix for diuresis of the volume expansion and spironolactone for suppression of excess mineralocorticoid secretion is recommended. If further pressure control is needed, captopril will control the overactivity of the renin-angiotensin system. β-blockade may be useful for increased sympathetic activity.[10]

Ultimately, treatment by removal of the underlying disorder must be attempted. Preoperative suppression of the hypercortisolism for a period of weeks will improve the risk and speed recovery. Currently, ketoconazole is the preferred drug.[3] Surgical removal of pituitary tumors using transsphenoidal microsurgery has become the method of choice, with cure rates approaching 80%.[41] Although pituitary irradiation has been used for primary treatment of Cushing's disease,[42] most authorities reserve radiation therapy for postsurgical recurrences. Bilateral adrenalectomy has also been used for pituitary resection failures when rapid symptom resolution is needed.[24] Likewise, resection of neoplasms of ectopic ACTH secretion or adrenalectomy (either unilateral or bilateral) is necessary for those forms of Cushing's syndrome. Replacement steroid therapy is needed following these surgical procedures. Small doses of fludrocortisone acetate (Florinef® 0.05 to 0.15 mg/day) along with adequate dietary sodium are sufficient for most afflicted young people.[21] Unfortunately, many of the tumors are malignant and postoperative chemotherapy is often required. Adrenocorticotrophic-dependent lesions have responded to ketoconazole and adrenal metastases to mitotane. However, in contrast to those with benign tumors, the prognosis is guarded for young patients with adrenal malignancies since most children succumb within 3 years of diagnosis.

Congenital Adrenal Hyperplasia

Congenital deficiencies of one or more of the hydroxylases involved in adrenal steroid biosynthesis are other, rather rare, disorders. Yet, such deficiencies lead to adrenal hyperplasia and an overabundance of secreted steroid from nonblocked pathways. Most common is the 21-hydroxylase deficiency which shifts steroid production toward the sex hormones with resultant virilization. It is not associated with hypertension.[43] However, individuals with either the 11-hydroxylase[44] or the 17-hydroxylase[45] deficiencies do become hypertensive. Renin production is suppressed and there is hypokalemia (Table 3). With the autosomal-recessive 11-hydroxylation defect, there is also a shift towards sex hormone production. Virilization in females and precocious sex development in males are found. The enzymatic block in the 17-hydroxylase deficiency stops sex hormone and cortisol production, thereby leading to lack of secondary sexual development in females and pseudohermaphroditism in males. These defects respond to glucocorticoid therapy of 10 to 30 mg/day of cortisol.

Pheochromocytoma

Probably the most common and most well-known endocrine form of hypertension is that associated with pheochromocytomas. Their significance lies with the fact that they can cause fatal hypertensive crises. Similar to the other endocrinopathies causing hypertension, pheochromocytomas are rare, affecting about one per 100,000 adults per year.[46] A little over 1% of children being investigated for hypertension may have the disorder.[47] Nevertheless, the consequences of a missed diagnosis are so grave that tumor must be considered in all severely hypertensive individuals.

Table 3.
Biochemical Findings in Congenital Adrenal Hyperplasia[7]

Deficiency	Plasma	Urine
11-β-Hydroxylase	↑ 11-Deoxycortisol ↑ Deoxycorticosterone	Tetrahydro-11-DOC Tetrahydro-deoxycorticosterone
17-α-Hydroxylase	↓ Renin, Hypokalemia ↑ Deoxycorticosterone ↑ Corticosterone	

Pathophysiology

Pheochromocytomas are functioning chromaffin-cell tumors originating from cells derived from the sympathetic chain, in turn derived from neural crest anlage. Accordingly, such tumors may be found in locations where there are cells of the sympathetic system, particularly the adrenal medulla. About 90% of pheochromocytomas occur in the adrenal. Some label the 10% of chromaffin tumors found outside the adrenal medulla as paragangliomata.[47]

Chromaffin cells synthesize and store catecholamines like dopamine and norepinephrine, as well as a number of other hormones including vasoactive intestinal peptide and ACTH.[48] In the adrenal medulla, these cells are unique in that they can convert norepinephrine to epinephrine. As a consequence, an excess of the urinary metabolite metanephrine is suggestive for a medullary pheochromocytoma with excess production of epinephrine. However, small medullary tumors may secrete only norepinephrine. Urinary vanillylmandelic acid (VMA) is another marker, albeit not as specific as to tumor location (Fig. 3). Other functioning tumors

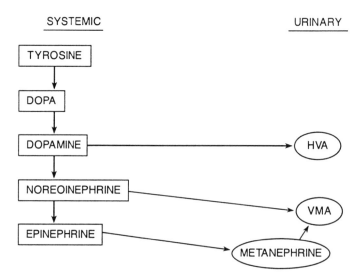

Figure 3: Substances in the pathways of catecholamine metabolism and their excretory products. HVA = homovanillic acid; VMA = vanillylmandelic acid. (Modified from Sheps et al[49]).

of the sympathetic system (like the benign ganglioneuroma or malignant neuroblastoma) produce mainly norepinephrine. Urine testing in these conditions will disclose excess homovanillic acid (HVA), the metabolite of norepinephrine's precursor, dopamine.[49]

Clinical Associations and Findings

Children are predisposed to have multiple tumors. These may be bilateral in the adrenal medulla or extra-adrenal along the sympathetic chain, bladder or in the organ of Zuckerkandl at the aortic bifurcation. Also, in young people the disease is often familial such as in the autosomal dominant multiple endocrine neoplasia (MEN) syndromes. Indeed, the diagnosis of pheochromocytoma has been made in some asymptomatic normotensive children on the basis of association with the MEN syndromes.[50] The MEN type 2 disorders commonly involve thyroid, parathyroid, and mucosal neuromas along with pheochromocytomas.[10] The individual with MEN type 3 seldom has hyperparathyroidism, but does have a marfanoid habitus.[51] Patients with pheochromocytomas must be observed for these features even after treatment for the tumor. The same holds true for those with thyroid carcinoma.[52]

Except for asymptomatic and normotensive patients with the MEN syndrome, almost all children with pheochromocytoma have significant hypertension (by task force criteria),[53] which is usually sustained. Elevated pressures are not as common in other tumors of sympathetic system origin. Less than 10% of young patients with pheochromocytoma have the "classic" paroxysmal hypertension. When part of the clinical picture, paroxysms can be brought on by stresses such as exercise, voiding, abdominal pressure, and drugs affecting catechols. One 17-year-old patient was reported to have a hypertensive crisis during childbirth.[50] Such spells may begin with anxiety and progress to tremors, palpitations, sweating, and lead to weakness. They may cause chest pain, pulmonary edema, encephalopathy, or even sudden death.

Associated cardiovascular disorders are common. Excessive cardiac muscle excitation-contraction coupling may lead to coagulation necrosis and myocarditis. With myocarditis there is contraction-band necrosis and inflammatory cell infiltration. The myocarditis may cause chest pain and mimic myocardial infarction with ECG findings compatible with coronary spasm. The disease process may be so severe as to cause pulmonary edema and has a high mortality.[54] Dilated cardiomyopathy may follow. Generally, resolution of the cardiac complications is found after the pheochromocytoma has been removed.[51]

Diagnosis

Sustained hypertension with severe headache is the most common presentation of young people with pheochromocytoma.[55] These symptoms may be coupled with significant sweating, flushing, and weight loss. Such findings should raise the question of whether a pheochromocytoma is present. A family history of such tumors or the MEN syndrome may be obtained in a number of pediatric cases. Nervousness, weakness, palpitations, polyuria, hematuria, gastrointestinal symptoms, postural hypotension, visual changes, and convulsions are also suggestive. The tumor is generally more common in males than females.

Biochemical support for the diagnosis of pheochromocytoma in children with suggestive symptoms should be sought first in the urine then in the plasma. One or more of the urinary screens for catecholamines will be positive in the majority of patients. Although difficult to obtain in many pediatric patients, 24-hour urine collections should be used if the patient is stable and off medication. While the metanephrine urine analysis is preferred by most, one should also measure VMA, HVA, and free catecholamine excretion (Table 4).[56] They may help characterize the tumor as epinephrine or norepinephrine secreting. However, false- positives do occur and may be found in patients on β-blockers or diuretics. Other medications such as clonidine may suppress catechol secretion.[48] Recently, measurement of urinary 3,4- dihydroxyphenylglycol (DHPG), a metabolite of norepinephrine, has been advocated for urinary catechol testing. The ratio of norepinephrine to DHPG is higher in pheochromocytoma than in other causes of hypertension.[57]

Plasma catecholamine determinations may also be of help in diagnosing pheochromocytoma (Table 4). When plasma determinations for epinephrine and norepinephrine are made, care must be taken to avoid endogenous catechol stimulation. An indwelling needle or catheter should be placed one-half hour prior to sampling in a resting child. False-negative serum values occur in as many as one third of individuals with documented tumors. Therefore, if a

Table 4.
Normal Screening Test Values for Catecholamines-Metabolites
(Modified from Gitlow)[56]

Age (y.)	<1	<5	<10	<18
Plasma epinephrine				<9.5µg/dL
Norepinephrine				<47.5µg/dL
Urine* VMA	<13.3	<7.3	<6.1	<3.5
HVA	<32.1	<14.8	<10.1	<6.5
Metanephrine	<4.2	<2.8	<2.7	<1.2
Free catechols				<0.1

VMA = vanillylmandelic acid; HVA = homovanallic acid.
*All values given as µg/mg creatinine.

normal serum catecholamine level is found and pheochromocytoma is still suspected, a glucagon provocative test preceded by an α-blocker may be used,[58] but perhaps it will be more efficacious to proceed with imaging examinations.

Previous technologies of pyelography and arteriography for diagnosis of pheochromocytoma have given way to computed tomography (CT) or magnetic resonance (MR) imaging and 131-I-metaiodobenzylguanidine (MIBG) scans used in complementary fashion. The radioactive isotope is taken up preferentially by adrenergic tissue. For abdominal tumors, these scans are highly accurate for tumors down to 1 cm in size. Tumors are rarely located elsewhere, for instance, in the heart[50] or neck. With a negative abdominal scan, a search of such tumor locations may be indicated.

Medical Treatment

Once the diagnosis of pheochromocytoma is confirmed and the lesion localized, medical treatment is initiated. The goals are to prevent the complications of pheochromocytoma and to prepare the patient for surgery. This translates into bringing the hypertension under control medically as an initial step. Usually, α-receptor blockade is begun first with phenoxybenzamine (Dibenzyline 0.4 to 2 mg/kg per day divided every 8 to 12 hours). Adverse reactions include postural hypotension which is experienced by most patients so treated.[55] Other side effects of dibenzyline treatment are tachycardia, syncope, and shock, as well as gastrointestinal disturbances.

The blood pressure consequences of dibenzyline treatment respond to volume expansion. If tachycardia and arrhythmias are a problem, a β-blocker like propranolol can be added. β-blockers should not be used alone. An unopposed α-pressor response or pulmonary edema may ensue. Prazosin has been proposed as a useful alternative to dibenzyline. Preferential blockage of postsynaptic blood vessel receptors preserves feedback inhibition of norepinephrine release so that tachycardia and the need for additional medication should not be a problem.[59]

The rare hypertensive crisis requires immediate control of the hypertension, usually with intravenous titration of sodium nitroprusside. As the pressure falls, volume expansion may be lifesaving. Arrhythmia monitoring and treatment are also vital.

Generally, preoperative preparation can be accomplished in a 1- to 2-week period. In-hospital therapy is best so that untoward catastrophic reactions can be recognized promptly and treated. When a rare patient is found with malignant pheochromocytoma and inaccessible metastases, medical measures may be needed indefinitely. Medications such as metyrosine[60] or 131-I-MIBG[61] may be successful in achieving tumor shrinkage.

Surgical Treatment

Operation is preferentially carried out through an extensive anterior abdominal approach. Since pheochromocytomas are frequently multiple in children, removal of the expected tumor must be followed by exploration for additional lesions which are then removed as found. The exploration includes a search of both adrenal areas, as well as along the sympathetic chain, the aortic bifurcation, and bladder. Bilateral adrenalectomy has been advocated for those with MEN syndromes due to the inevitable development of bilateral pheochromocytomas.[50] Expert anesthesiology with exact blood pressure control using phentolamine or nitroprusside, prompt volume expansion when the tumor is removed, and arrhythmia treatment with esmolol or lidocaine has made the operative outcome nearly uniformly successful. In a recent report of 77 patients (10% children) operated on at the Mayo Clinic, nearly 99% survived the intervention.[62] Those with benign tumors had a 96% 5-year survival. However, survival decreased to 44% in patients with malignant tumors.

Postoperatively, almost all patients become normotensive off medications. One must guard against transient hypoglycemia from sudden catechol decrease with resultant insulin increase. Those with adrenalectomy will need replacement therapy as discussed in the treatment for Cushing's syndrome. Postoperative urinary catecholamine levels should be checked for evidence of tumor recurrence or metastatic disease. A very few will have late recurrence of hypertension. This will also likely indicate tumor recurrence. In such cases, the outlined workup must be repeated. Isolated cases have been reported wherein renal artery compression by pheochromocytoma has caused renovascular hypertension either pre- or postsurgery to excise the pheochromocytoma.[44] Removal of the renal artery obstruction must then be attempted. However, with proper early diagnosis and treatment, most will be cured of their disease and have a favorable prognosis.

Hyperthyroid and Hyperparathyroid Conditions

Thyroid hormone is known to influence cellular metabolism in nearly every body tissue. Both tri- and tetraiodothyronine (T_3 and T_4) exert their biologic effects through nuclear binding, in turn, leading to increased protein synthesis and enhanced enzyme activity. With hyperthyroidism, cardiac contractility is increased and peripheral resistance decreased. In addition, blood volume may increase by as much as one fourth. As would be expected from these changes, in thyrotoxicosis about one third of patients have systolic hypertension. However, diastolic pressure remains low despite the associated tachycardia and increased cardiac output. Thus, the symptoms of hyperthyroidism predominate and the systolic hypertension is an associated finding only. With treatment of the hyperthyroid state, hypertension, if present, usually resolves.[63]

On the other hand, in hypothyroidism, heart rate and cardiac output are decreased while peripheral resistance is increased to maintain tissue perfusion. About one in five hypothyroid individuals becomes hypertensive.[63] Diastolic pressure is affected more commonly than systolic. In some, this may lead to myocardial hypertrophy. After treatment, return to the euthyroid state resolves the hypertension in over half of those involved.

Hyperparathyroidism has been found to be associated with a doubled frequency of hypertension.[64] The cause of hyperparathyroid-induced hypertension is obscure, but it is believed to be related to calcium metabolism. Hypercalcemia of such origin leads to increased peripheral resistance and hypertension. However treatment of the hyperparathyroidism in most instances does not resolve the hypertension.

Diabetes Mellitus

Hypertension has long been known to be a later-life event in adults with diabetes.[65] It appears to go hand-in-hand with diabetic nephropathy which is first marked by microalbuminuria.[66] However, most hold that the hypertension is not caused by the diabetic nephropathy; rather, the two conditions are found in association. Possibly they are related to genetic predisposition for such complications.[67] As a rule, hypertension associated with diabetes does not develop until the third or later decades of life. It is mainly systolic in nature and may be found in both type I and type II diabetes. The latter occurs in later life and may be related to obesity-induced hyperinsulinemia.[68] Blood pressure control affects diabetic nephropathy diminishing proteinuria. In fact, maintenance of blood pressure below the usual mean for age will delay the onset of microhematuria. A program for this purpose, applicable to young people, has been developed by Anderson and Rocchini.[69] It closely follows the measures outlined in Chapter 10.

Summary

Endocrine causes (Table 1) for hypertension are rare. Perhaps as much as 2% of pediatric hypertension can be traced to such disorders. Yet, hypertension caused by endocrinopathies are potentially curable. So consideration of hormonally induced hypertension is warranted in those with significant or severe hypertension of unknown cause. Most endogenous hormone excesses originate in the adrenal gland. Examples include Cushing's syndrome, aldosteronism, and pheochromocytoma. In childhood, diabetes mellitus, thyroid, and parathyroid conditions are rarely the origin for elevated blood pressure.

Mineralocorticoid disorders like aldosteronism are marked by hypokalemia, alkalosis, and kaliuria as well as high, albeit, variable blood levels of the steroid in question. Secondary aldosteronism is found in high renin states. In contrast, primary aldosteronism, often the result of adrenal hyperplasia, has low renin. A search for neoplastic origin must be made in all mineralocorticoid disorders using described biochemical and imaging techniques (Fig. 2). Effective medical or surgical treatments are available for most of these conditions.

Cushing's syndrome is the result of glucocorticoid excess. It is characterized by obesity and increased urinary free cortisol. Growth and behavior changes are frequent. About half the affected children have hypertension. When present, the hypertension can be controlled with lasix and suppression of glucocorticoid production with spironolactone. Surgical removal of an inciting neoplasm may be required. Complex diagnostic and localizing maneuvers are described to discover and isolate an inciting tumor whether it be pituitary, ectopic ACTH-producing, or adrenal. Unfortunately, the outcome is often uncertain and steroid replacement therapy may be needed. A Cushing-like syndrome may result from exogenous steroid therapy. Most cases, however, do not develop hypertension. Other adrenal steroid disorders may result from hydroxylase enzyme deficiencies and lead to hypertension and virilism. Often, they can be managed medically.

Pheochromocytomas are found in less than 1% of pediatric patients with serious hypertension. Yet, the catecholamines produced by the tumors may generate life-threatening situations. Children often have multiple tumors along the sympathetic chain in addition to in the adrenal medulla. Familial occurrence is known in the autosomal dominant multiple endocrine neoplasia (MEN syndromes).

While most children with pheochromocytoma hypertension have significant hypertension, the classic paroxysmal hypertension is uncommon and those with the MEN syndrome, diagnosed through familial occurrence, may be normotensive. Headaches and weight loss are common presenting symptoms. Measures of catechol excretion (Table 4) lead to the diagnosis. Various scans are then used to locate the tumor(s). Tumor removal may be treacherous with careful blood pressure control being necessary. In spite of successful surgery, those in whom the disease had a malignant origin have a guarded outlook.

References

1. Melby JC. Clinical review 1: endocrine hypertension. *J Clin Endocrinol Metab* 69:697-703, 1988.
2. Feld LG, Springate JE. Hypertension in children. *Curr Probl Pediatr* 18:317-373, 1988.

3. Biglieri EG, Irony I, Kater CF. Adrenocortical forms of human hypertension. In: Laragh JH, Brenner BM, eds. *Hypertension: Pathophysiology, Diagnosis, and Management.* New York: Raven Press; 1990.
4. Andersen GS, Toftdahl DB, Lund JO, Strandgaard S, Nielsen PE. The incidence rate of phaeochromocytoma and Conn's syndrome in Denmark, 1977-1981. *J Hum Hypertens* 2:187-189, 1988.
5. Kageyama Y, Bravo E. Hypertensive mechanisms associated with centrally administered aldosterone in dogs. *Hypertension* 11:750-753, 1988.
6. Gonzalez-Campoy JM, Romero JC, Knox FG. Escape from sodium-retaining effects of mineralocorticoids: role of ANF and intrarenal hormone systems. *Kidney Int* 35:767-777, 1989.
7. Guthrie GP Jr. Adrenal disorders causing hypertension in children. In: Kotchen TA, Kotchen JM. *Clinical Approaches to High Blood Pressure in the Young.* Boston: John Wright PSG Inc., 1983.
8. Young WF Jr, Hogan MJ, Klee GG, Grant CS, van Heerden JA. Primary aldosteronism: diagnosis and treatment. *Mayo Clin Proc* 65:96-110, 1990.
9. New MI, Baum CJ, Levine LS. Nomograms relating aldosterone excretion to urinary sodium and potassium in the pediatric population and their application to the study of childhood hypertension. *Am J Cardiol* 37:658-666, 1976.
10. Kaplan NM. *Clinical Hypertension,* 5th ed. Baltimore: Williams & Wilkins; 1990.
11. Conn JW. Presidential address, part I. Painting background, part II. Primary aldosteronism, a new clinical syndrome. *J Lab Clin Med* 45:3-17, 1955.
12. Ganguly A, Bergstein J, Grim CE, Yum MN, Weinberger MH. Childhood primary aldosteronism due to adrenal adenoma. Preoperative localization by adrenal vein catheterization. *Pediatrics* 65:605-609, 1980.
13. Brem AS, Oyer CE, Noto RB. Progressive hypertension associated with hypokalemic alkalosis. *J Pediatr* 118:479- 484, 1991.
14. Weinberger MH, Grim CE, Holfield JW, Kem DC, Ganguly A, Kramer NJ, Yune HY, Wellman H, Donohue WH. Primary aldosteronism: diagnosis, localization, and treatment. *Ann Intern Med* 90:386-395, 1979.
15. Ganguly A, Weinberger MH. Triamterene-thiazide combination: alternative therapy for primary aldosteronism. *Clin Pharmacol Ther* 30:246-250,1981.
16. Field ML, Roy S III, Stapleton FB. Low-renin hypertension in young infants. *Am J Dis Child* 139:823-825, 1985.
17. New MI. The role of steroid hormones in the development of low-renin hypertension in childhood. In: Loggie JMH, Horan MJ, Gruskin AB, Hohn AR, Dunbar JB, Havlik RJ. *NHLBI Workshop on Juvenile Hypertension: Proceedings from a Symposium.* New York: Biomedical Information Corp; 1984.

18. Stewart PM, Valentino R, Wallace AM, Burt D, Shackleton CHL, Edwards CRW. Mineralocorticoid activity of liquorice: 11-β- hydroxysteroid dehydrogenase deficiency comes of age. *Lancet* 2:821-824, 1987.

19. Farese RV Jr, Biglieri EG, Shackelton CHL, Irony I, Momez-Fontes R. Licorice-induced hypermineralocorticoidism. *N Engl J Med* 325:1223-1227, 1991.

20. Edwards CRW. Lessons from licorice. *N Engl J Med* 325:1242-1243, 1991. Editorial.

21. Jones KL. The Cushing syndromes. *Pediatr Clin North Am* 37:1313-1332, 1990.

22. Cushing H. The basophil adenomas of the pituitary body and their clinical manifestations. *Bull Johns Hopkins Hosp* 50:137-195, 1932.

23. Gomez Muguruza MT, Chrousos G. Periodic Cushing syndrome in a short boy: usefulness of the ovine corticotropin releasing hormone test. *J Pediatr* 115:273-278, 1989.

24. Carpenter PC. Diagnostic evaluation of Cushing's syndrome. *Endocrinol Metab Clin North Am* 17:445-472, 1988.

25. Sudhir K, Jennings GL, Esler MD, Korner PI, Blomberry PA, Lambert BW, Scoggins B, Whitworth JA. Hydrocortisone-induced hypertension in humans: pressor responsiveness and sympathetic function. *Hypertension* 13:416-421, 1989.

26. Whitworth JA. Mechanisms of glucocorticoid-induced hypertension. *Kidney Int* 31:1213-1224, 1887.

27. Handa M, Kondo K, Suzuke H, Saruta T. Dexamethasone hypertension in rats: role of prostaglandins and pressor sensitivity to norepinephrine. *Hypertension* 6:236-241, 1984.

28. Rebuffe-Serive M, Krotkiewski M, Elfverson J, Bjorntorp P. Muscle and adipose tissue morphology and metabolism in Cushing's syndrome. *J Clin Endocrinol Metab* 67:1122-1128, 1988.

29. Loeb JN. Corticosteroids and growth. *N Engl J Med* 295:547-552, 1976.

30. Kennedy L, Atkinson AB, Johnsone H, Sheridan B, Hadden DR. Serum cortisol concentrations during low dose dexamethasone suppression test to screen for Cushing's syndrome. *Br Med J* 289:1188-1191, 1984.

31. Crapo L. Cushing's syndrome: a review of diagnostic tests. *Metabolism* 28:955-977, 1979.

32. Rees L. ACTH, lipoprotein, and MSH in health and disease. *J Clin Endocrinol Metab* 6:137-153, 1977.

33. Kuhn JM, Proeschel MF, Seurin DJ, Bertagna XY, Luton JP, Girard FL. Comparative assessment of ACTH and lipotropin plasma levels in the diagnosis and follow-up of patients with Cushing's syndrome: a study of 210 cases. *Am J Med* 86:678-684, 1989.

34. Kaye TB, Crapo L. The Cushing syndrome: an update on diagnostic tests. *Ann Intern Med* 112:434-444, 1990.

35. Peck WW, Dillon WP, Norman D, Newton TH, Wilson CB. High-resolution MR imaging of pituitary microadenomas at 1.5 T: experience with Cushing's disease. *AJR* 152:145-151, 1989.

36. Fig LM, Gross MD, Shapiro B, Ehrmann DA, Freitas JE, Schteingart DE, Glazer GM, Francis IR. Adrenal localization in the adrenocorticotropic hormone-independent Cushing syndrome. *Ann Intern Med* 109:547-553, 1988.

37. Kazerooni EA, Sisson JC, Shapiro B, Gross MD, Driedger A, Hurwitz GA, Mattar AG, Petry NA. Diagnostic accuracy and pitfalls of [iodine-131] 6-β-iodomethyl-19-norcholesterol (NP-59) imaging. *J Nucl Med* 31:526-534.

38. Miller DL, Doppman JL. Petrosal sinus sampling: technique and rationale. *Radiology* 178:37-47, 1991.

39. Snow RB, Patterson RH Jr, Horwith M, Louis L, Fraser RA. Usefulness of preoperative inferior petrosal vein sampling in Cushing's disease. *Surg Neurol* 29:17-21, 1988.

40. Orth DN. Differential diagnosis of Cushing's syndrome. *N Engl J Med* 325:957-959, 1991. Editorial.

41. Pieters BFFM, Hermus ARMM, Meijer E, Smals AGH, Klopperborg PWC. Predictive factors for initial cure and relapse rate after pituitary surgery for Cushing's disease. *J Clin Endocrinol Metab* 69:1122-1126, 1989.

42. Sandler LM, Richards NT, Carr DH, Mashiter K, Joplin GP. Long-term follow-up of patients with Cushing's disease treated by interstitial irradiation. *J Clin Endocrinol Metab* 65:441- 447, 1987.

43. Fiet J, Gueux B, Raux-Demay MC, Kuttenn F, Vexiau P, Brerault JL, Couillin P, Galons H, Villette JM, Julien R, Dreux C. Increased plasma 21-deoxycorticosterone (21-DB) level in late- onset adrenal 21-hydroxylase deficiency suggest a mild defect of the mineralocorticoid pathway. *J Clin Endocrinol Metab* 68:542-547, 1989.

44. White PC, New MI, Dupont B. Congenital adrenal hyperplasia. *N Engl J Med* 316:1580-1586, 1987.

45. Winter JSD, Couch RM, Muller J, Perry YS, Ferreira P, Baydala L, Shackleton CHL. Combined 17-hydroxylase and 17,20-desmolase deficiencies: evidence for synthesis of a defective cytochrome P^{450}_{c17}. *J Clin Echocrinol Metab* 68:309-316, 1989.

46. Beard CM, Sheps SG, Kurland LT, Carney JA, Lie JT. Occurrence of pheochromocytoma in Rochester, Minnesota, 1950 through 1979. *Mayo Clin Proc* 58:802-804, 1983.

47. Dear JE, Sever PS, Barratt TM, Dillon MJ. Phaeochromocytoma: investigation and management of 10 cases. *Arch Dis Child* 65:269-274, 1990.

48. Benowitz NL. Diagnosis and management of pheochromocytoma. *Hosp Pract* June:163-177, 1990.

49. Sheps SG, Jiang NS, Klee GG. Diagnostic evaluation of pheochromocytoma. *Endocrinol Metab Clin North Am.* 17:397-414, 1988.

50. Caty MG, Coran AG, Geagen M, Thompson NW. Current diagnosis and treatment of pheochromocytoma in children. *Arch Surg* 125:978-981, l990.

51. Khairi MRA, Dexter RN, Burzynski NJ, Johnston CC Jr. Mucosal

neuroma, pheochromocytoma and medullary thyroid carcinoma: Multiple endocrine neoplasia type III. *Medicine* 54:89-112, 1975.

52. Gagel RF, Tashjian AH Jr, Cummings T, Papathanasopoulos N, Kaplan MM, DeLellis RA, Wolfe HJ, Reichlin S. The clinical outcome of prospective screening for multiple endocrine neoplasia type 2a. *N Engl J Med* 318:478-484, 1988.

53. Report of the second task force on blood pressure control in children: 1987. *Pediatrics* 79:1-25, 1987.

54. Imperato-McGinley J, Gautier T, Ehlers K, Zullo MA, Goldstein DS, Vaughan ED Jr. Reversibility of catecholamine-induced dilated cardiomyopathy in a child with a pheochromocytoma. *N Engl J Med* 316:793-797, 1987.

55. Benowitz NL. Pheochromocytoma. *Adv Intern Med* 35:195- 220, 1990.

56. Gitlow SE, Mendlowitz M, Wilk EK, Wilk S, Wolf RL, Bertani LM. Excretion of catecholamine catabolites by normal children. *J Lab Clin Med* 72:612-620, 1968.

57. Duncan MW, Compton P, Lazarus L, Smythe GA. Measurement of norepinephrine and 3,4-dihydroxyphenylglycol in urine and plasma for the diagnosis of pheochromocytoma. *N Engl J Med* 319:136-142, 1988.

58. Elliott WJ, Murphy MB, Straus FH II, Jarabak J. Improved safety of glucagon testing for pheochromocytoma by prior α- receptor blockade. A controlled trial in a patient with mixed ganglioneuroma/pheochromocytoma. *Arch Intern Med* 149:214-216, 1989.

59. Havlik RJ, Cahow E, Kinder BK. Advances in the diagnosis and treatment of pheochromocytoma. *Arch Surg* 123:626-630, 1988.

60. Serri O, Comtois R, Bettez P, Dubuc G, Buu NT, Kuchel O. Reduction in the size of a pheochromocytoma pulmonary metastasis by metyrosine therapy. *N Engl J Med* 310:1264-1265, 1984.

61. Sisson JC, Shapiro B, Beierwaltes WH, Glowniak JV, Nakajo M, Mangner TJ, Carey JE, Swanson DP, Copp JE, Satterlee WG, Wieland DM. Radiopharmaceutical treatment of malignant pheochromocytoma. *J Nucl Med* 25:197-206, 1984.

62. Sheps SG, Jiang N-S, Klee GG, van Heerden JA. Recent developments in the diagnosis and treatment of pheochromocytoma. *Mayo Clin Proc* 65:88-95, 1990.

63. Klein I. Thyroid hormone and blood pressure regulation. In: Laragh JH, Brenner BM. *Hypertension: Pathophysiology, Diagnosis, and Management.* New York: Raven Press; 1990.

64. Salahudeen AK, Thomas TH, Sellars L, Tapster S, Keavey P, Farndon JR, Johnston ID, Wilkinson R. Hypertension and renal dysfunction in primary hyperparathyroidism: effect of parathyroidectomy. *Clin Sci* 76:289-296, 1989.

65. Hitzenberger K. Uber den Blutdruck bei diabetes mellitus. *Arch Intern Med* 2:461, 1921.

66. Mogensen CE, Chachati A, Christensen CK, Close CF, Deckert T, Hommel E, Kastrup J, Lefebvre P, Mathiesen ER. Microalbuminuria:

an early marker of renal involvement in diabetes. *Uremia Invest* 9:85-95, 1985-1986.

67. Viberti GC, Keen H, Wiseman HJ. Raised arterial pressure in parents of proteinuric insulin-dependent diabetics. *Br Med J* 295:515-517, 1987.

68. Simonson DC. Etiology and prevalence of hypertension in diabetic patients. *Diabetes Care* 11:821-827, 1988.

69. Anderson J, Rocchini AP. Hypertension in individuals with insulin-dependent diabetes mellitus. *Pediatr Clin North Am* 40:93-104, 1993.

Chapter 8

Hypertension in the Newborn

Introduction

While hypertension is uncommon in newly born infants, when present it can cause and/or compound problems especially in low-birth weight infants. The definition of hypertension in early life, particularly in those with low-birth weight, has been the subject of a number of investigations. Pressures have been shown to vary by method of recording. Direct intra-arterial pressures are considered the "gold standard." General agreement, however, of what constitutes hypertension in the first hours and days of life remains to be settled. Nonetheless, it seems clear that age and weight as well as gestational maturity are major determinants of newborn blood pressure. In the first days of life a useful rule is that resting-mean pressures in excess of 75 mm Hg in the term infant, and in excess of 60 mm Hg in the premature infant are high and deserve further consideration. This chapter will review methods of pressure recording in these newborns and their normal pressure values, then consider causes and findings of pressure elevation as well as review treatments.

Blood Pressure Measurement

Blood pressure cuff size is most important in newborn infants. A cuff that is too small will give a false impression of hypertension and lead to over treatment. Conversely, a cuff that is too large may result in falsely low readings.[1] A cuff bladder width which covers two thirds of the arm and a length of three fourths of the midarm circumference will result in reasonable measurements. An alternative criterion is that cuff bladder width to arm circumference ratio should be 0.4 to 0.5.[2]

Auscultation pressure measurements are usually difficult. Auscultation over a small antecubital fossa for Korotkoff sounds is not readily accomplished. Korotkoff sounds are quite soft in the newborn and difficult to hear. For this reason, other methods are in use today.

Blood pressure by palpation of pulses distal to the blood pressure cuff may be possible and, indeed, has a history of being used extensively. However, weak pulses not uncommonly obviate this technique. The method measures systolic pressure only and has largely been replaced by Doppler or oscillometric methods. Yet, the method provides a simple way of following trends in systolic pressure.[3]

The flush technique of determining blood pressure furnishes a near the mean pressure. Moss and Adams found a wide range of values between direct measurements of systolic and diastolic pressure.[4] When a cuff deflation rate of 5 mm Hg per second was used, the pressure obtained approximated directly measured arterial mean blood pressure. Formerly, the method was the standard for pressure determination in newborns. It depends on adequate peripheral perfusion and may not be accurate in newly born babies. While not in use in the newborn intensive care units, the method remains useful for estimating pressure in other clinical settings.

Doppler pressure measurement devices have found favor in situations where conventional blood pressures are difficult to record, as is the case in newborns. Black and coworkers, in 1972, compared arterial and Doppler pressures in 28 infants weighing between 2.0 and 5.0 kg.[5] Deviations of 2.5–2.0 mm Hg for systolic pressures were reported. Pressures so measured tend to be lower than direct arterial pressure measurements and diastolic pressures are less reliable.[3] Doppler systems in which transducers are separated from the cuff tend to be more accurate than systems with integrated cuff-transducers.[6] Doppler devices are disadvantaged by time-consuming methodology, inability to record pressures continuously, and inaccuracy of diastolic pressure readings. An additional drawback is that the transducers are subject to easy breakage.

Oscillometric pressure measurement is the only noninvasive method that directly estimates mean arterial pressure. The method in current use was reported by Ramsey in 1979,[7] and has been refined by the Dinamap Corporation (Critikan, Tampa, FL). Kimble and colleagues found that by using proper-sized disposable cuffs, the automated system can provide accurate systolic and mean pressure readings.[8] The 95% confidence limit for a single Dinamap measurement was 7.7 mm Hg. Sonesson and Broberger compared intra-arterial and oscillometric pressures in 15 very low-birth-weight neonates.[9] When a cuff width to arm circumference ratio of 0.44 to 0.55 was used, nonsignificant differences of greater than 1 mm Hg between invasive and oscillometric pressures were found. Likewise, Colan and coworkers found that 94% of differences between arterial and oscillometric pressures did not exceed 10 mm Hg in 32 young patients.[10] They noted that physiologic stability was required for accurate measurements, as patient movement led to faulty determinations.

Direct blood pressure measurement by way of indwelling arterial catheters is a common method of obtaining blood pressures in newborn intensive care units. The catheter is most often inserted through the umbilical artery and passed to the aorta. There is debate as to whether or not placement of the catheter tip above the renal arteries is harmful. Fanaroff has presented data indicating more perfusion changes (loss of pulse or distal limb cyanosis) with low catheters (18%) than with high ones (9%).[11] While a large number of infants have been so monitored, normative data are somewhat sparse. On the other hand, renal artery thrombosis ranks high on the list of causes for neonatal hypertension.[12]

Blood pressure data from a number of reports are summarized in Table 6. Direct arterial pressure recordings can be compared with pressures obtained by other methods. In normal, term newborn infants, mean intra-arterial pressures generally range between 40 and 70 mm Hg. Pressures obtained by other techniques may show more variability.

Factors Influencing Blood Pressure in Neonates

Age of the newborn, maturity or gestational age, and *size* or weight profoundly influence blood pressure. Bucci and colleagues developed a regression equation based on these parameters to predict systolic blood pressure:

$$\text{mm Hg SBP} = 23.20 + 8.13w + 0.50ga + 0.23pa - .0016(ga^2) \quad 1.$$
$$(w = \text{body weight in kg, } ga = \text{gestational age in weeks,}$$
$$pa = \text{postnatal age in hours})^{13}$$

The formula gave a reasonable fit to pressures actually measured in their study of 189 low-birth weight infants less than 97 hours old.

Physical activity of the newborn also affects blood pressure. Sucking and crying infants have higher pressures. Awake but quiet infants may have lower pressures than sleeping infants. Diseases and treatments such as ventilator support for hyaline membrane disease generally result in lower pressures.

Little data is available concerning *familial aggregation* of blood pressure in newborns in contrast to the plethora of information available on older children and adults. Among others, Svensson reported on the long-term effects on blood pressure of progeny born to hypertensive mothers.[14] Blood pressure correlations between mother and child were not seen until the age of 6 years. However, Ibsen and Gronbaek found significant correlation between the systolic blood pressure in infants aged 4 to 5 days and the blood pressure of their mothers.[15] None of the mothers were being treated for hypertension. Thus, familial aggregation of blood pressure may begin early in life. More data are awaited.

Measurement site does not seem to influence blood pressure level. A number of studies of limb site for blood pressure recording have demonstrated that little or no significant difference exists between pressures taken in the upper extremity versus those obtained in the lower extremity.[2,16,17] Likewise, no significant differences were found between pressures in the right arm and left arm.

Several studies of *continuous direct arterial pressure* recordings have been analyzed by computer.[18,19] These techniques allow the detection of brief but significant fluctuations of pressure and correlation of these events with other events such as time of day. With the availability of noninvasive devices to record pressures on a near continuous basis, study of circadian variability of newborn blood pressure has been undertaken.[20] New analytic methods have been proposed which may detect risk for hypertension in later life.

Measurement techniques will affect blood pressure. Small or narrow cuff size has been noted to give falsely high values. Doppler devices result in higher blood pressure values. When direct intra-arterial methods are used, equipment factors such as tubing length (use short as possible), width and stiffness (wide bore stiff tubing and few stopcocks are preferred) must be considered. Frequency response of the system is another consideration and should be five times higher than the highest significant frequency in the signal imposed on the system.

"Normal" Blood Pressure Values

In *current practice*, pressure measurements in newborn intensive care units are obtained either by the direct intra-arterial method or by an automated oscillometric method. In most other newborn care situations, the oscillometric method is used. Recently, Park and Menard suggested recording blood pressures routinely in those younger than 3 years of age if an oscillometric device is available.[21]

Comparative newborn data is presented in Table 1. In the term-resting 1-day-old infant weighing over 2500 gms, direct arterial systolic/diastolic pressures vary between 50/33 and 92/61 mm Hg.[22] Oscillometric pressures range between 49/23 to 92/66 mm Hg in such infants.[2,23]

In "sick," very *low-birth-weight* newborns (< 1000 gms) in the first hours of life, direct intra-arterial blood pressure may be as low as 20/12 mm Hg with a mean of 15 mm Hg.[18] Conversely, in relatively well very low-birth-weight day-old-infants, the direct mean pressure may be as high as 49 mm Hg.[19] Tan reported oscillometric mean blood pressure as high as 83 mm Hg in day-old sleeping low-birth-weight infants.[24] The reason for the large difference between the direct arterial and oscillometric mean pressure is not clear, and the latter data must be viewed with circumspection.

There is a *rise in blood pressures* in all studies to about the age of 6 weeks, regardless of absolute blood pressure values. The rise is about 1 to 2 mm Hg per day for the first week of life, then 1 to 2 mm Hg per week until age 6 weeks.[25] After the age of 6 weeks, both term and preterm infants have similar pressures. Little increase in pressure is seen from then until 5 or 6 years of age.[21] Thus, age is a prime consideration in defining hypertension, even in early life.

Causes of Hypertension in the Newborn

From a *historic* standpoint, few cases of neonatal hypertension were reported prior to 1960.[12] Most of the early known cases involved renal thrombi. Subsequent burgeoning knowledge of newborn care as well as blood pressure values and ease of pressure measurement led to the recording of many more cases of hypertension. It is believed that there is a true increase in the number of hypertensive newborns, largely related to thromboembolic occlusions of the renal vasculature. Hypertension from such events is estimated to occur in

Table 1.
Blood Pressure Report Summary
(Summary of Reported Blood Pressure Values)

Source		Method	Age	Wt	(N)	Systolic	Diastolic	Mean
Moss[22]	1963	IA	Term	Resting	(74)	72 ± 10	47 ± 7	Calc 55.3 +/8
				Crying		94 ± 13	72 ± 14	
			Premature	Resting	(26)	64 ± 10	39 ± 8	Calc 47.3 +/8
				Crying		81 ± 15	57 ± 14	
Kitterman[51]	1969	IA	1 h	1001–2000 gms	(16)	49	26	35
			3 h			51	28	37
			6 h			52	31	40
			12 h			50	30	
			1 h	2001–3000 gms	(11)	59	32	43
			3 h			60	32	43
			6 h			58	34	43
			12 h			59	35	42
			1 h	3000 gms	(17)	70	44	53
			3 h			65	39	50
			6 h			66	41	50
			12 h			66	41	50
Adams[19]	1971	Continuous IA	to 12 h	820–1500 gms	(15)			39 (28–49) (± 1.6–4.5)
			to 24 h		(15)			37 (29–49) (± 2.0–4.6)
			to 36 h		(10)			38 (32–46) (± 2.2–7.9)
			to 48 h		(9)			39 (35–46) (± 2.9–9.0)

Table 1.
Blood Pressure Report Summary
(Summary of Reported Blood Pressure Values) (Cont.)

Source	Method	Age	Wt	(N)	Systolic	Diastolic	Mean
Versmold[52] 1981	IA	1st 12 h	750 gms		44 (14–34)	24 (14–34)	33 (24–42) 25
			1000 gms	(16)	49 (39–59)	26 (16–36)	35 (25–44) *29
			3000 gms	(45)	63 (50–73)	36 (27–45)	47 (37–56) *37
Moscoso[18] 1983	Continuous IA	2 & 3rd h	1000 gms	(9)	35 ± 7.4	21 ± 4.5	26.0 ± 5.4
		7 & 8th h			40.9 ± 4.9	25 ± 2.8	30.0 ± 3.3
		11 & 12th h			40.5 ± 5.5	24.7 ± 4.7	30.0 ± 4.5
	in "sick" babies	2 & 3rd h	1000–1250 gms	(10)	35.3 ± 2.8	20.9 ± 2.6	25.9 ± 2.7
		7 & 8th h			42.6 ± 4.0	25.3 ± 3.4	31.2 ± 3.1
		11 & 12th h			42.7 ± 5.2	26.8 ± 3.7	33.0 ± 3.2
Shortland[53] 1988	IA	1 day/m	1000 gms (650–1210)	(20)	46 ± 3.5	32 ± 3.5	35 ± 3.5
		3 d			53 ± 7.5	34 ± 7.0	38 ± 7.5
		6 d			52 ± 8.0	32 ± 3.5	37 ± 5.0
Cabal[56] 1992	IA	1st 24 h		90th%	90th%	90th%	90th%
			750 gms	(120)	43 (37–49)	22 (16–28)	28 (22–34)
			1000 gms		45 (39–51)	24 (18–30)	36 (30–42)
			2500 gms		58 (52–74)	37 (31–43)	44 (38–50)

*Low nl limit

Table 1.
Blood Pressure Report Summary
(Summary of Reported Blood Pressure Values) (Cont.)

Source	Method	Age	Wt	(N)	Systolic	Diastolic	Mean
Tan[24]	1988 Oscillometer Dinamap	1 d	1221 ± 171	(45)			
			Awake		67.9 ± 15.4	43.5 ± 14.4	57.7 ± 15.9
			Asleep		65.0 ± 13.6	41.4 ± 13.6	55.8 ± 13.6
		3 d	Awake		74.3 ± 15.7	49.3 ± 15.8	63.7 ± 15.1
			Asleep		77.0 ± 15.7	52.7 ± 16.0	64.8 ± 17.1
		10 d	Awake		72.8 ± 15.3	46.7 ± 13.9	59.2 ± 15.2
			Asleep		74.7 ± 16.1	50.0 ± 15.1	59.9 ± 14.2
		28 d	Awake		78.0 ± 16.8	48.7 ± 15.4	65.0 ± 16.8
			Asleep		80.9 ± 18.5	50.9 ± 17.3	64.7 ± 18.5
Lee[55]	1976	Term	Sleep		73 ± 10	46 ± 8	Calc 55.0 ± 8
		Active	Sleep		77 ± 10	46 ± 8	
			Awake		79 ± 9	52 ± 8	
			Awake + Sucking		85 ± 10	55 ± 7	
De Swiet[56]	1980 Doppler	Term	Awake	(4)	72 ± 6		
		3 d		(71)	74 ± 9		
		4 d		(44)	77 ± 10		
		5 d		(42)	77 ± 10		
		6 d		(9)	82 ± 9		
		7 d		(4)	88 ± 17		
		8–10 d					
		Term	Asleep	(72)	68 ± 7		
		3 d		(681)	70 ± 8		
		4 d		(426)	72 ± 8		
		5 d		(322)	72 ± 9		
		6 d		(47)	72 ± 9		
		7 d		(18)	72 ± 9		
		8–10 d					

Table 1.
Blood Pressure Report Summary
(Summary of Reported Blood Pressure Values) (*Cont.*)

Source	Method	Age	Wt	(N)	Systolic	Diastolic	Mean
Lagler[57] 1980	Doppler	3–13 min	>2500 gms (2500–4000)	(65)	56.8 ± 9.0		
		60 min		(71)	59.4 ± 8.8		
		360 min		(72)	61.5 ± 8.8		
Shaftel[49] 1983	Doppler	"Admission"	1933.4	(79)	49.5 ± 1.9		
Piazza[16] 1985	Oscillometer	1 d	2500–3000 gms	(20)	72.3 ± 12.5		
			3001–3500	(35)	72.3 ± 12.8		
			3501–4000	(45)	72.2 ± 8.0		
Tan[23] 1987	Oscillometer (Dinamap)	1 d	3330 ± Awake	(46)	70.5 ± 9.1	42.7 ± 9.8	55.3 ± 8.6
			Asleep		70.4 ± 9.6	42.3 ± 12.0	55.5 ± 11.4
		3 d	Awake		71.1 ± 12.3	49.3 ± 9.7	63.4 ± 12.9
			Asleep		74.5 ± 11.3	47.5 ± 10.3	58.8 ± 9.3
		6 d	Awake		75.8 ± 10.1	48.6 ± 11.0	62.1 ± 11.8
			Asleep		73.0 ± 11.2	45.5 ± 12.3	57.5 ± 12.0
Park[2] 1989	Oscillometer (Dinamap)	36 h/3273 2320–4580)		(140)	62.6 ± 6.9	38.9 ± 5.7	48.0 ± 6.2
		36 h CALF		(79)	68.4	43.5 ± 6.2	53.0 ± 7.3
		36 h		(140)	61.9 ± 5.3	39.6 ± 5.3	47.6 ± 6.0
		36 h		(79)	66.8 ± 10.1	42.5 ± 7.3	51.5 ± 9.0

about 1 per 1000 births,[26] and almost all newborn hypertension is secondary or associated with a known cause. On the other hand, at this time little is known of primary hypertension in the newborn. Few reports of unexplained newborn hypertension are available.[27] It is likely that more information about primary hypertension will accrue when studies are undertaken of neonates with blood pressure over the 95th percentile.

Definition of Hypertension

The definition of hypertension in the full-term newborn is elusive and it is even more difficult to define hypertension for the preterm infant. Some authorities consider pressures in excess of 90/60 mm Hg or a mean of 70 mm Hg on 3 separate days hypertensive in the term newborn.[26,28] However, these levels do not consider the previously demonstrated importance of age. Perhaps it would be more realistic to consider the 95% confidence limits about the mean curve as advocated by Fanaroff.[11] Use of percentiles as presented by Park deserves consideration in defining hypertension by the presence of three readings on separate days outside the 95th percentile.[21] Guideline blood pressure values for term newborns have been published by the Second Task Force on Blood Pressure Control in Children.[29] According to their guidelines, significant hypertension exists at 7 days of age if the systolic pressure is equal to or greater than 100 mm Hg. Thereafter, systolic pressures of 110 mm Hg or over are labeled as significant hypertension. Similar graphs are awaited for the preterm and low-birth-weight infant. In the meantime, use of the proposed mean pressure of 60 mm Hg on 3 separate days will have to suffice in these tiny babies.

Ophthalmoscopy

Ophthalmoscopy in infants labeled hypertensive by the above criteria provides a noninvasive look at the pressure effects on the vascular system. Skalina and coworkers found changes such as narrowed arterial caliber, spasm, and hemorrhages in 11 of 21 hypertensive newborns.[28] Nine of these babies had the respiratory distress syndrome and three had suffered asphyxia. Persistence of fetal circulation, transposition of the great arteries, phrenic nerve palsy, bilateral vocal cord paralysis, hemolytic disease, necrotizing enterocolitis, group B streptococcal septicemia, congenital hyper-thyroidism, and unilateral dysfunctional polycystic kidney were each found in one infant. Presumably, intra-arterial catheters were used for monitoring many of these infants. Some developed heart enlargement or failure as well as abnormal renal function. Follow-up revealed resolution of the retinopathy.

Incidence

Incidence figures for newborn hypertension are not readily available. Ingelfinger noted that, in the Boston area, about 0.2% of 10,000 births had recorded blood pressure elevation each year.[27] Eight of 12 newborns referred to her for hypertension had vascular causes, mainly renovascular. Central nervous system causes were found in two, one had a tumor, and another had coarctation of the aorta. This group of patients, while small, suggests a distribution of causes for hypertension. Based on the limited information available, Table 2 has been developed as a best guess estimate on the frequency of various types of secondary newborn hypertension.

Renal Causes

As in older individuals, renal causes account for most of the hypertension in newborns. Over half of the elevated blood pressures found in this age group have been related to intravascular cannu-lation, mainly from renal artery thrombosis. Prior note has been made of the infrequency of neonatal hypertension in the first half of the twentieth century. Coincident with the widespread use of indwelling umbilical lines for infant monitoring and treatment, there has been a rise in the frequency of hypertension. Among babies undergoing umbilical artery catheterization, the incidence of hyper-tension is about 3%.[26]

Renal Artery Thrombosis

Actually, the incidence of renal artery thrombosis is probably much higher. In a report of an angiographic search for thrombotic complications of umbilical catheters, Goetzman and coworkers found thrombi in 23 of 98 intensive care infants (24%).[30] Others have

Table 2.
Causes of Secondary Neonatal Hypertension

% * (Estimated)	Organ System	Disease
80	Renovascular	
75		Renal artery/vein thrombosis
1		Renal artery stenosis
1		Polycystic/parenchymal disease
1		Renal hypo/dysplasia
1		Obstructive uropathy
1		Other
10	Central Nervous	
		Hemorrhage
		Infection
		Congenital defect
5	Coarctation of the aorta	
5	Oncologic	Neural crest tumor
	Endocrine	Adrenogenital syndrome/Cushings disease/primary hyperaldosteronism/hyperthyroidism
	Infection	
	Medication	Ocular phenylephrine/steroids/theophylline/calcium/fluid and electrolyte overload
	Other	Abdominal surgery/pneumothorax

*(based on data from references[25–27,44]).

reported similar findings.[31,32] Not all neonates with thrombi will have symptoms. Neal and associates discovered thrombi in 18 of 19 babies just prior to withdrawal of their umbilical artery catheters.[33] Only one of these babies had clinical evidence of the thrombosis. Similarly, in older patients, hypertension develops in about 25% of those with renal artery thrombosis.[34]

Adelman maintains that the *catheter-tip location* is an important factor in the etiology of renal arterial thrombosis. At his institution, the catheter tip is always withdrawn to a point below the renal arteries.[12] In that way, if there is embolization from the catheter tip, it will be downstream, away from the renal arteries. On the other hand, Fanaroff, as already mentioned, has found no difference in the incidence of hypertension from high catheters.[11] He has noted, however, that low-catheter-tip placements result in more adverse effects on the distal circulation such as cyanotic distal lower extremities or loss of arterial pulsation.

Catheter-Related Hypertension

It is unlikely that catheter-related hypertension in the newborn will decrease in the near future. There is widespread use of neonatal intensive care units which per se favor umbilical vessel cannulation. Also, it is common for inexperienced house officers to effect umbilical artery cannulation in these units. However, technical advances may decrease the need for invasive monitoring. For the present, the rule should be to avoid umbilical vessel cannulation whenever possible.

There is a curious association between *patent ductus arteriosus* and renal artery thrombosis. Gross first reported this association in 1945.[35] Since nearly half of preterm infants have a persistently patent ductus arteriosus and most of these babies are now surviving, some of those who develop hypertension may be from embolization of a ductal thrombus to the renal arteries.[36] Parenthetically, it should be noted that some neonates with a large patent ductus were found to have low arterial pressures.[37] With ductal ligation, the pressures promptly returned to usual values.

Renal Artery Stenosis

Renal artery stenosis is an infrequent cause of neonatal hypertension. There is an association of rubella[38] and idiopathic hypercalcemia[39] with renal arterial narrowing. While these are rare events, they should be considered in hypertension of undiagnosed cause.

Parenchymal and Structural Renal Disorders

A number of parenchymal and structural renal disorders may be associated with newborn hypertension. Grouped together, they probably account for less than 1% of the elevated pressures found at that age. Of these disorders, infantile polycystic kidney disease is the most common and may improve in time with blood pressure control.[27]

Congenital renal hypoplasia-dysplasia are also known and expected albeit rare causes of newborn hypertension.[26] Little data are available in the literature concerning these conditions.

Obstructive uropathies have been reported to cause hypertension in early life. The importance of such disorders lies in the fact that they may respond to surgical intervention.[40] Other renal disorders such as infection, immune nephropathies, and the like are extraordinarily rare causes of newborn hypertension. However, these and the listed renal disorders may cause renal failure. Hypertension can be expected in about 10% to 20% of those with renal failure.[41]

Neurologic Disorders

Hypertension with newborn neurologic disorders is a relatively common occurrence.[42] Of the disorders in question, cerebral hemorrhage is most common. Whether or not the blood pressure elevation precedes the bleed is unknown. However, at least in some instances, hypertension is a likely antecedent of the hemorrhage.[43] As a result of undeveloped cerebral autoregulation, rises in blood pressure may lead to bleeding in cerebral capillaries which lack a firm glial structure support. With maturation, the incidence of hemorrhage becomes less. Less commonly, defects such as those resulting in hydrocephalus may be associated with hypertension. Neonatal central nervous system infections may also be associated with blood pressure elevation. For example, hypertension is seen in meningitis, especially if there is obstruction to cerebrospinal fluid flow.

Coarctation of the Aorta

Coarctation of the aorta, as described in Chapter 5, may not be obvious at birth. An associated patent ductus arteriosus may allow adequate perfusion to the lower body, particularly to the kidneys. Thus, the coarctation may be masked. Not surprisingly, Thoele and coworkers, in their study of coarctation recognition, found that hypertension was not the reason for referral in any of 36 neonates with the defect.[44] More commonly, these babies present with congestive heart failure or an arm-leg pulse/pressure difference or even just a heart murmur. Coarctation in the newborn is often complicated by other cardiac defects. When newborns with coarctation are referred, over 60% will be found to be hypertensive. Certain babies with coarctation are ductal-dependent and, in these infants, sudden ductal closure may result in a shock syndrome.

Among *medications* causing elevated blood pressure, the commonly used mydriatic, phenylephrine, exemplifies the need to monitor pressure when such medications are given. Lees and Cabal found a mean systolic pressure increase of over 5 mm Hg with mydriatic use in seven low-birth-weight neonates.[45] Although their pressures were not in the hypertensive range the researchers cautioned about adverse effects in these fragile infants. Other medications that bear watching include steroids and theophylline. Likewise, some concern must be given to infusions of fluids and electrolytes, although dietary sodium is not an apparent problem.[46] Along these lines, calcium infusion for neonatal hypocalcemia has been shown to increase systolic pressure transiently by over 7 mm Hg.

Endocrine Conditions

Various endocrine conditions known to produce hypertension may rarely make their appearance in the newborn period. Of these, perhaps the adrenogenital syndrome is most common and infants with findings of the syndrome should have frequent determinations of their blood pressure. Hyperthyroidism, Cushing's syndrome, and primary aldosteronism also occur in the newborn, but are rare causes of hypertension in that age group.

Other Causes

Miscellaneous other causes of newborn hypertension include extracorporeal membrane oxygenation (ECMO), abdominal surgery, and pneumothorax. Systolic blood pressure over 100 mm Hg for 4 or more hours was found in 18 of 31 cases of ECMO by Boedy and colleagues.[47] The hypertension was not related to increased plasma-renin activity (PRA), colloid or sodium loads, or infusion rates. Their patients did not have an increased incidence of intracranial hemorrhage (ICH). On the other hand, while Sell and coworkers also found hypertension common in babies on ECMO, they noted significant ICH in 11 of their 41 ECMO babies.[48] Those with ICH had a greater proportion of total ECMO time with blood pressures over 90 mm Hg than others without ICH. With aggressive blood pressure treatment using captopril, two of 23 patients developed clinically significant ICH, whereas nine of 18 without such treatment had significant ICH. Their babies had elevated levels of PRA, aldosterone, epinephrine, norepinephrine, prostaglandin E_2, thromboxane, and antidiuretic hormone.

Findings-Diagnosis in Hypertensive Newborn Infants

About 25% to 50% of those newborns with hypertension will have no symptoms.[12] They will simply have three or more recordings of blood pressure in the previously defined hypertensive range. Most will have a history of having had an umbilical artery catheter in place. Others will have cardiac, respiratory, or neurologic symptoms and then such patients can be detected as hypertensive. In such instances, the hypertension will be found to cause the difficulty rather than result from an intrinsic cardiac, pulmonary or neurologic disorder. The majority of those with newborn hypertension are discovered in the first week of life. It should be noted that as many as 9% of newborn intensive care unit "graduates" will be detected to be hypertensive in their early postdischarge examinations.[49] Blood pressure determination, therefore, becomes an important component of the examination when reassessing these babies.

Certain treatments can, as previously noted, result in hypertension. Therapy to expand volume and medications such as theophylline or mydriatic agents are known offenders. History of their use should be sought when hypertension is found. Babies born to mothers who had hypertension during pregnancy may be at risk for later-life hypertension but do not appear to have newborn hypertension.[14]

Newborn hypertension can result in tachypnea from heart failure. Mottling, weak pulses, and even cyanosis may also be present with hypertension-induced cardiac decompensation. Presence of a heart murmur may be a sign of a patent ductus arteriosus causing the hypertension.

Neurologic symptoms like lethargy, tremors, opisthotonos, seizures, apnea, and hemiparesis have all been described in newborn hypertension. These and the other described findings are nonspecific and may be due to concomitant medical processes such as sepsis, hypoxia, or metabolic derangements. Further evaluation generally allows determination of the symptom cause.

Physical examination commonly does not reveal abnormal findings save for the blood pressure elevation. Many will still have an umbilical artery catheter in place or evidence of its recent removal. Rarely, a flank mass or bruit may be detected. In those with cardiorespiratory symptoms, cardiomegaly, pulmonary rales, and hepatomegaly may be found. Others with neurologic symptoms may be seen to be floppy or hypertonic and have altered reflexes and/or sensorium. Some will have systolic or continuous ductal murmurs. Arterial pulses may be strong or weak. Mottled skin, cool extremities, and distal cyanosis may be present. When specifically checked, differences in arm-leg pulse and blood pressure may be found in those with aortic coarctation.

Laboratory evaluation will reveal hematuria and proteinuria in about one third of hypertensive newborns.[12] About half of these infants will have serum creatinine levels above 0.7mg/dL and BUN levels above 15 mg/dL. Likewise, elevation of plasma-renin activity is common. A few may have abnormal coagulation profiles. Abdominal aortography in those hypertensive newborns with umbilical artery catheters still in place will reveal abnormal findings in over two-thirds of the cases. Radioisotope scans, which may be performed without a catheter in place, will be positive in a slightly smaller number. Computerized scans can evaluate each kidney separately.[25] When a scan is nondiagnostic, an abdominal aortogram can be done via the femoral route in those without umbilical catheters.

Diagnosis of neonatal hypertension depends on confirmation of high blood pressure. Thus, it is paramount to take blood pressures in the course of newborn evaluations, especially in those of low-birth weight. Once hypertension is detected, most will have either no or nonspecific findings. However, a careful search is necessary for causes such as coarctation of the aorta or for vasoactive therapies. Laboratory evaluations should concentrate on determining whether or not a renal disorder is at fault.

Treatment of Hypertension Found in Newborns

As in older children, where possible *preventive measures* should be used to obviate the occurrence of hypertension. Thus, the use of umbilical artery catheters should be restricted to those absolutely requiring such monitoring. When umbilical artery catheters are used, they should be removed as soon as feasible. Likewise, medications affecting blood pressure such as catecholamines, theophylline, and steroids should be avoided where possible. Cautious use of electrolyte infusions is also important to avoid iatrogenic hypertension in newborns.

In a similar vein, when mild elevations of blood pressure are discovered, an initial trial of *nonpharmacologic* measures to reduce the elevated pressure may be warranted. Such measures as lowering the intake of fluid and sodium, provision of adequate potassium intake, ensuring a quiet, euthermic, nonnoxious environment may be helpful. If one is treating a very low-birth-weight neonate, lowering a mildly elevated pressure with a diuretic may prevent cardiovascular or cerebral complications.

On the other hand, more aggressive treatment may be in order for newborns with higher blood pressure. Little information is available concerning blood pressure levels requiring therapy in the first days of life. A useful rule is to treat those infants medically with pressure elevations consistently above the 99th percentile for age (above 3 standard deviations).[27] Accordingly, based on Table 1 data, it appears reasonable to consider pharmacologic intervention when a term newborn repeatedly has systolic Doppler pressures of 95 to 100 mm Hg. By 6 weeks of age, the level of Doppler systolic blood pressure requiring treatment consideration increases to over 120 mm Hg. In the low-birth-weight newborn a mean blood pressure in excess of 65 mm Hg may signal a need for treatment.

Medical treatment varies according to the severity of the newborn hypertension. For mild to moderate pressure elevation, hydralazine or diuretics (Table 3) are used by titrating doses to achieve pressure control. Persistent hypertension or poorly control-led blood pressure may require addition of another medication such as propranolol. In most instances when moderate to severe pressure elevation is found, captopril has been used to control the hyperten-sion. This useful medication must not be given to those with bilateral renal artery stenosis or to those with stenosis of the renal artery to

Table 3.
Useful Medications for Treatment of Neonatal Hypertension

Medication	Dose/Range	Route/Frequency
Chlorothiazide	10–25 mg/kg	P.O./q12h
Furosemide (Lasix)	1–4 mg/kg	I.V.,P.O./q6–12h
Hydralazine	0.25–3.0 mg/kg	I.V.,P.O./q8h
Propranolol	0.5–1 mg/kg	P.O./q6h
Captopril	0.05–0.4 mg/kg	P.O./q8h
Nitroprusside	0.5–5.0 μg/kg/min	I.V. drip

a single kidney. In such instances, complete suppression of the renin-angiotensin system may occur with associated circulatory collapse.[50] Rarely, extreme systolic pressure elevation to over 150 mm Hg in the term, or 120 mm Hg in the preterm newborn will cause fulminating heart failure. Such life-threatening emergencies require treatment with carefully titrated doses of intravenous nitroprusside. When the pressure has been reduced to tolerable levels, treatment can be changed to oral-gastric tube captopril.

For the most part, antihypertensive therapy is successful in controlling the disorder and preventing newborn mortality.[12] However, relatively high medication doses may be needed. Treatment is continued for at least several months after blood pressure has been normalized. At that point, medication can be slowly withdrawn. In most instances, hypertension will not recur. These infants can be expected to remain normotensive, at least in the near-term future.

Once hypertension control is achieved, consideration can be given to removal of the cause, such as by resection of a coarctation of the aorta. In the few cases that do not respond well to medical treatment or who experience drug intolerance, early operative intervention, if available, may be necessary. This is especially likely if a single diseased kidney or stenosis of a renal artery is responsible for the hypertension. In such cases, surgical relief of the narrowed vessel or even nephrectomy should not be delayed.

Summary

Much information remains to be learned about hypertension in the newborn, especially in those of low-birth weight. At present, current practice calls for measuring blood pressure with an oscillometric device using a proper cuff size. The cuff should occupy at least two thirds of the limb length to which it is applied. Pressures vary with age and size. In the term newborn under the age of 1 week, a systolic pressure over 90 mm Hg is high. Pressure over 100 mm Hg is considered significant hypertension, generally requiring investigation and treatment. Most commonly the cause is a renal problem, but neurologic disorders, coarctation of the aorta, and tumors are considerations. Therapy should be directed at the cause if known. Medical management with nonpharmacologic and pharmacologic measures may be indicated. Use of a diuretic may suffice. Captopril has been proven to be useful for nonresponsive patients, provided the infant does not have renal artery stenosis. In the low-birth-weight infant, mean arterial pressure of over 60 mm Hg is cause for concern and evaluation. In such newborns, hypertension is often due to indwelling arterial catheters. Thus, avoiding arterial line placement may avoid hypertension. Careful use of the outlined measures will control the problem in all but a few patients. Over time, most of these babies can be weaned from treatment.

References

1. Lum LG, Jones MD Jr. The effect of cuff width on systolic blood pressure measurements in neonates. *Pediatrics* 91:963-966, 1977.
2. Park MK, Lee DH. Normative arm and calf blood pressure values in the newborn. *Pediatrics* 83:240-243, 1989.
3. Darnall RA. Noninvasive blood pressure measurement in the neonate. *Clin Perinatol* 2:31-49, 1985.
4. Moss AJ, Adams FH. Flush blood pressure and intra-arterial pressure. *Am J Dis Child* 107:489-491, 1964.
5. Black IFS, Kotrapu N, Massie H. Application of Doppler ultrasound to blood pressure measurement in small infants. *J Pediatr* 81:932-993, 1972.
6. Reder RF, Dimich I, Cohen CL. Evaluating indirect blood pressure measurement techniques: a comparison of three systems in infants and children. *Pediatrics* 62:326-330, 1978.
7. Ramsey M III. Noninvasive automatic determination of mean arterial pressure. *Med Biol Eng Comput* 17:1-18, 1979.
8. Kimble KJ, Darnall RA Jr, Yelderman M, Ariagno RL, Ream AK. An automated oscillometric technique for estimating mean arterial pressure in critically ill newborns. *Anesthesia* 54:423-425, 1981.
9. Sonesson SE, Broberger U. Arterial blood pressure in the very low birth weight neonate. *Acta Paediatr Scand* 76:338-341, 1987.
10. Colan SD, Fujii A, Borow KM, MacPherson D, Sanders SP. Noninvasive determination of systolic, diastolic and end-systolic blood pressure in neonates, infants and young children: comparison with central aortic pressure measurements. *Am J Cardiol* 52:867-870, 1983.
11. Fanaroff AA, Stork EK, Carlo W, Kliegman R. Neonatal hypertension. *88th Ross Conf Report* 85-89, 1985.
12. Adelman RD. Neonatal hypertension. *Pediatr Clin North Am* 25:99-110, 1978.
13. Bucci G, Scalamandre A, Savignoni PG, Mendicini M, Picece-Bucci S, Piccinato L. The systemic systolic blood pressure of newborns with low weight. *Acta Paediatr Scand* 229(suppl):1- 26, 1972.
14. Svensson A. Hypertension in pregnancy. *Acta Medica Scand* 695(suppl):1-44, 1985.

15. Ibsen KK, Gronbaek M. Familial aggregation of blood pressure in newly born infants and their mothers. *Acta Paediatr Scand* 69:109-111, 1980.

16. Piazza SF, Chandra M, Harper RG, Sia CG, McVicar M, Huang H. Upper- vs lower-limb systolic blood pressure in full-term normal newborns. *Am J Dis Child* 139:797-799, 1985.

17. Uhari M, Isotalo H, Kauppinen R, Kouvalainen K. Difference between upper and lower limb blood pressure in newborns. *Acta Paediatr Scand* 70:941-942, 1981.

18. Moscoso P, Goldberg RN, Jamieson J, Bancalari E. Spontaneous elevation in arterial blood pressure during the first hours of life in the very low-birth-weight infant. *J Pediatr* 103:114-117, 1983.

19. Adams MA, Pasternak JF, Kupfer BM, Gardner TH. A computerized system for continuous physiologic data collection and analysis: initial report on mean arterial blood pressure in very low-birth-weight infants. *Pediatrics* 71:23-30, 1983.

20. Cagnoni M, Tarquini B, Haglberg F, Marz W, Cornelissen G, Mainardi G, Panero C, Shinoda M, Scarpelli P, Romano S, Bingham C, Hellbrugge T. Circadian variability of blood pressure and heart rate in newborns and cardiovascular chronorisk. *Prog Clin Biol Res* 227B:145-151:1987.

21. Park MK, Menard SM. Normative oscillometric blood pressure values in the first 5 years in an office setting. *Am J Dis Child* 143:860-864, 1989.

22. Moss AJ, Duffie ER, Emmanouilides G. Blood pressure and vasomotor reflexes in the newborn infant. *Pediatrics* 32:175-179, 1963.

23. Tan KL. Blood pressure in full-term healthy neonates. *Clin Pediatr* 26:21-24, 1987.

24. Tan KL. Blood pressure in very low birth weight infants in the first 70 days of life. *J Pediatr* 112:266-270, 1988.

25. Bloway DL, Warad BA, Alon U. Hypertension in the neonatal period. *Child Nephrol Urol* 12:113-118, 1992.

26. Adelman RD. Neonatal hypertension. In: Loggie JMH, Horan MJ, Gruskin AB, Hohn AR, Dunbar JB, Havlik, RJ, eds. *NHLBI Workshop in Juvenile Hypertension*. New York: Biomed Information Corp; 267-282:1984.

27. Ingelfinger JR. *Pediatric Hypertension*. Philadelphia: WB Saunders; 229:1982.

28. Skalina MEL, Annable WL, Kliegman RM, Fanaroff AA. Hypertensive retinopathy in the newborn infant. *J Pediatr* 103:781-786, 1983.

29. Report of the Second Task Force on blood pressure control in children. *Pediatrics* 79:1-25.1987.

30. Goetzman BW, Stedalnik RC, Bogren HG, Blankenship J, Ikeda RM, Thayer J. Thrombotic complications of umbilical artery catheters: a clinical and radiographic study. *Pediatrics* 56:374-379, 1975.

31. Ford KT, Teplick SK, Clark RE. Renal artery embolism causing neonatal hypertension. *Radiology* 113:169-170, 1974.

32. Plummer LB, Kaplan GW, Mendoza SA. Hypertension in infants: a complication of umbilical arterial catheterization. *J Pediatr* 89:802-805, 1976.

33. Neal WA, Reynolds JW, Jarvis CW, Williams HJ. Umbilical artery catheterization: demonstration of arterial thrombosis by aortography. *Pediatr* 50:6-13, 1972.

34. Lessman RK, Johnson SF, Coburn JW, Kaufman JJ. Renal artery embolism. *Ann Intern Med* 89:477, 1978.

35. Gross RE. Arterial embolism and thrombosis in infancy. *Am J Dis Child* 70:61-73, 1945.

36. Siassi B, Blanco C, Cabal LA. Incidence and clinical features of patent ductus arteriosus in low-birth weight infants: a prospective analysis of 150 consecutively born infants. *Pediatrics* 57:347-351, 1976.

37. Ratner I, Perelmuter B, Toews W, Whitfield J. Association of low systolic and diastolic blood pressure with significant patent ductus arteriosus in the very low birth weight infant. *Crit Care Med* 13:497-500, 1985.

38. Menser MA, Sydney MB, Reid RR, Dorman RC, Reye RDK. Renal-artery stenosis in the rubella syndrome. *Lancet* 1:790-792, 1966.

39. Bliddal J, DuPont B, Melchior JC, Ottesen, OE. Coarctation of the aorta with multiple artery anomalies in idiopathic hypercalcemia of infancy. *Acta Paediatr Scand* 58:632-637, 1969.

40. Carella JA, Silber I. Hyperreninemic hypertension in an infant secondary to pelviureteric obstruction treated successfully by surgery. *J Pediatr* 88:987-989, 1976.

41. Reimold EW, Don TD, Worthen HG. Renal failure during the first year of life. *Pediatrics* 59:987-994, 1977.

42. McCormick WF, Rosenfield DB. Massive brain hemorrhages: a review of 144 cases and an examination of their causes. *Stroke* 4:946-957, 1973.

43. Lou HC, Lassen NA, Friis-Hansen B. Is arterial hypertension crucial for the development of cerebral hemorrhage in premature infants? *Lancet* 1:1215-1217, 1979.

44. Thoele DG, Muster AJ, Paul MH. Recognition of coarctation of the aorta. *Am J Dis Child* 141:1201-1204, 1987.

45. Lees BJ, Cabal LA. Increased blood pressure following pupillary dilation with 2.5% phenylephrine hydrochloride in preterm infants. *Pediatrics* 68:231-234, 1981.

46. Lucas A, Morley R, Hudson GJ, Bamford MF, Boon A, Crowle P, Dossetor JFB, Pearse R. Early sodium intake and later blood pressure in preterm infants. *Arch Dis Child* 63:656-657, 1988.

47. Boedy RF, Goldberg AK, Howell CG Jr, Hulse E, Edwards EG, Kanto WP Jr. Incidence of hypertension in infants on extracorporeal membrane oxygenation. *J Pediatr Surg* 25:258-261, 1990.

48. Sell LL, Cullen ML, Lerner GR, Whittlesey GC, Shanley CJ, Klein MD. Hypertension during extracorporeal membrane oxygenation: cause, effect, and management. *Surgery* 102:724-730, 1990.

49. Sheftel DN, Hustead V, Friedman A. Hypertension screening in the follow-up of premature infants. *Pediatrics* 71:763-766, 1983.
50. Colavita RD, Gaudio FM, Siegel NL. Reversible reduction in renal function during treatment with captopril. *Pediatrics* 71:839, 1983.
51. Kitterman JA, Phibbs RH, Tooley WH. Aortic blood pressure in normal newborn infants during the first 12 hours of life. *Pediatrics* 44:959-968, 1969.
52. Versmold HT, Kitterman JA, Phibbs RH, Gregory GA, Tooley WH. Aortic blood pressure during the first 12 hours of life in infants with birth weight 610 to 4220 grams. *Pediatrics* 67:607-613, 1981.
53. Shortland DB, Evans DH, Levene MI. Blood pressure measurements in very low birth weight infants the first week of life. *J Perinat Med* 16:93-97, 1988.
54. Cabal LA, Siassi B, Hodgman JE. Neonatal clinical cardiopulmonary monitoring. In: Fanaroff AA, Martin RJ, eds. *Neonatal-Perinatal Medicine: Diseases of the Fetus and Infant.* St. Louis: Mosby Year Book; 437-455:1992.
55. Lee YH, Rosner B, Gould JB, Loew EW, Kass EH. Familial aggregation of blood pressures of newborn infants and their mothers. *Pediatrics* 58:722-729, 1976.
56. DeSwiet M, Fayers P, Shinebourne EA. Systolic blood pressure in a population of infants in the first year of life: The Brompton study. *Pediatrics* 65:1028-1034, 1980.
57. Lagler E, Duc G. Systolic blood pressure in normal newborn infants during the first 6 hours of life: transcutaneous Doppler ultrasound technique. *Biol Neonate* 37:243-245, 1980.

Chapter 9

Clinical Features and Evaluation for Hypertension in the Young

Introduction

Most young people with hypertension will not have any symptoms until adulthood when their hypertension is far advanced. Therefore, it is with good reason that hypertension has been labeled the "silent disease." Indeed the challenge is to find risk factors so that those who are destined to become victims of persistent hypertension might be forewarned and appropriately treated. Because of this situation, health-care agencies have recommended that blood pressures be taken periodically. In the young, the United States Task Force advises that pressures be recorded yearly, beginning at age 3 years.[1] Thus, most hypertensives will simply be discovered on the basis of a casually obtained blood pressure.

In this chapter, the clinical features of persistent hypertension are presented with the realization that most often the only finding will be elevated blood pressure. Of course the higher the pressure the more likely it is that there will be associated symptoms. Also, with higher pressures, an underlying cause for the pressure elevation is more likely to become evident. Causes for hypertension vary by age, and workup for hypertension is therefore discussed by age groups. In pediatrics there does not seem to be much of a sex or racial difference in the incidence of hypertension. As can be seen, in most instances a minimal workup is all that is necessary. Some

209

of the information presented here is elaborated upon in other chapters, such as that on the newborn. In this chapter, an effort is made to bring together the findings of hypertension in the young.

Clinical Features

Primary Hypertension

It is now recognized that most persistent hypertension, even in childhood, is without known cause. With confession of etiologic ignorance, this form of hypertension has been labeled primary or essential hypertension. In reality, this disease category likely represents a number of different disorders, most remaining to be further elaborated upon. Fortunately, a majority of young people afflicted with primary hypertension do not have a severe elevation of blood pressure. Rather, they are at risk for later-life target organ damage from the pressure elevation. These young patients are believed by their family and friends to be completely healthy. Their hypertension is first suspected on the basis of a casual blood pressure measurement. It is then confirmed by several subsequent pressure measurements. When all are found to be elevated, the definition of hypertension is fulfilled. With few exceptions, the pressure elevation is at a level between the 95th and 99th percentile for age by the United States Task Force standards.[1] In other words, they have significant but mild to moderate hypertension. In contrast, those with secondary hypertension (see below) will usually have severe hypertension.

Generally, even on close questioning, young patients with primary hypertension are asymptomatic. Perhaps the infant will have increased fussiness. The child or adolescent may admit to a few headaches or fatigue, but these are common complaints and no more frequent in patients having high rather than normal blood pressures. Those with high pressures tend to be overweight and may have had epistaxis or a slight increase in heart rate. Their cardiac apex beat may be strong and peripheral pulses brisk. Third heart sounds are common. Again, these findings are not unusual. The examination of a child with primary hypertension most often is not different from the normotensive youngster, save for the pressure elevation. There are some age-specific considerations.

Newborns and Infants

Newborns and infants with primary hypertension are asymptomatic in most cases. In others, the infant may be irritable, have feeding problems, and grow slowly. Those failing to thrive should have their blood pressure measured; this perhaps will lead to the discovery of hypertension. All hospitalized infants should have their blood pressures taken, at least on admission, using the methodology described in Chapter 8. After the first month of life, blood pressures in excess of 112/74 mm Hg are cause for concern.[1] Admittedly the diagnostic yield of blood pressure measurement will be small, but it is in proportion to the time spent and may be rewarding in following clinical progress.

Toddlers and Children

Toddlers and children should have their blood pressures measured on a yearly basis, beginning at age 3. At most, 1% or 2% will be found to have persistent hypertension with pressures at or above 122/78 mm Hg in midchildhood.[1] Almost all will be asymptomatic save for the previously noted nonspecific findings.

Adolescents and Young Adults

Adolescents and young adults appear less often for routine evaluations. When they do, their blood pressure should be taken. Many will have pressures measured only on entry to high school or sports participation. While about 10% will have high blood pressure at the time of first measurement, at most only 1% or 2% will be found to have persistent significant hypertension (all pressures in excess of 136/86 mm Hg). These young people will ordinarily be asymptomatic. In a blood pressure survey of over 8000 high school ninth-graders in Pasadena, California, less than 1% had first systolic pressures over 150 and/or diastolic pressures over 98 mm Hg.[2] So it can be seen that those with elevated blood pressures on an initial measurement will likely have a mild to moderate pressure elevation. Severe pressure elevations are uncommon. Underlying disease was not evident in any of the Pasadena students with high blood pressure.

Secondary Hypertension

Secondary hypertension is uncommon, occurring in perhaps one in a thousand children. However, these young patients tend to have marked pressure elevation, i.e., over the 99th percentile.[1] They often have serious complaints. In these children, hypertension is not so much a disease but rather a finding complicating another disorder. Young people with symptomatic hypertension are likely to seek medical care in clinics or physicians' offices or even emergency rooms. They may be hospitalized for treatment of seizures or heart failure. Many of the diseases causing hypertension are listed in Table 1. As with primary hypertension, the clinical picture varies by age group.

Newborn and Infants (see also Chapter 8).

The distressed newborn monitored with umbilical arterial catheterization is at special risk for hypertension as are those requiring extracorporeal membrane oxygenation. They require special attention to rule out hypertension. Blood pressures are not taken routinely in infants after hospital discharge. However, certain clinical conditions may be the result of hypertension and suggest the need for pressure measurement (Table 2). Failure to thrive may herald other symptoms. Rarely unexplained seizures or respiratory difficulty leading to the diagnosis of heart failure may be found to result from hypertension. After the first week of life, babies with secondary hypertension usually have systolic blood pressures in excess of 110, and at 1 month, pressures over 118/82 mm Hg (see Table 2, Chapter 10).

Toddlers and Children

A number of renal conditions become manifest in childhood and together they are the most common cause for secondary hypertension in pediatric patients (Chapter 6). Renal disorder and the other less common diseases listed in Table 1, are the major considerations when a child is found to have severe hypertension. Children with these problems are commonly symptomatic with blood pressures in excess of 130/86 mm Hg.[1] Their difficulties may be acute or chronic.

Table 1.
Causes of Secondary Hypertension in Childhood[3–6]

Disease	Frequency		Primary Manifestations (with Severe Hypertension)
Renal	74%		(Chapter 6)
		% of Renal	
Acute renal disease		45	edema, hemat- proteinuria, creatinine $\leq$ 3X normal
Renal scarring		27	urinary reflux, bacturia
Chronic glomerular disease		19	failure to thrive, marked increased creatinine (Cr)
Hemolytic uremic syndrome		4	oligo/anuria, hemolytic anemia, DIC, increased Cr
Polycystic disease		2	flank mass, abnormal scans
Other renal		3	(Chapter 6)
		100%	
Coarctation (coarc) of Aorta	15		BP/pulses rt arm > leg, coarc by echocardiogram or aortogram (Chapter 5)
Renovascular disease	7		abd bruit, nl/incr PRA, abnl angiogram (Chapter 6)
Adrenal disorders	1		electrolyte disorders, sex $\pm$ weight changes (Chapter 7)
CNS disorders	1		+ neuro findings, abnl scan
Systemic disorders	1		failure to thrive, abnormal lab
Nonadrenal tumors	1		mass, wt loss, abnormal scans
	100%		

They may complain of severe morning headaches, usually occipital, perhaps associated with visual disturbances. They may be edematous or have respiratory difficulty. Others may have neurologic symptoms such as dizziness or even seizures. Not all patients, however, have overt symptoms. A few may be discovered on the basis of a routine examination, for example, patients who have undiagnosed coarctation of the aorta, with previously undetected absent femoral pulses.

Adolescents and Young Adults

Secondary hypertension is far less common in this age group than in younger patients. Many of the disorders listed in Table 1 are considerations in the etiology of hypertension in adolescents.

Table 2.
Clinical Findings which may Indicate the Presence of Hypertension
in the Infant or Child[1,20]

Finding	Suspected Disorder
Abdominal masses or murmurs	Wilms' tumor or neuroblastoma renal artery stenosis
Weak distal pulses	Coarctation of the aorta
Heart murmur	Patent ductus arteriosus ± coarctation of aorta
Gonadal hypertrophy/dysgenesis	Adrenal hyperplasia Turner's syndrome
Salt loss/electrolyte imbalance	Adrenal disorders
Burns/large fractures	Secondary hypercalcemia from bone demineralization
Failure to thrive	Primary or secondary renal disorders
Neurofibromatosis	Renal artery stenosis
History of umbilical artery catheterization	Renal artery thrombosis
Orbital tumor	Neuroblastoma
Steroid therapy	Cushing's syndrome
Unexplained heart failure	Hypertensive cardiomyopathy
Unexplained seizures	Hypertensive encephalopathy

With severe hypertension, the blood pressure is over 144/92 mm Hg.[1] Some will be obese. A number will have end-stage renal disease perhaps with cardiac manifestations. A few of the females will be on oral contraceptives. Other patients will be taking medications or drugs which can elevate blood pressure. Trauma and orthopedic hypertension related to bone demineralization during immobilization are also problems in this age group.

Evaluation

Once hypertension is discovered, workup is required to rule out specific causes of the disorder. With severe resting pressure elevation, for example, greater than or equal to 160 mm Hg systolic and/or greater than or equal to 100 mm Hg diastolic in an older child or adolescent, a specific etiology is likely. In such situations, a diligent search should be made for a cause of the hypertension. Most important is a good history (Appendix) and physical examination. The differential diagnosis includes the entities listed in Tables 1 and 2. On the other hand, most young people will have a mild to moderate pressure elevation only. Their workups generally should be kept to a minimum, first considering the conditions listed in Table 3.[3-6] Since etiology of hypertension varies by age, workups should be focused on the main age groups, carefully considering the above mentioned information.

History (Appendix)

The duration of the hypertension is a primary consideration. Initial onset and treatment set the stage for further evaluation. The goal is to obtain maximal historical information so that minimal testing will be required. In symptomatic patients, the presence of acute disease, especially renal disorders and/or infections, will narrow the diagnostic possibilities. Some patients may have a history of treatment for previous renal or other disease likely to be associated with hypertension.

As stated, most pediatric patients with hypertension are asymptomatic. When symptoms are elicited in the history of a hypertensive patient, the majority are nonspecific. Nevertheless, probing can add diagnostic clues. For example, headaches occur with many problems such as stress, infection, or migraine. When the headaches are

Table 3.
Estimated Age-Related Hypertension Causes[2-6,13,17]

Age Group	Neonate	Infant	Toddler	Child	Adolescent	Young Adult
CONDITION	%	%	%	%	%	%
Congenital (incl coarc)	14	10	5	3	<1.0	<0.1
Renovascular (incl thrombosis)	50	30	5	2	1	<0.4
Renal parenchymal disease	1	20	30	25	6	<4.0
Primary hypertension	15	30	50	65	91	95
Other	20*	10	10	5	2	1
	100	100	100	100	100	100

*incl central nervous system

frequent and occipital in location, their association with blood pressure elevation warrants a hypertensive workup. The same is true for a history of swelling or edema in the presence of hypertension. In a small number of cases, certain groups of symptoms will suggest specific disorders. Most common are symptoms referable to the urinary tract which include hematuria, dysuria, fevers, frequency, and/or edema. Pheochromocytoma is a consideration with complaints of palpitations and excessive perspiration, particularly if episodic, along with unexplained fever and nondietary weight loss. Muscle cramps and weakness with constipation are found in hyperaldosteronism. Altered menarche may suggest adrenal malfunction.

Dietary history is of concern to evaluate failure to thrive on the one hand and obesity on the other. Food frequencies at meals and snacks should be assessed. While excess electrolyte ingestion seldom is implicated in pediatric hypertension, inquiry into dietary cation intake, may provide diagnostic clues in a few instances. Inquiry should also be made into medication usage. Teenage girls should be asked if they use contraceptive pills. Likewise, while questions about smoking and alcohol consumption do not furnish direct etiologic information for hypertension in young people, they may point at other causes like substance abuse.

In all age groups, careful inquiry should be made into the family history. This includes grandparents, uncles, and aunts as well as the nuclear family. Not only is it important to note whether hypertension exists in family members but also at what age it was found and with what degree of severity. Then inquiry should be made as to whether specific treatment was needed. In this manner the importance of a blood pressure elevation can be assessed and a likely course predicted for those with primary hypertension. The same type of questioning should be carried out for other cardiovascular diseases in family members. Information should also be sought concerning a family history of tumors, renal disease, and maternal toxemia, as each has been related to a propensity for hypertensive disorders.

A painstaking history is required to elicit the information described. Yet when everything is considered, most inquiries will be negative. That is, no causal clues will be found for the hypertension. But for the small number of positives, the questioning can lead to life-saving measures. To aid in this activity a self history is presented in an Appendix at the end of this chapter. Use of this questionnaire may save hours of time and quickly lead to a working diagnosis.

Physical Examination

In the examination of the hypertensive patient, it is stressed that blood pressure in both upper and at least one lower limb must be carefully taken according to the principles outlined in Chapter 2.

Inspection in most instances will reveal either a completely normal appearance or obesity. In those with generalized obesity, primary hypertension is likely. An occasional patient will have pallor with edema suggestive of renal disease. Pallor with excessive perspiration, on the other hand, especially if associated with flushing, suggests pheochromocytoma. Others with renal disease may simply have failure to thrive or evidence of weight loss. A small number of rare pediatric disorders have a characteristic appearance. In Cushing's syndrome, moon facies, obesity confined to the trunk with a buffalo hump, and striae are found. Williams and Turner's syndromes are distinguished by elfin facies in the former and short stature, web neck with low posterior hair line and prominent epicanthal folds in the latter. Patients with these syndromes often have developmental delay. Hypertension in Turner's syndrome is from coarctation of the aorta, while patients with William's syndrome have renal arterial narrowing. Another uncommon disorder with renal artery stenosis is von Recklinghausen's disease. It is marked by cafe-au-lait spots and neurofibromas. Assessment of sexual development may reveal a rare endocrinopathy.

Evidence of unilateral mouth droop and failure of eyelid closure of Bell's palsy or a stroke are other rare findings in hypertension.

Inspection of the optic fundi seldom reveals abnormalities. Nevertheless, it is one of the few ways to assess end organ damage of hypertension and should be carried out on all patients with severe hypertension. An occasional child will have arterial "silver wire" spasm (grade 1) or even arteriovenous nicking (grade 2 changes). Fundal hemorrhages (grade 3) and papilledema (grade 4) are rare.

Palpation may reveal an enlarged thyroid, but thyroid disease is an uncommon cause of hypertension in the pediatric age group. Prominent arterial pulsations are common, but are nonspecific unless confined to one or both upper limbs; then coarctation of the aorta must be considered. Likewise, absent femoral pulses usually signal coarctation. A forceful cardiac apex beat is another nonspecific finding. With leftward displacement, it may indicate cardiac enlargement in the few with end-organ impact of hypertension. A search for abdominal masses, especially in the flank regions, may reveal renal cysts or tumors. Other abdominal tumors such as Wilms' tumor in early childhood or neuroblastoma may cause hypertension but are rare.

Auscultation over the heart may reveal a basal heart murmur. This finding should lead to the consideration of coarctation of the aorta, or possibly patent ductus arteriosus, which may be associated with hypertension in the newborn. Murmurs of both conditions must be differentiated from commonly heard normal murmurs. Third heart sounds may signal ventricular hypertrophy, but are often heard in normal young people. Abdominal auscultation is required to aid in the diagnosis of renal artery stenosis. It must be recognized that only about a third of the cases will have murmurs. Rarely, an abdominal coarctation will cause a murmur in the abdomen. Auscultation over the carotid arteries has been advocated to detect arterial disorders. However, it must be recalled that benign carotid bruits are far more frequent in young people than is arterial disease. In young people, such ausculation may do more harm than good.

A neurologic examination is important to evaluate for signs of a previous stroke, which may be manifested by hemiparesis. On extraordinary occasions facial paralysis may be found.

Laboratory Studies

Once the initial history and physical examination have been completed with confirmation of the diagnosis of hypertension, patients can be separated into two groups. Group 1 consists of patients likely to have primary hypertension on the basis of being asymptomatic, having blood pressure elevation below the 99th percentile, and no abnormalities found on examination. The vast majority of pediatric hypertensives will fit into this category (Table 3). Group 2 encompasses those likely to have secondary hypertension. In this category, the young will have blood pressures over the 99th percentile and/or symptoms and/or significant findings on the examination. Relatively few pediatric patients with hypertension will be found in this group. Both groups of patients should undergo a basic laboratory workup. For group 1 no further testing is indicated unless the basic laboratory investigation reveals some abnormality. In group 2, the basic laboratory tests will tend to confirm or point to another etiologic diagnosis requiring additional laboratory workup.

In some, the level of hypertension will have decreased by the time of referral or follow-up. If the history and/or physical examination findings are suggestive of a recurrent problem, ambulatory blood pressure measurements may be indicated. Likewise, if the blood pressure is repeatedly found to be elevated, but the history and examination are unrevealing, "white coat" hypertension may be present. In the latter situation, ambulatory blood pressure monitoring is also useful in distinguishing truly persistent hypertension.

Basic tests which should be done on all pediatric patients undergoing evaluation for hypertension include a sedimentation rate, hematocrit, hemoglobin, urinalysis, and blood chemistry panel with electrolytes (sodium, potassium, chloride, carbon dioxide content), creatinine, and uric acid. In addition, group 2 patients should have an echocardiogram for determination of left ventricular (LV) mass, as well as coarctation of the aorta if that is suspected. Left ventricular mass is another measure of end-organ effect of hypertension and marks the effect of persistent blood pressure elevation. It is usually increased with severe hypertension and thus tends to verify the impression of severe secondary hypertension. Additionally, group 2 females with unexplained hypertension or suspected renal disease should have a urine culture.

In all likelihood the advocated basic tests will be normal. In those with blood pressures below the 99th percentile, no further testing is needed, although it is important to keep under observation patients having risk factors for future hypertension. If high-normal or mild to moderate hypertension persists over time, it may be worthwhile to consider performing some of the stress tests described in Chapter 4 on risk.

The experience on which this approach is based goes back to that reported by Londe and coworkers.[7] They performed extensive testing in a clinical research center on 41 asymptomatic, persistently hypertensive children with completely negative results. Others have had similar experiences. Levine and colleagues failed to find positive laboratory findings or an explanation for blood pressure elevation in 28 hypertensive high school students identified in a 1975 New York City screening program.[8] In a similar manner, we evaluated 80 black teenage students whose blood pressure values were in the upper half for all Pasadena high school ninth grade students' pressures.[9] In all 80 students, extensive biochemical testing failed to reveal a cause for upper level pressures.

Should the minimal outlined workup fail to reveal a curable

form of hypertension when one actually exists, there is little danger of harm.[10] The treatment advised for a diagnosis of primary hypertension, when in fact secondary hypertension exists, will control the disorder. In time, the actual diagnosis will become evident. On the other hand, when an expansive workup is launched, there is always a possibility of false-positive findings. These, may lead to further testing which might place the patient in some degree of jeopardy. For example, if indications for renal arteriography are equivocal, performance of the test would subject the patient to a small but definite risk. Additionally, patient discomfort and cost are considerations. Simply following a patient over time could make it possible to avoid the arteriography altogether. In other words, treatment of hypertension does not necessarily await a completed workup. Once blood pressure is controlled, patients can be followed safely and evaluated further if necessary.

More diagnostic laboratory tests are needed in only a few hypertensive pediatric patients. By and large these are group 2 individuals in whom the etiology of the hypertension is not clear, or extent of disease causing hypertension is unknown. Plasma-renin determinations (PRA) may provide etiologic clues and are obtained mainly in those with severe unexplained hypertension. Peripheral vein PRA values may be suggestive of renal disease if they are high. On the other hand, if the value is low, aldosteronism may be a consideration.

Plasma-renin value per 24-hour sodium excretion (renin-sodium profile) expresses renin activity as a function of sodium intake (mirrored by excretion). Negative sodium balance stimulates renin production whereas positive sodium balance results in decreased renin production. Renin-sodium profile has been used to distinguish adults with high profile values. These patients have vasoconstricted hypertension and reduced cardiac output. In contrast, those with low profile values have less vasoconstriction and have elevated plasma volume and cardiac output.[11] The 24-hour urinalysis required for the profile determination also has some fallout benefits. In the same process, urinary protein is quantified for assessment of renal damage (if any), and quantified electrolyte excretion may aid in the diagnosis of an endocrinopathy. These determinations are not commonly performed in children, for little relationship between renin-sodium profile and casual blood pressure determination has been found. More recently, renin-sodium profiles have been linked to differences in ambulatory blood pressures in young people.[12]

Those with high profile values (perhaps vasoconstricted) had larger awake-sleep systolic pressure differences as well as higher and a more variable sleeping diastolic pressure. Despite these findings, at present it is felt that the renin-sodium profile does not add materially to the diagnostic workup for pediatric hypertension and cannot be widely advocated.

Many sophisticated, rather specific, other tests are available to assess pediatric hypertension. The goal of such testing is to find a curable form of hypertension. The use of a further laboratory evaluation should be based on historical and/or physical findings and/or basic laboratory tests suggesting a particular disease entity. It is helpful to consider systematically the diagnoses listed in Table 1 when reviewing the results of the initial assessment. For example, coarctation of the aorta usually is apparent by arm-leg pulse and blood pressure differences. Echocardiography with color Doppler-flow mapping will confirm the diagnosis sufficiently well to permit relief by surgery or aortoplasty as described in Chapter 5.

When renal disease is suspected, appropriate laboratory investigation should be considered from the list in Table 4 as recommended in Chapter 6. Alternatively, when an endocrine disorder is a consideration, the hypertension workup should include the schemes presented in Chapter 7. Various tumors may cause hypertension. Short of a palpable mass, they may be difficult to discover, even with computer tomography or magnetic resonance imaging

Table 4.
Diagnostic Test Used to Assess Renal Disorders
(Details noted in Chapter 6)

Imaging Studies	Biochemical Studies
Excretory urogram	Urine sodium and chloride
Abdominal/renal ultrasound	Plasma renin activity
CT/MR scan of kidneys	Glomerular filtration rate
DMSA/DTPA scans	ACE inhibition test
Digital subtraction angiography	
Invasive Testing	
Voiding cystourethrogram	Renal vein renin sampling
Renal arteriography	

CT = computer tomography; MR = magnetic resonance; DMSA = di-mercaptosuccinic acid; DTPA = diethylenetriamine-penta-acetic acid; ACE = angiotensin-converting enzyme.

scans. In these instances, biochemical testing (Chapter 7) may provide the needed clues.

Finally, there may be an individual in whom no apparent etiology for the hypertension can be discovered. If the hypertension is severe, segmental renovascular disease must be ruled out prior to labeling the patient as having primary hypertension.[13] The scheme outlined in Figure 3, Chapter 6, may be helpful for this purpose.

The question arises as to who is best suited to perform the workup for the pediatric patient casually discovered to have sustained hypertension. It is the opinion of this author that those furnishing primary pediatric care should provide an initial thorough evaluation by history and physical examination. Then the basic laboratory tests should be obtained, after which the same practitioner is in a position to treat most children with the disorder. However, if the hypertension is at a level above the 99th percentile and the etiology is unclear, an early referral to a specialist in pediatric hypertension is indicated. Referral is also indicated for evaluation and initial treatment if a more rare form of hypertension is suspected.

Summary

Most often, the features of the young hypertensive patient are nonspecific. The infant may fail to thrive, the child and adolescent may complain of headaches, and commonly the latter are obese. Yet, all will have repeatedly elevated blood pressures on examination. Blood pressure elevation discovered on an incidental pressure recording is how most hypertension is discovered in the pediatric age group. Evaluations of young patients are largely dependent on a thorough history and physical examination. Blood pressures must be carefully determined in at least three limbs. Most patients evaluated because of high blood pressure will have primary hypertension. Their pressures tend to be mildly to moderately elevated. They may have a positive family history of hypertension. In certain instances, findings will point to a cause of (secondary) hypertension. For instance, there may be a history of a renal disorder. In others, characteristic weak or absent femoral pulses may indicate coarctation of the aorta. In rare cases, central obesity with "buffalo hump" and striae may suggest Cushing's syndrome.

A basic set of laboratory tests including urinalysis, sedimentation rate, hemoglobin, hematocrit, and blood chemistry panel are recommended for all persistently hypertensive patients. The degree of pressure elevation as compared to standards set by the United States Task Force on hypertension[1] will point to the need for more elaborate testing. Patients with pressures above the 99th percentile should have an echocardiogram to assess the severity of their disease. Additional sophisticated bacteriologic, biochemical, and/or imaging studies will assist in the discovery of renal, vascular, endocrine, or other potentially curable causes of the hypertension. For this purpose, the diagnoses listed by frequency in Table 1 may be helpful.

Cost containment in terms of patient time, physician effort, and fiscal need should be considered. Most patients will need minimal workup prior to application of treatment measures (Chapter 10). They can and should be treated by their primary health-care person or resource. Only those with uncommon or serious disorders require prompt specialty consultation/treatment.

References

1. National Heart Lung and Blood Institute Task Force on Blood Pressure Control in Children: Report of the second task force on blood pressure control in children. *Pediatrics* 79:1-25, 1987.
2. Hohn AR. The Pasadena study. Unpublished data, 1992.
3. Leumann CP. Blood pressure and hypertension in childhood and adolescence. *Ergenbnisse der inneren Medizin und Kinderheilkunde* 43:111-183, 1979.
4. Dillon MJ. Hypertension. In: Postlethwaite RJ, ed. *Clinical Paediatric Nephrology*. Bristol: Wright; 1-25:1986.
5. Broyer M, Bacre JL, Royer P. Renal forms of hypertension in children: report on 238 cases. In: Giovannelli G, New MI, Gorini S, eds. *Hypertension in Children and Adolescents*. New York: Raven Press; 1981.
6. Lieberman E. Clinical assessment of the hypertensive patient. In: Kotchen TA, Kotchen JM, eds. *Clinical Approaches to High Blood Pressure in the Young*. Boston: John Wright; 237- 248:1983.
7. Londe S, Bourgoignie JJ, Robson AM, Goldring D. Hypertension in apparently normal children. *J Pediatr* 78:569-577, 1971.
8. Levine LS, Lewy JE, New MI. Hypertension in high school students: evaluation in New York City. *NY State J Med* 76:40-44, 1976.
9. Dwyer JH, Dwyer KM, Scribner RA, Hohn AR. Effect of calcium supplementation on blood pressure in African American youth. *33rd Annual Conference on Cardiovascular Disease Epidemiology*. Santa Fe, 1993. Abstract.
10. Kaplan NM. Argument for a minimal evaluation of the hypertensive

patient. In: Buhler FR, Laragh JH, eds. *The Management of Hypertension: Handbook of Hypertension.* 13:145- 153, 1990.

11. Laragh JH, Sealey JE, Niarchos AP, Pickering TG. The vasoconstriction-volume spectrum in normotension and pathogenesis of hypertension. *Fed Proc* 41:2415-2423, 1982.

12. Harshfield GA, Pulliam DA, Alpert BS, Stapleton FB, Willey ES, Grant WS. Ambulatory blood pressure patterns in children and adolescents: influence of renin-sodium profiles. *Pediatrics* 87:94-100, 1991.

13. Deal JE, Snell MF, Barratt TM, Dillon MJ. Renovascular disease in childhood. *J Pediatr* 121:378-384, 1992.

14. Adelman RD. Neonatal hypertension. In: Loggie JMH, Horan MJ, Gruskin AB, Hohn AR, Dunbar JB, Havlik RJ. *NHLBI Workshop in Juvenile Hypertension.* New York: Biomed Information Corp; 267-282:1984.

15. Rudnick KV, Sackett DL, Hirst S, Holmes C. Hypertension in a family practice. *Can Med Assoc J* 117:492-497, 1977.

16. Danielsson M, Dammstrom BG. The prevalence of secondary and curable hypertension. *Acta Med Scand* 209:451-455, 1981.

17. Sigurdsson JA, Bengtsson C, Tibblin E, Wojciechowski J. Prevalence of secondary hypertension in a population sample of Swedish women. *Eur Heart J* 4:424-433, 1983.

18. Lewin A, Blaufox D, Castle H, Entvisle G, Langford H. Apparent prevalence of curable hypertension in the Hypertension, Detection and Followup Program. *Arch Intern Med* 145:424-427, 1985.

19. Sinclair AM, Isles CG, Brown I, Cameron H, Murray GD, Robertson JWK. Secondary hypertension in a blood pressure clinic. *Arch Intern Med* 147:1289-1293, 1989.

20. Loggie JMH. Evaluation of the hypertensive child and adolescent. In: Loggie JMH, ed. *Pediatric and Adolescent Hypertension.* Boston: Blackwell Scientific Pub; 112-118:1992.

APPENDIX

Self History for Evaluation of Hypertension

(To be completed by parent or primary caregiver or involved young person if mature enough)

High Blood Pressure Preevaluation Questionnaire

To parent (or patient):

Please complete the applicable parts of this form as much as possible. This information will help us in our evaluation of your child (or yourself) for a possible problem with high blood pressure.

Child's (patient's) name: _____

Birth date:_____ /_____ /_____Current age_____ yrs. (mons.)

Person completing this form: Mother (_) Father (_) Other, specify:

Why has your child been brought in for this evaluation? _____

Name and address of referring health care provider (if any): _____

Have you ever been previously told that your child has high blood pressure?
    yes (_) no (_)

Does your child have a kidney problem? yes (_) no (_)

Has your child had any special tests for high blood pressure?
    yes (_) no (_)
If yes, where and when? _____

Is your child taking any medicine? yes (_) No (_) If yes, please specify the medication and its dose: _____

I. PREGNANCY (Complete only if patient less than 7 years old):

A. Are you this child's natural mother? yes (_) no (_). if not, relation
B. Mother's age at time of pregnancy:____ years.
    Length of the pregnancy:__months.
C. Did the natural mother have high blood pressure during the pregnancy? yes (_) no (_).

D. Did the natural mother require any medications during the pregnancy? yes (__) no (__). If yes, list the medications taken and the reason why they were taken, include any vitamins and iron: _____

E. Was the natural mother X-rayed before or during the pregnancy? yes (__) no (__)

F. Did the mother have flu during the pregnancy? yes (__) no (__).

G. Did the mother have any other infection during the pregnancy? yes (__) no (__). If yes what kind?_____

H. Were there any special or difficult problems during the pregnancy? yes (__) no (__). If yes, what? _____
_____
_____

II. DELIVERY PERIOD (Complete if patient less than 7 years old):

A. How long was the labor?_____hours.

B. What kind of delivery was this? Vaginal (__) C-Section (__).

C. If C-Section was done, what was the reason? _____

D. What was the baby's birth weight?_____/_____ pounds/ounces.

E. Was this child normal at birth? yes (__) no (__).

F. If not, did this child have breathing problems after birth? yes (__) no (__). If yes, please describe: _____

G. Were there any birth injuries or problems in the delivery room? yes (__) no (__). If yes, please describe: _____

III. NEWBORN TO INFANCY PERIOD (Complete if patient under 7 years):

A. Was this baby kept in an incubator? yes (__) no (__). If yes, how long?___days. What was the reason? _____

B. Were any abnormalities of the baby noted in the newborn nursery? yes (__) no (__). If yes, please describe: _____

C. Did the baby have a catheter (tube) inserted into the umbilical vein or artery? yes (__) no (__).

D. Was the baby's blood pressure monitored or taken in the newborn period? yes (__) no (__).

E. Did the baby have high blood pressure? yes (__) no (__).

F. Was her/his color bluish? yes (__) no (__); or yellow (jaundice) in the newborn nursery? yes (__) no (__).

G. Did the baby have blood exchange transfusions? yes (__) no (__) If yes, how many?_____.

H. Was the baby on ECMO (extra corporeal membrane oxgenation)? yes (__) no (__).

I. Were you told of any feeding problem? yes (__) no (__).

J. Is/was the baby breast fed? yes (__) no (__). If yes, were you taking any medicine during the period you were breast feeding? yes (__) no (__). If yes, type/dose _____

K. If your child is less than 2 years old, please answer the following:
1. Does she/he still take bottle feedings? yes (__) no (__).
2. If yes, what formula are you using?_____
3. How many bottles are fed each day? _____
4. How many ounces are taken in each feeding?_____ounces.
5. How long does it take to feed one bottle?_____minutes.
6. How much spitting up is there? _____

IV. DEVELOPMENT:

A. At what age did your child:
Sit alone?____months.
Walk?____months.
Talk?____months.
2. Toilet training:
Dry by day___years.
Dry by night___years.
Bowel trained___years.

B. What grade is she/he in at school?_____grade.

C. Has she/he ever failed to be promoted in school? yes (__) no (__). If yes, please describe. _____

D. Does the child attend special classes or a special school? yes (__) no (__).

E. Are there any particular problems in school? yes (__) no (__). If yes, please describe: _____

F. Does the child play any sports? yes (__) no (__). If yes, please name: _____

G. How does this child compare to brothers/sisters and other children? same (__) different (__). If different, please describe:_____

H. Does this child have behavior problems? yes (__) no (__). If yes, please describe: _____
_____
_____

V. OTHER PREGNANCIES:

A. Did the natural mother have any other pregnancies? yes (__) no (__) not known (__). If yes, how many?_____.

B. Number of living children:__. Ages of living children_____
_____

C. Has the mother ever miscarried? yes (__) no (__). If yes, how many times?____. Please list the cause(s) _____
_____

VI. FAMILY HISTORY:

A. Mother's age____years. Father's age____years.
B. Mother's health: good (_) If not, explain: _____
   _____
   Smoke? no (_) yes (_) ____packs per day.
   Blood pressure normal? yes (_) no (_). If no, taking any blood pressure
   medicine? no (_) yes (_) type/dose: _____

C. Father's health: good (_) If not, explain: _____
   _____
   Smoke? no (_) yes (_) ____packs per day.
   Blood pressure normal? yes ( ) no ( ). If no, taking any blood pressure
   medicine? no (_) yes (_) type/dose: _____

D. Mother's mother alive and well? yes (_) no (_) explain _____
   _____
   Was/is blood pressure normal? yes (_) no (_) took (takes) medicine for
   blood pressure control? yes (_) no (_).
E. Mother's father alive and well? yes (_) no (_) explain _____
   _____
   Was/is blood pressure normal? yes (_) no (_) took (takes) medicine for
   blood pressure control? yes (_) no (_).
F. Father's mother alive and well? yes (_) no (_) explain _____
   _____
   Was/is blood pressure normal? yes (_) no (_) took (takes) medicine
   for blood pressure control? yes (_) no (_).
G. Father's father alive and well? yes (_) no (_) explain _____
   _____
   Was/is blood pressure normal? yes (_) no (_) took (takes) medicine
   for blood pressure control? yes (_) no (_).
H. Other relatives with high blood pressure? yes (_) no (_)
   alive and well? yes (_) no (_) list relative(s)_____
   _____
   took (takes) medicine for blood pressure control? yes (_) no (_)
   don't know (_).
I. Are there any health problems in brothers or sisters? no (_) yes (_)
   type and age _____
J. Other health problems in relatives (name):
   1. Birth defects (cleft lip/palate, clubfoot, heart defect etc.)_____
   _____
   2. Down syndrome _____
   3. Heart murmur _____
   4. Heart attack _____
   5. Stroke _____
   6. Rheumatoid disease _____
   7. Lupus_____
   8. Cancer_____
   9. Diabetes _____

    10. Thyroid or gland disease_____

    11. Mental illness _____

    12. Migraine headaches_____

    13. Tuberculosis_____

    14. Allergies (including asthma, hay fever, eczema etc.)_____

K. Do any other illnesses run in the family? no (__) yes (__)
    If yes, specify _____

L. Have any of the children in the family died? no (__) yes (__)
    If yes, cause _____

M. Have any relatives died prior to age 50 years? no (__) yes (__)
    If yes, cause _____

VII. SOCIAL HISTORY:

A. Parents' present marital status? married (__) divorced (__)
    never married (__)

B. Are there any financial concerns? no (__) yes (__)
    If yes, describe _____

C. Are there transportation problems? no (__) yes (__)

D. Who is this child's primary caretaker? mother (__) father (__) other (__)
    who is _____

VIII. PAST MEDICAL AND SURGICAL HISTORY

A. Has this child ever been hospitalized? no (__) yes (__) If yes, when and
    why? _____

B. Has this child ever had any operations? no (__) yes (__) If yes, what
    kind, when and where _____
    Any problems or complications from surgery no (__) yes (__) If yes,
    explain: _____

C. Does this child have any allergies? no (__) yes (__) type _____

D. Indicate if this child had any of the following by checking box:
    1. Strep throat (__)
    2. Scarlet fever (__)
    3. Impetigo (infected skin rash) (__)
    4. Mumps (__)
    5. Chicken pox (__)
    6. Measles (10 day) (__)
    7. German measles (3 day) (__)
    8. Rheumatic fever (__)
    9. Diabetes (__)
    10. Other illness (specify) _____

E. Has this child had the following immunizations (check box):
    1. DPT (diphtheria-pertussis-tetanus) series (__)
    2. Polio series (__)

3. MMR (measles-mumps-rubella) (__)
4. Hepatitis (__)
F. Is this child's vision normal? yes (__) no (__) If no, describe _____

G. How many colds does this child get each year?_____
H. How many ear infections each year_____

IX DIET HISTORY (Please check foods eaten and how often they are eaten):

	Daily	2–3 X/week	Weekly	Monthly	Rarely
Fresh/frozen					
Beef any cut	__	__	__	__	__
Pork or Ham	__	__	__	__	__
Chicken/Turkey	__	__	__	__	__
Fish	__	__	__	__	__
Eggs	__	__	__	__	__
Shellfish	__	__	__	__	__
Vegetables	__	__	__	__	__
Fruits	__	__	__	__	__
Prepared foods					
Canned soups/meats	__	__	__	__	__
Canned vegetables	__	__	__	__	__
Pizza	__	__	__	__	__
Spaghetti/pasta	__	__	__	__	__
Chips/nuts	__	__	__	__	__
Soft drinks	__	__	__	__	__
Fried foods					
Potatoes	__	__	__	__	__
French fries	__	__	__	__	__
Hamburgers/hotdogs	__	__	__	__	__
Food from grains					
Cereal	__	__	__	__	__
Bread	__	__	__	__	__
Cake/pie etc.	__	__	__	__	__
Dairy products					
Whole milk	__	__	__	__	__
Lowfat milk	__	__	__	__	__
Butter	__	__	__	__	__
Ice cream/shakes	__	__	__	__	__
Yogurt	__	__	__	__	__
Dairy substitutes					
Margarine	__	__	__	__	__
Mayonnaise/salad dressing	__	__	__	__	__
Other snacks					
Chocolate	__	__	__	__	__
Candy	__	__	__	__	__
Any not mentioned	__	__	__	__	__

X SYSTEM REVIEW:

Check if this child has any of the following:
1. Headaches (__)

2. Dizziness or fainting (__)
3. Seizures or convulsions (__)
4. Nose bleeds (__)
5. Hearing problem (__)
6. Trouble breathing or breathing fast (__)
7. Frequent colds or respiratory infections (__)
8. Chronic cough (__) snoring at night (__)
9. Tires more easily than friends (__)
10. Blueness (__)
11. Chest pain or palpitations (__)
12. Constipation (__)
13. Fevers (__)
14. Burning or pain on urination (__)
15. Passes urine frequently (__)
16. Joint pain or swelling (__)
17. Muscle weakness (__)
18. Skin rashes (__)
19. Excessive sweating (__)
20. Weight loss (__)
21. Obesity/excess weight gain (__)
22. Bleeding tendency (__)
23. Consume licorice (__) alcohol (__) excess salt (__)
24. Take steroids (__) oral contraceptives (__)
25. Other problem(s) (__) If checked, explain: _____

XI. RACIAL IDENTIFICATION (High blood pressure is more common in some racial groups)

A. With what race do you identify this child? Asian (__) Black (__)
    Hispanic (__) Native American (__) Non Hispanic White (__)
    Mixed (parents of different races) (__) Other (__) list:_____
B. If Asian check: Chinese (__) Filipino (__) Japanese (__)
    Other (__) list: _____

This is the conclusion of the history form. Thank you for answering all the applicable questions for which you have information.

Chapter 10

Treatment of Pediatric Hypertension

Introduction

By now it has become clear that the disorders considered under the label of hypertension actually are a number of diseases, some known, and others awaiting discovery. In reality, as already mentioned, hypertension is a physical finding. Because, in most cases the etiology is unknown, hypertension is commonly thought of as a disease itself. Treatment in these cases therefore is symptomatic. That is, therapy is aimed at blood pressure control.

Although treatment of certain forms of pediatric hypertension has been mentioned in foregoing chapters, a summary of the problems facing those who would treat hypertension and an overall approach to therapy is believed warranted in this chapter. Since most young people suffering from hypertension will not have a specific etiology attached to their disorder, it is necessary to decide whether it is beneficial to attempt blood pressure control. Both nonpharmacologic and, if necessary, pharmacologic means are available for this purpose. These modalities will be presented and elaborated upon in this chapter. At the same time, it is believed that hypertensive disorders have their beginnings in the pediatric age range. It is intriguing to consider whether or not at least some forms of hypertension can be prevented or delayed in their expression. Early intervention, preferably nonpharmacologic, in those predisposed to develop high blood pressure might afford at least some control of the disorder.

233

Prevention (A Hope!)

Medical care of pediatric patients, by nature, involves an orientation for maintaining wellness. Public and private infant and child health programs are provided to immunize the young against an array of potentially disabling diseases. These programs also prevent, detect, and treat other threatening conditions, such as hypertension. Despite its beginning in early life, relatively little in the way of preventive programs is available for hypertension. The interested practitioner is left with dispensing general nutritional advice. Animal models exist for hypertension prevention.[1,2] Unhappily, the results are not transposable to children. The problem is that, unless overt symptoms present themselves, it is difficult or nearly impossible to diagnose patients during early life who are destined to become hypertensive. However, there are some diagnostic clues and there are some therapeutic generalizations. These, in some subgroups, may lead in the direction of prevention or delay of onset of hypertension. It is helpful to recognize the risk factors for hypertension (see Chapter 4).

While it is recommended that blood pressures be taken on a yearly basis from age 3 onward,[3] perhaps a more realistic start for recording blood pressure would perhaps be at school age. Little would be lost by the 2-year delay in asymptomatic individuals. Should high blood pressure be discovered, patients can be placed under observation and/or managed according to a modified task force scheme (Fig. 1). When yearly blood pressures are obtained they should be plotted on the task force grids and the tracking observed (maintenance of rank or percentile order over time). High trackers (in the top one fourth of normal pressures for age) and upward trackers (higher blood pressure rankings over years) may be at increased risk. These individuals could benefit from counseling and closer follow-up.

Those with a family history of hypertension, particularly when more than one member has the disorder, must be considered at risk and observed accordingly. A family history of hypertension in young blacks is a strong risk factor.[4] It may be of benefit to these people to emphasize a diet rich in potassium and calcium. Those who show evidence of obesity need appropriate counseling and treatment. Patients with diabetes mellitus present a special concern and warrant careful blood pressure monitoring.[5] Promotion of healthy

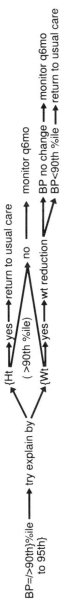
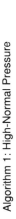

Algorithm 1: High-Normal Pressure

BP=/>90th}%ile ⟶ try explain by {Ht ⟶ yes ⟶ return to usual care
to 95th}   (>90th %ile)
                                 ⟶ no ⟶ monitor q6mo
                                {Wt ⟶ yes ⟶ wt reduction ⟶ BP no change ⟶ monitor q6mo
                                                            ⟶ BP<90th %ile ⟶ return to usual care

Algorithm 2: Significant Hypertension

BP > 95th to =/<99th %ile ⟶ obese ⟶ yes ⟶ wt reduction ⟶ BP =/<95th %ile ⟶ yes ⟶ monitor q6mo till BP < 90 %ile
                                                                            ⟶ no ⟶ Basic workup* ⟶ Nonpharm Rx
                            ⟶ no ⟶ Basic workup* ⟶ BP =/<95th %ile ⟶ yes ⟶ monitor q6mo
                                                                      ⟶ no ⟶ Nonpharm Rx

•Basic workup assumed negative if positive follow leads given•

Algorithm 3: Serious Hypertension without symptoms or proteinuria/left ventricular hypertrophy

BP > 99th %ile ⟶ Basic workup* ⟶ BP level reduced ⟶ yes =/>95th to 99 %ile ⟶ proceed as in Algorithm 2
                                                   ⟶ no ⟶ if DBP =/>12 or SBP > 25 mm Hg over 99th %ile begin medical Rx at once
                Diagnostic workup   if DBP <12 or SBP <25 mm Hg over 99th %ile begin nonpharm Rx
                Further Rx per outcome of workup

Algorithm 4: Serious hypertension with symptoms or with proteinuria/left ventricular hypertrophy

BP > 99th %ile ⟶ Begin Rx at once, when controlled workup beginning with basic tests

Basic workup* = urinalysis, sed rate, Hgb, Hct, bld chem with 'lytes (see Chapter 9)

Figure 1: Algorithms for workup/treatment of persistent BP = > 90th percentile (AV of 2 measures repeated on next two visits. These four algorithms are intended to guide the practitioner through the evaluation and treatment of four levels of blood pressure elevation: high normal pressure (90th to 95th percentile), significant hypertension (pressure in the 95th to 99th percentile), serious hypertension (pressure above the 99th percentile), and hypertensive emergencies (pressure above the 99th percentile with findings or symptoms). Pharmacologic therapy is used only if systolic or diastolic pressures are consistently above the 99th percentile at rest. A cause for hypertension should be vigorously sought in this group of patients, but all those with pressures above the 95th percentile should have the listed basic workup.

lifestyles, including exercise and stress control as well as avoidance of alcohol and smoking, is advocated for all, but especially for those at risk for hypertension (Table 1). Unfortunately, lifestyle recommendations may not be popular. A new attitude and motivation by society may be necessary.

Some promise to indicate that prevention of hypertension is feasible was shown in a 5-year trial involving 201 adult men and women with high normal blood pressures.[6] Lifestyle changes involving 5% reduction in overweight, reduction in sodium intake to 1800 mg daily, limitation of alcohol consumption to two drinks daily, and an increase in exercise were promoted in 102 subjects in the intervention group, but not in a control group. At the conclusion of the trial, the incidence of hypertension in the control group was 19.2% but only 8.8% in the intervention group. In addition, both workplace and office blood pressures were lower in the intervention group. A summary of these and other primary preventive measures for hypertension has recently been published.[7]

Making the Diagnosis

Meticulous attention to detail in blood pressure measurement, as outlined in Chapter 2, is vital to avoid falsely stigmatizing a young individual as hypertensive. Home pressure recording and ambulatory blood pressure monitoring show promise to avoid false diagnoses. Unfortunately, at the present time, neither home pressure

---

Table 1.
Children at Risk for Hypertensive Disorders

*List of Those in Need of Regular Blood Pressure Monitoring**

1. Those with blood pressures persistently between the 90th and 95th percentile
2. Those with blood pressure tracking in upward direction
3. Those with blood pressures occasionally ≥ 95th percentile
4. Those with significant (more than 2 members) family history of treated hypertension, especially blacks
5. Those who are obese, especially if parent(s) are obese
6. Those with family history of stroke or coronary artery disease
7. Those with hyperlipidemia or family history of same
8. Those with diabetes mellitus

*Blood pressure should be taken at least at yearly intervals.

recording data nor ambulatory blood pressure monitoring information are available upon which to base the diagnosis of pediatric hypertension and corresponding treatment decisions. It is therefore necessary for this purpose to use carefully taken office or clinic measurements related to the similarly taken task force standards.[3] Significant hypertension is diagnosed when blood pressures are repeatedly between the 95th and 99th percentile. Serious hypertension is felt to exist when blood pressures are at or above the 99th percentile. The pressures should be at those levels on three or more separate occasions to be considered diagnostic (Table 2).

While the process for diagnosing hypertension and the degree of severity is lengthy and involved, finding the etiology is even more difficult. The vast majority of hypertensive pediatric patients will have primary hypertension (Table 4, Chapter 9). That is, they have hypertension from, as yet, unknown cause(s). Their hypertension will be significant but not severe, i.e., blood pressure below the 99th percentile. Those with serious hypertension are suspect for secondary hypertension, and must be evaluated for a curable form of hypertension.

Workup and Need for Treatment

Many in the pediatric community believe that most children who are hypertensive prior to school age have a recognizable cause for their disorder.[3,8] On closer perusal, what is meant are patients

Table 2.
Diagnosis of Hypertension by Age
(Modified from Task Force Report[3])

	Systolic BP = (mm Hg)		Diastolic BP = (mm Hg)	
Age	*Signif**	*Serious+*	*Signif*	*Serious*
Newborn (8–30 d)	104	110		
Infant (<2 y)	112	118	74	82
Child (2–5 y)	116	124	76	84
Child (6–9 y)	122	130	78	86
Child (10–12 y)	126	134	82	90
Adoles (13–15 y)	136	144	86	92
Adoles (16–18 y)	142	150	92	98

Adoles = adolescent;
*Signif = significant hypertension = BP > 95th percentile;
+Serious = serious hypertension = BP > 99th percentile.

who come to the physician's attention because of symptomatic (serious) hypertension. The prevalence of persistent, serious hypertension in the pediatric age group is probably less than one in a thousand children. Undoubtedly for every infant or young child found to have symptomatic hypertension there are at least several others who have undetected significant (mild to moderate) hypertension. Perhaps as many as one in a hundred have mild to moderate pediatric hypertension. Thus, it is important to be specific about the degree of hypertension. One should qualify the diagnosis of hypertension as mild to moderate ($\geq$ 95th percentile to the 99th percentile) or severe (> 99th percentile).

Once categorized, workup and decision making for treatment can be initiated along the lines of the Task Force scheme (Fig. 1).[3] Obese pediatric patients with mild to moderate (but not serious) hypertension should first have a trial at weight reduction. Most will have a decrease in blood pressure to normotensive values with successful weight loss and will require nothing more than medical follow-up. Regrettably, many will not maintain the weight loss and face a continuing battle with their problems. Only the one third or so of the obese patients who do not have a fall in blood pressure with weight reduction should have a basic workup. The workup includes a urinalysis, blood sedimentation rate, hemoglobin and hematocrit, and blood chemistry panel including creatinine and electrolytes.

The basic workup is also recommended for the nonobese, mild to moderate hypertensive. In all likelihood, the workup will be unrevealing. However, in the course of the workup some patients will be found to have a spontaneous fall in blood pressure to below the 95th percentile. They will then require subsequent blood pressure monitoring only. Others, obese or not, with continued pressure in the mild to moderate hypertensive range are advised to begin a program of nonpharmacologic treatment (see below). By following the recommended procedures, less than 1% of children in a medical-care program will be treated for hypertension. This, however, does not mitigate against advising prudent health habits for all young people, especially those just evaluated and those potentially at risk for later-life onset hypertension.

In every child health-care program or practice there are likely to be one or two individuals who have severe hypertension. When confronted with such a child, the scheme outlined in Figure 1 is again recommended. In the course of the evaluation, some may have regression of blood pressure levels. Those who do not should have a diagnostic workup for a treatable cause of the hypertension based on historical and examination findings as well as basic laboratory results. Among such causes renal disease is found in over 75%. Far less often, coarctation of the aorta or renovascular disease are at fault. Endocrine and other causes are rare. In most cases with severe hypertension, using the diagnostic workup scheme proposed in Chapter 9 should lead to the cause of the hypertension.

In any event, if the blood pressure is very high (ie., DBP > 12 mm Hg or SBP > 25 mm Hg above the 99th percentile), initiation of antihypertensive treatment should not await the outcome of sophisticated laboratory procedures. Such tests often require special facilities and are time consuming. Drug therapy for emergencies as described below should be started at once. Delay in treatment may place the child in jeopardy from seizures or heart failure. Medical treatments are discussed later and may be interrupted as needed in the course of the workup. The ultimate goal is to find a treatable cause of the hypertension and take the necessary steps to effect a cure. Thus, for example, if renal arterial narrowing is the cause of the high blood pressure, surgical or angioplastic elimination of renal artery stenosis will relieve the hypertension.

Nonpharmacologic Treatment of Hypertension

There is a recognized tendency for blood pressures under observation to become lower over time. This is the so-called "regression toward the mean," and is the reason to wait a short while prior to instituting therapy for individuals with high pressures, provided the pressure elevation is not very severe. With a demonstrated, persistent moderate or mild degree of blood pressure elevation, a decision should be made whether or not to initiate treatment. It must be recognized that the value of treatment in mild to moderate hypertension in young people has not been extensively investigated. Information is also lacking on any harm such treatment might evoke. Nevertheless, since nonpharmacologic treatment mainly involves generally advocated good health measures, it is worth using for those with mild hypertension and as a first measure in treating moderate hypertension. Those with severe hypertension will also benefit from nonpharmacologic intervention as drug-dose requirements are lessened.

Major nonpharmacologic treatments include weight control, sodium restriction, exercise promotion, and limitation of alcohol consumption. Adjuncts to these are increasing potassium consumption, relaxation therapy, and the restriction of dietary fat while increasing fiber. The use of calcium and magnesium supplements are controversial and not recommended at this time. When employing these therapeutic measures, patient motivation becomes a problem. The use of paramedical assistance to motivate adherence to the program can provide the necessary boost for success. It must be borne in mind that not all patients will respond to the outlined measures and that the battle with recidivism is constant. To help combat the latter and to provide rationale for treatment, certain specifics of the nonpharmacologic program components are noted in the following paragraphs.

Weight Control

There has been much material written about obesity and hypertension. Nearly two thirds of children with hypertension are obese.[9] A number of adult studies have demonstrated that weight reduction toward ideal weight as an isolated intervention, lowers blood pressure.[10,11] Several mechanisms appear active for this effect including natriuresis,[12] reduction in blood volume and cardiac output,[13] fall in sympathetic nervous system activity,[14] fall in plasma insulin,[15] and calcium homeostasis.[16] While pediatric information on weight loss and blood pressure reduction are scarce, data from the Muscatine Study indicate that weight reduction tends to lower blood pressure in children as well.[17] Although weight control is advocated, care must be taken not to induce an eating disorder in the involved young person. Rather, the advice should be to slow the velocity of weight gain so that the maturing patient will "grow into" the proper ideal weight channel. A balanced diet with modest caloric restriction is generally adequate for this purpose. A weight loss program such as outlined by Rocchini may be useful.[18] Patient and family motivation is the challenge. It must be remembered that it is extremely difficult to maintain a weight control process. However, a large portion of the counseling and follow-up support can be performed by dietary personnel.

Low Fat–High Fiber Diet

The restriction of dietary fat alone does not seem to result in decreased blood pressure in adults.[19] However, when combined with a high fiber-low sodium diet, a significant fall in blood pressure is achieved.[20] On the other hand, increasing plant fiber alone has been reported to lower adult blood pressure.[21] Likewise, hypertensive adults who were given 15 gms/day of fish oil had a reduction in blood pressure of greater than 6/4 mm Hg.[22] Information is lacking in children. However, a food frequency questionnaire study of 9-year-old children found blood pressure inversely related to fiber intake along with potassium, protein, complex carbohydrate.[23] It would seem reasonable to ensure a diet containing sufficient fiber and avoidance of very fatty foods. While it is known that those on vegetarian diets have lower blood pressures than those on omnivorous diets,[24] vegetarian diets are generally not recommended for children.

Sodium Restriction

Despite an increasing sentiment that sodium consumption is linked to blood pressure level,[25] the value of sodium restriction is still debated.[26] Grudgingly, some authorities on adult hypertension recommend moderate sodium restriction either as part of a nonpharmacologic regimen or in conjunction with drug therapy for hypertension.[27-29] Others are more enthusiastic about sodium restriction.[30] The compelling study of MacGregor and associates of adults with mild essential hypertension provides additional evidence for sodium restriction for hypertensive patients.[31] They demonstrated that as sodium intake was reduced, a corresponding change in blood pressure was seen. The lowest sodium intake group (about 50 mmols/day) had a blood pressure reduction of 19/9 mm Hg. The effect persisted for the duration of the 1-year study.

For adults, a modest reduction of sodium to about 70 mmols/day, or about 4 gms of table salt, is usually recommended.[28] Whether or not normotensives at risk for hypertension can benefit from dietary sodium reduction is an unanswered question. However, the Hypertension Prevention Collaborative Research Group recently demonstrated that reduction of sodium intake was effective in lowering blood pressure a small but significant amount (− 1.7 ± 0.9 mm Hg) in 2182 men and women with high-normal pressures.[32]

Sodium reduction as an adjunct to drug therapy is held to be very helpful. A comparison of an angiotensin-converting enzyme inhibitor plus either a diuretic or sodium restriction revealed a similar reduction in blood pressure in 25 moderately hypertensive adults.[33] Thus, monodrug therapy can be used in situations where two medications were previously felt to be needed. Restriction of sodium intake may also permit a decrease in antihypertensive drug-dosage requirement as well as allowing some patients to be weaned from medication altogether.[28]

There is some evidence that hypertensive pediatric patients, will have blood pressure reduction from sodium restriction, similar to adults.[34] Compliance is a major problem for such therapy in young people. By having high school students who have borderline hypertension monitor their urinary sodium with a "salt titrator tape," Tochikubo and colleagues were able to motivate the young people to comply with their nonpharmacologic antihypertensive program.[35] The students achieved a mean urinary sodium (equals intake) of 52 mmols/day with corresponding blood pressure decrease of 12/7 mm Hg. The students also lost an average of 1.7 kg in weight. In another study of mostly boarding students, at two high schools, Ellison and colleagues varied the institutional food-salt content.[36] Those students on a 15% to 20% lower sodium diet had slightly but significantly decreased blood pressures (−1.7 ± 1.5 mm Hg). Thus authorities on pediatric hypertension, like their adult counterparts, recommend modest sodium restriction as one of the useful nonpharmacologic interventions for children.[37-39]

Potassium Increase

While a number of epidemiologic studies of adults have shown an inverse relationship of dietary potassium to blood pressure,[40-45] and animal data support the value of potassium supplementation,[46-48] the results of potassium supplementation in the diets of adults have been labeled as unconvincing.[27] This is particularly true of potassium supplementation to normotensive adults, even those with high normal blood pressures.[32,49,50] On the other hand, when potassium supplements are given to mildly or moderately hypertensive individuals, in most instances a lowering affect is seen on blood pressure.[51] This may be especially true for black hypertensives[52] and those with diuretic-induced hypokalemia.[53] Because potassium therapy is potentially hazardous, most supplementation studies have been kept to less than 3 months in duration.

In a summary of supplementation studies, it was noted that

about 60 mmol of potassium were given, mainly as the chloride salt, to each adult hypertensive. A modest reduction in blood pressure of about 7/2 mm/Hg was found.[51] However, the chloride ion has been implicated in the development of hypertension and might have counteracted the effect of the potassium.[54] To avoid the possible negative effect of chloride on potassium blood pressure reduction, Miller and colleagues gave a potassium gluconate-citrate mixture, but still found no change in blood pressure after potassium administration to normotensive adults and children.[50] Their study of twin children is one of the few such pediatric investigations in the literature. These researchers caution that the results should not be extrapolated to other races or susceptible subgroups.

The mechanism of potassium action remains obscure, with natriuresis being an evident consequence of potassium administration. Effects on the renin-angiotensin system with suppression of renin release and a direct vascular effect with vasodilation are also noted.[55] Regardless of the mechanism, there is evidence that a long-term (12 years) high dietary intake of potassium reduced stroke-associated mortality by about 40% in a group of whites over 50 years of age.[56] The investigators recommended increasing dietary potassium by about 10 mmols/day by the addition of one or two servings of fruits or vegetables similar to those listed (Table 3). They noted that this addition did not produce any harm.

The lower sodium diet recommended for children with, or at risk for, hypertension is likely to result in a higher intake of potassium. In addition, authorities on pediatric hypertension also recommend increasing dietary potassium.[37,38] The simple inclusion of an extra serving of one of the foods listed in Table 3 will provide 7 to 10 mmols more potassium per day without hazard to the

Table 3.
Foods Containing 7–10 mmol Potassium per Serving*

Juices	Raw Fruit	Vegetables	Dairy Product
1 glass orange	1 banana	$\frac{1}{2}$ c beans	1 c milk
1 glass tomato	1 orange	1 baked potato	1 c yogurt
1 glass grapefruit	$\frac{1}{2}$ avocado	1 tomato	
1 glass pineapple	$\frac{1}{4}$ c raisins		
	$\frac{1}{6}$ cantaloupe		

*modified from.[38]

recipient. Supplemental potassium in the form of pills or liquid, particularly of the chloride salt, is not advisable unless there is a deficiency such as that from chronic diuretic therapy.

Calcium Supplementation

Epidemiologic studies relate calcium intake (like that of potassium), negatively to blood pressure with the principal source being dairy products.[57-60] The relationship has been demonstrated in a number of cultures with different eating patterns, making it unlikely to be due to a confounding effect from other nutrients. The apparent benefit of calcium in decreasing blood pressure has been tested by supplementation studies. These show conflicting results.[61-66] It appears that those with a calcium deficiency, whether it be from aging,[67] pregnancy,[68] or inadequate intake,[69] benefit from calcium supplements. The improvement appears to be mainly from the decrease in diastolic pressure. Others with the disorder or at risk for hypertension generally do not benefit from supplementation or may even show an increase in pressure.

In our Pasadena study of black high school students with blood pressures ranging in the upper half of the class, interim results of the double-blind 1.5 gm/day calcium supplementation were a lower diastolic blood pressure of 2.5 mm Hg.[69] A dietary deficiency of calcium was presumed due to low consumption of dairy products. Those students who were also deficient in potassium intake (by food-frequency questionnaire) had a greater decline in diastolic blood pressure.

A paradox seems to exist, in that increased calcium intake can both promote and reduce hypertension. The spectrum of responses to calcium administration are reminiscent of the sodium story wherein only those sensitive to salt appear to benefit from restriction. Accordingly, the varied responses to calcium should not be a surprise. The mechanism appears to originate with the increased calcium excretion found in certain hypertensives. In turn this leads to alterations in calcium-regulating hormones (increased parathyroid hormone secretion, decreased calcitonin, increased 1,25-dihydroxyvitamin D) with all their consequences, including the involvement of the renin-angiotensin system.[70] The problem is to identify those who could benefit from calcium supplementation. Aside from the previously mentioned instances, the solution to the problem is not yet at hand. Those with low-renin activity (like most blacks) and increased parathyroid hormone with low serum ionic calcium levels may be a group to consider.[71,72] As a rule, however, calcium supplements are not advocated for the treatment of hypertension.[51,66] Rather, consumption of enough dairy products to insure a daily intake of 800 to 1000 gms calcium is usually all that is needed.

Exercise

Young people who are physically fit have lower blood pressures.[73,74] It would seem that maintenance of fitness would especially be beneficial for those at risk for or with high blood pressure. Despite the widespread belief that regular exercise is beneficial for hypertensives, the evidence is somewhat limited.[27,75] Many reports on the use of exercise therapy in hypertension (mostly of adults) suffer from lack of controls. Yet the few well-designed studies give credibility to the use of isotonic (endurance) exercise as a therapeutic modality for the disorder.[76-79]

In dynamic or isotonic (endurance) exercise such as by treadmill, jogging, or bicycle, systolic blood pressure in normotensive individuals becomes elevated usually to levels less than 200 mm Hg. There is little change in diastolic pressure. In hypertensives, peak exercise systolic pressure is elevated to over 200 mm Hg and diastolic pressure is mildly elevated also. Those who undergo endurance training may have a decrease in blood pressure averaging 4/4 mm Hg if normotensive, and 11/6 mm Hg if hypertensive. An ambulatory pressure monitoring study showed that the pressure reduction effect occurred during the day but not during monitored sleep.[80]

In contrast, static or isometric (weight-training) exercise pressures may become markedly elevated to as much as 300 mm Hg systolic with corresponding increases in diastolic pressures. In normotensive adolescents, there is little reported change in blood pressure induced by weight training.[81] However, in the hypertensive adolescents, pressure reduction has been noted with weight training.[82] Long-term effects on blood pressure are unknown in these young people.

When endurance training is undertaken, it is recommended to be for periods of at least one-half hour three times a week. The exercise should increase the heart rate about 60% of predicted maximum.[82] There is an increased risk of sudden death in adults during exercise due to prevalence of ischemic heart disease.[75] This does not appear to be the case in young people, and endurance exercise can be regarded as safe for them. Accordingly, exercise stress testing is usually not needed prior to beginning an exercise training program for a youngster.

Sports participation is a concern for those caring for young hypertensives. Consequently, it is somewhat consoling that sudden athletic death is unknown for hypertensive young athletes.[83] However, some do recommend that workup, according to the scheme in Figure 1, be followed for hypertensive athletes as in other hypertensive individuals. Those with severe, symptomatic hypertension should be excluded from competitive sports until their disease is controlled.[84] All other hypertensive children and adolescents should be allowed full sports participation with appropriate medical supervision and follow-up.

Another problem for those advising young hypertensives on exercise concerns expectations when medications are prescribed. Diuretics, by virtue of volume depletion, impact negatively on exercise capacity. Endurance may be reduced by almost 20%.[85] Nonselective β-blockers prevent the blood pressure-lowering effect of exercise and blunts exercise capacity over 10%.[86] However, selective β-blockade will allow a conditioning program to proceed relatively unhampered. Commonly used vasodilators do not impact on exercise training at all.[87,88]

The therapeutic benefit of exercise for hypertension is clear from the foregoing. In addition, there is some information that regular exercise may help prevent the onset of hypertension. A large group of Harvard alumni were found by Paffenbarger and coworkers to have more than a one-third greater incidence of hypertension if they did not engage in vigorous physical activity.[89] These findings were confirmed by Blair and colleagues in a study of over 6000 men and women whose risk for hypertension varied directly with fitness over time.[90] In school children, increased leisure time activity resulted in lower blood pressures.[91] Thus, it is important that an exercise habit be instilled in young people that will benefit them throughout their lives.

Relaxation

The fact that stress is related to hypertension is both self evident and documented in a number of studies.[92,93] It would seem that relaxation would be beneficial for reducing blood pressure in individuals stressed by natural and wartime disasters as well as those suffering socioeconomic or job-related stress. Certainly, relaxation during sleep results in blood pressures that are lower than while awake and during exercise.[94] A number of studies have been carried out to assess the blood pressure effect of relaxation responses.[32,95-97] Unfortunately, these responses are difficult to measure and subject to many confounding influences. Even such techniques as "paranormal healing" (healing by thought projection or laying on of hands) have been espoused as resulting in blood pressure reduction.[98] Thus, conflicting information exists as to the worthiness of relaxation responses in the treatment of hypertension. The long-term effects have been described as "not very promising".[99]

Three main types of relaxation techniques have been used: biofeedback,[95] relaxation response,[100] and progressive muscle relaxation.[97] While each has its proponents, the relaxation response advocated by Benson is simple, suitable for home use, and achieves results equal to the other methods.[100] In the latter, the patient with eyes closed, is told to become progressively limp from the feet up. While concentrating on breathing through the nose he/she is instructed to remain passive and say the word "one" during expiration, ignoring extraneous thoughts. Twice daily 20-minute sessions commonly lead to a reduction in sympathetic nervous system responsivity and lower blood pressure.[97]

The relaxation response may be pertinent to adolescents with high blood pressures, especially minority groups suffering from socioeconomic stress. The teen years are particularly vulnerable times for the maturing individual who may have difficulty in coping with illness or risk of illness. Therefore compliance with any program of behavior modification will tax the provider of this patient's health care as well as the family unit.[92] Despite the challenge and uncertain benefit, this author believes the relaxation response is worth attempting in young people with persistent mild to moderate hypertension.

Avoidance of Alcohol Excess, Medications, Drugs

Hypertension related to consumption of excessive amounts of alcohol has been called the most common form of treatable hypertension in adults.[27,101] Once the threshold of two ounces of alcohol per day is passed, blood pressure, especially systolic, rises in a more or less linear fashion with increasing consumption to six to eight ounces, where it levels off. This effect is seen in all races and in both sexes, although not equally.[45,101,102] Reduction in alcohol intake results in a lowering of the blood pressure in most reported instances.[27,101] However, as Kaplan points out, there is some merit to moderate alcohol consumption (i.e., one or two ounces per day[103]).

The effect of alcohol on blood pressure appears to increase with age.[104] Little data are available for the pediatric age group. Adolescents and young people apparently do not suffer from the pressor effects of alcohol. Still, the other problems for teen drinkers including accidents, entry to substance abuse, and cardiomyopathy are very real. Avoidance is the best policy for young people. Again peer and even family pressure requires strength of coping through support of caregivers.

Certain medications like sympathomimetic amines, steroids, and oral contraceptives may result in hypertension. When these medications are used, blood pressures should be monitored. In instances when the blood pressure becomes elevated, reduction in dose or complete withdrawal usually is all that is needed to return the blood pressure to normal. On the other hand, hypertension from abused drugs often goes unnoticed until the abuser requires medical attention, occasionally in a hypertensive crisis. Needless to say, treatment may be difficult because of the multiple factors involved. Again, avoidance is the only answer but may be extremely difficult to achieve.

Smoking

The major adverse effects of smoking on adults are common knowledge. It is less well known that adult smokers do not have hypertension more often than nonsmokers,[105] although they are much more likely to have the malignant form of the disease.[106] Well-justified standard advice is to "quit smoking!" Paradoxically, after smoking cessation more individuals are hypertensive than those who continue to smoke, probably on the basis of weight gain.[107]

Like their adult counterparts, children and adolescents who smoke have no greater incidence of high blood pressure than nonsmokers. In fact, their blood pressures actually tend to be lower than the nonsmokers.[108,109] Apparently, from a hypertension standpoint, smoking is not a consideration. However, recent unpublished studies of ambulatory blood pressures taken during smoking are said to show transient pressure increases with each encounter. The sum of these is probably a considerable period of pressure elevation. However, there are so many documented adverse events from smoking that even if the impact of smoking on blood pressure is not significant, every effort should be made to discourage beginning the smoking habit. Individuals of pediatric age are the right people to focus upon.[92]

Specific Treatments for Curable Forms of Hypertension

When secondary hypertension is suspected and, if urgently necessary, the blood pressure controlled, a search must be made for a curable form of the disorder. If the cause has escaped detection it may be found, in most instances, by using Algorithm 3 in Figure 1. Once the cause is known, specific treatment should be considered. Unfortunately, many causes of secondary hypertension are not amenable to curative treatments and require symptomatic treatment. In some, the disorder will become less burdensome or even resolve over time, as is the case in newborns with catheter thrombus induced hypertension (Chapter 8).

Of those with a specific cause, some may be cured by the simple withdrawal of an inciting substance like licorice or a medication such as an oral contraceptive. A few endocrine conditions will improve with specific pharmacologic therapy, for example, spironolactone for aldosteronism due to adrenal hyperplasia. Then there are conditions like coarctation of the aorta (Chapter 5), and renovascular hypertension (Chapter 6), as well as certain other renal and endocrine (Chapter 7) forms of hypertension which may resolve with surgical intervention or interventional techniques like balloon arterioplasty. Organ transplantation, especially renal, may give rise to another set of problems requiring constant attention to medical therapy.

The best treatment for any form of hypertension is specific treatment of the underlying disorder. An elaboration of specific cause-oriented treatments can be found in the chapters devoted to the underlying disorders noted above. The critical part of the process is the recognition of the underlying disorder. Once recognized, those with surgically treatable hypertensive disorders warrant early surgical intervention even in infancy.

Pharmacologic Treatment of Hypertension

Pharmacologic treatments are mentioned in the various chapters devoted to differing aspects of hypertension and the disease processes causing the disorder. However, it is pertinent to bring the information together in one place and perhaps, in a new light, add some details. The repetition is hoped to be beneficial.

Treatment Goals

Fortunately, few young people will require medicines to treat their hypertension. With maximized nonpharmacologic treatment, it has been estimated that far less than 1% of pediatric hypertensives will need drug therapy to control their blood pressure.[3] This means that the average provider of pediatric health care will probably have less than one in a thousand patients requiring antihypertensive medication. As outlined in Figure 1, in all save those with severe hypertension, nonpharmacologic treatment is recommended as initial therapy. Only when the patient is symptomatic, or the response to nonpharmacologic measures is judged inadequate, are medicines started. If there is any doubt, and the patient is asymptomatic with no proteinuria, cardiomegaly or echocardiographic evidence of left ventricular hypertrophy,[110] it would be reasonable to procrastinate with drug therapy.

There is much uncertainty about long-term drug treatment in young people.[111] There is little pediatric data available, and adult information indicates increased lipids and hypoglycemia are found with long-term diuretic or β-blockade treatment (see below[112,113]). Further help on deciding whether or not to begin drug treatment is available in the form of ambulatory blood pressure monitoring.[114] If most of the blood pressures are below the 95th percentile and none above the 99th percentile, drug treatment may be postponed or avoided altogether. Of course, other compelling reasons for treatment might exist. That is, positive renal, cardiac, or other organ system findings might require treatment at lower levels of blood pressure in order to prevent further damage.

Once the decision is made to begin drug therapy, it should be recognized that nonemergent cases do not require a rapid decrease in blood pressure. Rather, a slow reduction in blood pressure is desirable. The ultimate goal is a high-normal blood pressure or a pressure below the 95th percentile. For a 15-year-old, this would be below 136/86 mm Hg.[3] Parenthetically in the same case, pressure reduction below 144/92 (99th percentile) by a combination of low drug dose and nonpharmacologic means might also suffice. Blood pressure will likely continue to fall slowly by natural regression toward the mean, and complications may accompany more aggressive treatment.

First Drug and Substitutions–Combinations

A variety of "first drug" programs are in use. The long advocated "stepped-care" approach may be giving way to an individualized approach.[3,115-117] The "stepped-care" approach, although still labeled as such, is more individualized. An increased number of choices and steps may be offered than are in the 1993 fifth revision of the Joint National Committee on Detection, Evaluation, and Treatment of High Blood Pressure report,[117] (Fig. 2). For example, the initial drug treatment may begin with a calcium entry blocker (CEB), such as nifedipine or an angiotensin-converting enzyme (ACE) inhibitor, like enalapril. In contrast, the former pediatric scheme suggested only the initial choice of a diuretic or β-blocker.[3] It is generally recommended that initial drug dosages be kept low, particularly with diuretics.[118] With lack of response it is felt that adding a second drug is better than increasing the dose of the first. In that way side effects, which often are dose-dependent can be minimized.

In selecting the initial drug certain individual features should be kept in mind. Blacks tend to have a low renin, volume-dependent hypertension. Accordingly, thiazide diuretics are often prescribed for backs as a first medication. If there is no response, the addition of the cardioselective β-blocker, metoprolol, may be particularly effective in controlling the blood pressure.[119] Those with renal disease also respond well to diuretics if the glomerular filtration rate is not too low.

Those with high renin hypertension respond to β-blockers but because of side effects the trend now is to use ACE inhibitors as the first drug.[120] Angiotensin-converting enzyme inhibitors are particularly useful in hypertensives with heart failure. α-blockers are used in those with hypercholesterolemia. Likewise, both ACE inhibitors and CEB do not appear to have a hyperlipidemic effect nor do they appear to cause hyperglycemia.[121,122] Calcium entry blockers are advocated for those with coronary artery disease and are also effective in hypertensive emergencies.[38]

The standard way of assessing the effect of initial therapy in nonurgent cases is by casual office blood pressure measurements

Step 1: Nonpharmacologic Treatment

1. Weight Control
2. Sodium Restriction
3. Adequate Dietary Potassium & Calcium
4. Low fat-high fiber diet
5. Exercise & Relaxation Response
6. Avoidance of alcohol, medications, drugs
7. No Smoking

(if pressure not controlled progress in steps but continue nonpharmacologic treatment in all steps)

Step 2: Initial Drug Treatment (Single Drug)

1. Calcium Entry Blocker (CEB) or
2. ACE inhibitor or
3. β-Blocker or
4. Diuretic

} Use Low Dose

(if pressure remains uncontrolled)

Step 3: Add 2nd Drug of Different Class + Or Substitute Another Drug of Same Class

+ (Diuretic or   (α$_1$-Blocker or
  (β-Blocker or   (Vasodilator or
  (Calcium Antagonist or (Central Acting α$_2$-Agonist
  (ACE Inhibitor or

(if pressure still not controlled)

Step 4: Add 3rd Drug of Different Class Or Substitute 2nd Drug

(failure of pressure control)

Step 5: Further Evaluation or Referral Or Add 3rd or 4th Drug

Stepdown Program   (trial after prolonged pressure control)

Figure 2: Individualized step-care approach to hypertension therapy. Therapy of hypertension may be individualized according to this scheme based on information in the text. Should nonpharmacologic treatment (Step 1) not control a blood pressure elevated beyond the 99th percentile, drug treatment may be added to the regimen (Step 2). Other drugs may be substituted or added for therapeutic failures (Step 3 and 4) but the practitioner would be well advised to seek consultation from an expert in pediatric hypertension if blood pressure is not reduced to a point below the 99th percentile.

taken at perhaps weekly intervals. These may overread the degree of residual pressure elevation. Home blood pressure monitoring may give a more accurate idea of the effectiveness of the antihypertensive treatment regimen.[123] Ideally, 24-hour ambulatory pressure evaluations would give the most accurate assessment,[124] but such measurements are expensive and time consuming. They may best be reserved for the most difficult or refractory cases.

Once again, it is emphasized that nonpharmacologic therapy must be rigorously pursued along with any drug treatment program. In that manner, drugs and doses usually can be minimized. If the initial drug response is deemed inadequate, another drug can be added or substituted as indicated in Figure 2. It is important to titrate medicines to the individual patient. This may require a number of changes or additions to the regimen. If, in spite of a careful medication regimen, the pressure remains outside the 99th percentile in a young person without obvious cause for the hypertension, a repeat workup may be in order. Since it is uncommon for the provider of general pediatric care to have much experience in antihypertensive therapy, in most instances polydrug therapy and further workups are best left to a center specializing in pediatric hypertension.[110]

Hypertensive Emergencies

Infrequently, blood pressure surges, either from a known hypertensive disorder, most likely renal, or de novo from a yet undiscovered cause, create a life-threatening situation. The blood pressure is extraordinarily high, usually greater than 1.3 to 1.5 × the 95th percentile.[112] The rapidity of rise rather than the baseline pressure seems to be the main factor. Those having high pressures to begin with reach the highest pressures with crisis. These hypertensive crises are characterized by cerebral, cardiac, or neurologic symptoms. It is paramount to begin antihypertensive therapy at once. Others, with nonspecific complaints only, may be found to have extremely high blood pressure as well. They may have headaches, somnolence, or fatigue. The dangerous symptoms of encephalopathy or heart failure will be absent. They too must be treated urgently lest a full-blown emergency symptom complex ensues which may lead to retinal or intracranial hemorrhage, or other life-threatening consequence. On rare occasions, a hypertensive crisis may result from withdrawal of antihypertensive drugs, such as clonidine or α-methyldopa.[125] Pheochromocytoma (Chapter 7) and the use of monoamine oxidase (MAO) inhibitors are rare causes of hypertensive emergencies.[126]

Regardless of the cause, these blood pressure-related crises are true emergencies. Immediate reduction in blood pressure is essential to the outlook of the affected patient. The patient must be hospitalized and an intravenous line placed at once. For those with encephalopathic symptoms, intravenous treatment either with sodium nitroprusside or labetalol is given carefully to guard against a too rapid reduction in pressure. (Table 4).[127] In that way, further compromise in cerebral circulation can be avoided. For those able to cooperate, sublingual nifedipine is the choice, although some

Table 4.
Drugs for Treatment of Hypertensive Emergencies[110,127]

Drug	Route/to Time Act	Dose	Recommendation	Side Effects
Sodium Nitroprusside	I.V./ immed	0.5–10.0 µg/kg/min	Choice if obtunded	use in ICU, hypotension, cyanide toxicity
Labetalol	I.V./in min	1–3 mg/kg/h	2nd choice if obtunded	orthostatic hypotension ht fail, broncho spasm, GI Sx
Diazoxide	I.V./in min	0.25–5 mg/kg/min	3rd choice if obtunded	hyperglycemia hypotension salt/ water retention
Nifedipine	sublingual 10–20 min	0.25–0.5 mg/kg q30min (max 1 mg/kg)	Choice if not obtunded	flushing, hypotension, tachycardia, edema, GI Sx
Hydralazine	I.V./in 30 min	0.1–0.5 mg/kg	back-up drug	tachycardia, flush hypotension
Captopril	sublingual or oral/ 20–30 min	1.0–3.0 mg/kg	useful (See Ref[127])	hypotension espec if prev diuretic,
or Enalapril	I.V./in 20–30 min	5µg/kg for infant up to 625 µg/kg for adoles	Same as Captopril	in renovasc dis → reversible renal failure

believe that captopril is equally effective and may have fewer side effects.[128] More recently, we have used intravenous enalapril for this purpose. The emergency treatment of pheochromocytoma, as presented in Chapter 7, includes a peripherally acting α-adrenergic antagonist.

As with the treatment of hypertension in general, a relatively slow reduction of blood pressure in hypertensive emergencies is safest. One must guard against acute hypotension in an already circulatory state. That is why the sublingual route of antihypertensive medication is preferred where possible. The drug is absorbed somewhat more slowly than from the enteral route. It is suggested that the pressure be decreased towards the desired pressure by not more than one third in the first half day.[110] On the next day, an additional one-third step can be taken toward the goal pressure. Thereafter, the medication can be changed to a usual blood control regimen and, over the next 3 or 4 days, titrated to the desired blood pressure, generally below the 95th percentile for age.

Pharmacopeia

Among the various drug groups available for treatment of hypertension are diuretics, adrenergic inhibitors, centrally acting agonists, calcium entry blockers, converting-enzyme inhibitors, and vasodilators. The pediatric pharmacopeia in hypertension is more limited than in adult medicine as a result of fewer patients needing treatment. Thus, as in so many instances, therapeutic advances come slowly to pediatrics and many practitioners prescribe a relatively few well-known drug regimens. Perhaps it is just as well as it is usually best to use medications that are familiar to the prescriber. In special pediatric situations, like treatment of hypertension, this means the use of a few medicines. The pharmacopeia herein described will make no effort to be all inclusive or even "up to date"; rather, a description of several well-known drugs of each category will follow.

Diuretics

Diuretics have been in use for over 3 decades[129,130] (Table 5). They have been effective by increasing sodium excretion, thereby reducing fluid volume. A variety of diuretics, acting at different sites of the collecting system, are available for use (Table 5). From a practical standpoint, if diuretics are to be used, it is common to begin antihypertensive therapy with hydrochlorothiazide (HydroDIURIL®) 1 mg/kg per day. Other diuretics are used as additional therapy as needed. A consideration of the main diuretic groups follows.

Thiazide Diuretics: Acting on the early segment of the distal tubule, the thiazide diuretics function mainly through volume depletion. The diuretic response to the thiazides is not entirely dose-related. That is, increasing doses do not necessarily result in increasing diuresis. Thiazide diuretics were formerly the mainstay of antihypertensive therapy in the young. Their image became somewhat tarnished as it was found that the thiazides, and perhaps the loop diuretics, result in altered lipid, uric acid, and glucose metabolism. Elevated lipid levels, especially triglyceride, but LDL cholesterol as well, are a concern for the development of coronary artery disease. This may be a reason why, in some adult studies, mortality from all causes was not altered with diuretic therapy despite control of blood pressure.[129] The uric acid elevation mentioned has rarely resulted in gout. However, elevated glucose levels affect diabetics adversely. Increased death rates have been reported in diabetics receiving thiazide diuretics.[131]

Other concerns of chronic thiazide diuretic use have surfaced, mainly in the adult literature. Increased potassium excretion is well known and is commonly counteracted by the addition of a potassium-sparing diuretic such as spironolactone. Less well known is

Table 5.
Diuretics for Pediatric Antihypertensive Treatment[109,,126]

Drug Type & Name	Initial Oral Dose (mg/kg)	Interval (qh)	Max Dose (mg/kg)
Thiazide Diuretics			
hydrochlorothiazide	0.5	12	2
chlorthalidone	0.5	24	2
metolazone	0.2	24	0.4
Loop Diuretics			
furosemide	0.5	6–12	6
ethacrynic acid	1	12–48	3
Potassium-Sparing Diuretics			
spironolactone	1	24	3

the fact that calcium excretion is decreased. Additionally, skeletal muscle tissue may suffer both potassium and magnesium depletion.[132] In hypertensives with renal damage, thiazide diuretics did not appear to protect against progression of the disease process, whereas an ACE inhibitor did.[133]

The noted adverse effects have been found to be dose-related.[134,135] Thus, with low doses, thiazide diuretic therapy is again occupying an important place in the treatment of hypertension. Thiazides may be used alone or in combination with another class of drug. In the latter situation, the low-dose diuretic often potentiates the additional medication, enabling a lower dose of both medications to be used. Indeed, the pharmaceutical industry has recognized this and produced combination medications such as Capozide® (captopril and hydrochlorothiazide).[136] Thiazide diuretics, except for metolazone (Zaroxolyn®), evoke little response when the GFR is very low, i.e., less than 30%.

Loop Diuretics: Furosemide (Lasix®) is a powerful diuretic acting on the ascending loop of Henle by inhibiting chloride reabsorption. It is not generally used for initial therapy because of side effects. Unlike thiazide diuretics, response to furosemide is dose-related. The response is also related to uric acid level, high levels decreasing the diuresis.[137] Sometimes rather high doses of the medication are used (Table 5), particularly in the treatment of hypertension from chronic renal disease when the GFR is below 30%. As a result of its effectiveness, furosemide may cause dehydration and metabolic alkalosis with hyponatremia and hypokalemia.[127] It also causes hyperglycemia through suppression of insulin secretion.[138] Hyperlipidemia, similar to that found with thiazide usage, and ototoxicity are other unwanted effects. Should the patient become refractory to furosemide and diuresis be required to control the blood pressure, a trial of ethacrynic acid may be worthwhile. Because of the nonreversible hearing loss caused by its use, ethacrynic acid is reserved for use only when hypertensives become unresponsive to other diuretics.

Potassium-Sparing Diuretics: Spironolactone (Aldactone®) is a relatively safe drug principally used for its potassium-sparing effect in combination with other more powerful diuretics. It is also useful in the treatment of aldosteronism. Side effects of prolonged use include gynecomastia and hirsutism.[127] Hyperkalemia may develop if potassium balance is not observed carefully. The other drugs in this group, amiloride and triamterene, have not seen much pediatric usage.

β-Adrenergic Receptor Blockers

This group of adrenergic inhibitors (Table 6) became available about 3 decades ago, when propranolol (Inderal®) was introduced for β-blockade.[139] A myriad of uses were found for it and its adverse cardiac, pulmonary, and metabolic effects became well known. Propranolol was found to cause or increase cardiac failure, particularly in babies; worsen bronchospasm; cause hypoglycemia in infants or exaggerate hypoglycemia in diabetes as well as blunt the warning signs of hypoglycemia, such as hunger and tachycardia. As a rule it should not be used in such circumstances. In addition to the previously described effects, propranolol causes adverse changes in lipid metabolism with decreased HDL cholesterol. Raynaud's phenomenon and gastrointestinal disturbances are other unwanted effects of β-blockade.[140] Propranolol also suffers from a first-pass effect. That is, it is metabolized readily by the liver and, accordingly, propranolol doses must be increased to compensate for the early hepatic removal of the medication.

Recently, longer acting and more selective β-blocking compounds such as atenolol (Tenormin®) and metoprolol (Lopressor®) have been developed and, like propranolol, are useful in the treatment of hypertension.[141] This selective group of drugs principally block β-1 (cardiac) or β-2 (smooth muscle) adrenergic receptors at low to moderate doses, but with increased dosage will "cross over" to block both receptors. Thus, at high doses even β-1 blockers may produce bronchospasm, a β-2 blocking effect.[142] Some β-blockers like propranolol and, to a lesser extent, metoprolol are lipid soluble and can cross the blood-central nervous system barrier. The result may be a central nervous system disorder, usually, involving sleep. A weakly soluble β-blocker such as atenolol can obviate such effects, because atenolol does not cross the blood-brain barrier in any significant amount.

β-blockade has been proposed as a first-line drug therapy in high renin hypertension, especially in young people with rapid heart rates.[3,] but β-blockers may be useful even in the low renin hypertension found in blacks,[143] particularly in combination with a diuretic. When β-blockers are used, it is best to begin with a low dose and make upward adjustments as necessary (Table 6). However, if high doses are required it is better to add another drug. Because of prolonged biologic effect, twice daily dosing may be sufficient when propranolol is used and once daily dosing if atenolol or metoprolol

Table 6.
Adrenergic Inhibitors Currently in Use[3,110,127]

Drug Class / Drug	mg/kg/Dose	Route	Doses/Day	Usage	Comment/Toxic (see Txt)
β-**Blockers** Nonselective Propranolol	0.5–2. max 8–10	Oral	2–4	high-renin hypertension	often used in combo Rx with a diuretic
Selective (β-₁) Atenolol	1.–2.0	Oral	1	same; β_2 effect avoided	not cross bld-brain barrier; withdraw slowly
Metoprolol	1.–2.0 max 5.0	Oral	2	same	crosses bld-brain barrier
α-**Blockers** Prazosin	0.05 1st dose max 1st dose 0.1 mg to max total 0.5 mg/kg	Oral	2–3	in heart fail; bronchospsm; hyperlipidem; diabetes	1st dose, syncope or orthostatic hypotension; fluid retention
Peripheral α-**Inhibitors** Reserpine	.001–.003	Oral	1	infreq used: with diuretic	depression; nasal stuffiness

is used. Since atenolol is metabolized in the kidneys, dosage every other day is used when creatinine clearance is reduced.[127]

α- Antagonists (α-Receptor Blockers)

α-blockade with phenoxybenzamine and phentolamine were used for some time in the treatment of pheochromocytoma. More recently, the α-adrenergic blocker prazosin (Minipres®) has been used. It has fewer side effects and has a beneficial effect on lipid metabolism. It decreases total cholesterol, and LDL cholesterol while increasing HDL cholesterol.[144] Prazosin can be used in heart failure, diabetes mellitus,[145] and in the presence of bronchospastic disorders. It may be used in combination with diuretics and β-blockers. Prazosin may cause orthostatic hypotension and syncope when first given, especially in diuresed (fluid-depleted) individuals. This "first dose" orthostatic symptomatology is found in 1% to 4% of patients and is self-limited. It disappears on further dosage. With appropriate caution, this and other side effects should not be major problems.[110]

When beginning prazosin therapy, a small first dose is used (50 mu/kg—Table 6.)[127] Hypotension, should it occur, usually is seen about 90 minutes after the first dose. Placing the patient in the recumbent position and, if needed, adding supportive treatment will resolve the condition. It should be noted that the hypotension may recur with each initial upward adjustment of the dosage or addition of another drug. A small number of other side effects do not cause major difficulties and are mainly those resulting from the reduction in blood pressure such as dizziness, drowsiness, headache, palpitations, and nausea. Prazosin is somewhat short-acting. Other α-blocking drugs are available, such as doxazosin (Cardura®)[146] and terazosin (Hytrin®). They have similar effects and require one daily dose only. However, there are other side effects, particularly syncope, with doxazosin and no pediatric experience has been reported with either drug.

Another type of adrenergic blocker acts on peripheral nerve endings, reducing sympathetic tone and resulting in decreased peripheral resistance.[147] Peripheral adrenergic inhibitors include reserpine and guanethidine. Both have central effects, but their main impact on blood pressure is peripheral. Both have seen long usage, but with more effective agents these drugs are not widely used at present. Reserpine (Serpasil®) is still regarded as effective, safe, and inexpensive. It is most effective if used with a diuretic. Centrally mediated side effects of depression and sleep disturbance, along with nasal stuffiness and fluid retention are usually not severe with the low-dose therapy needed for hypertension.[148]

α-Agonists

These centrally acting agonists include methyldopa, widely used prior to the advent of β-blockers, and clonidine which by $α_2$-receptor stimulation reduce sympathetic activity. Clonidine (Catapres®) use suffers from rebound hypertension which may create a hypertensive emergency as described previously. This may be a problem for pediatric patients whose compliance is always in question.[110] Methyldopa (Aldomet®) is not generally used for pediatric patients with hypertension because of effects on mood and propensity to cause hypersensitivity reactions.[110] It is, however, widely used for chronic hypertension in pregnancy,[149] where follow-up data indicate its safety with little fetal impact. The usual dose for a pregnant young person is 250 to 500 mg 2 to 3 times a day up to 3 gms a day.[127]

Calcium-Entry (Channel) Blockers

A relatively recent addition to the antihypertension armamentarium, calcium-channel blockers like nifedipine have rapidly become one of the mainstays in the treatment of hypertension and are used as an alternative initial therapy.[117]

Their net effect is to decrease vascular smooth muscle tone thereby resulting in a lower blood pressure. For treatment in pediatric hypertension, nifedipine (Procardia®, Adalat®) is started at 0.25 mg/kg per day and increased to a maximum of 1 mg/kg per day divided into three or four doses (Table 7). As previously noted, nifedipine is especially effective in hypertensive emergencies (Table 4). Nifedipine not only decreases systemic hypertension but also appears to be useful in pulmonary hypertension including that which results in high altitude pulmonary edema.[150] The drug also has been found useful in pregnancy-induced hypertension.[149] Nifedipine is a dihydropyridine derivative. Its short action has prompted the development of the longer acting compounds like nifedipine XL (Procardia XL®) (Table 7), and analogs like nicardipine (Cardene®) and felodipine.[151]

Table 7.
Other Drugs for the Treatment of Hypertension in the Young[127]

Drug Class/Name	Route	Age	1st Dose (mg/kg)	Max Dose (mg/kg/day)	Interval (qh)
Calcium-Entry Blockers (1st-line Rx)					
Nifedipine	Oral/sublingual	Child	0.25	1.0	6–8
		Adolesc	*10/30	#180/120	6–8/qd
Angiotensin-Converting Enzyme Blockers (1st-line Rx)					
Captopril	Oral	<2 mo	0.1–0.25	2.0	6–24
		>2 mo	0.5	6.0 (to 75mg/d)	6–24
		Adolesc	**25	**150	8–12
Enalapril	Oral	Inf/Child	0.1	0.5	24
		Adolesc	2.5–5	10–40	12–24
	I.V.	Inf/Child	0.005	0.01–0.03	8–12
		Adolesc	0.625	2.5–5	6
Vasodilators (3rd-line Rx)					
Hydralazine	Oral	Child	0.75	7.5 (to 200/d)	6–12
		Adolesc	10.0	300	6
	I.V.	Child	0.1	20	4–6
		Adolesc	10.0	240	4–6

* = mg per dose/mg per sustained release form per day;
# = total mg per day/total mg per sustained release form per day;
** = mg per dose.

Calcium-channel blockers also have cardiac effects both on impulse formation-transmission and as an inotropic agent. Nifedipine acts mainly on vascular smooth muscle while another channel blocker, verapamil (Calan®, Isoptin®) has strong cardiac action with use in tachyarrhythmias and hypertrophic cardiomyopathies.[152] Side effects are mainly those of reducing blood pressure such as dizziness, hypotension, flushing, and headaches, as well as hypersensitivity-type reactions including connective tissuelike disorders with positive ANA.[110,127] Nifedipine is thought to improve renal function in those with renal disease,[153] but may not slow the progression of the underlying disorder even though blood pressure is controlled.[154]

Angiotensin Converting Enzyme (ACE) Inhibitors

As another relatively recent entrant in the therapy of hypertension this group of drugs has been proven to be very effective in lowering blood pressure with few side effects. Over the last decade, these drugs have gone from being used in the most severe hypertension cases only to use as an initial drug for individualized therapy of hypertension.[117] The ACE inhibitors decrease production of angiotensin II and at the same time decrease bradykinin breakdown.[155] As a result, prostaglandin secretion is promoted. Both factors lead to vasodilation and blood pressure reduction. Reduced levels of angiotensin II also lead to a decrease in aldosterone secretion with resultant natriuresis.

The ACE inhibitors' effects protect the brain, heart, and kidneys. Coronary circulation is enhanced while heart rate and output are not significantly changed. In hypertensives with left ventricular hypertrophy (LVH), regression of the hypertrophy has been shown with ACE inhibitor treatment.[156] Cerebral blood flow is maintained while sympathetic nervous system activity is decreased. In the kidneys, there is preferential dilation of the efferent arteries with reduction of intraglomerular pressure. Protection is furnished against progressive renal damage from glomerular hypertension.[157] In contrast to other antihypertensive agents, ACE inhibitors do not change serum lipid patterns and improve insulin sensitivity.[158]

Side effects are uncommon with ACE inhibitors, occurring in 1% or 2% of cases. Freedom from adverse central nervous system effects is noteworthy. Development of a dry hacking cough is perhaps the most frequent side effect.[159] Other side effects include excessive hypotension, correctable by salt repletion; tachycardia and azotemia, reversible upon withdrawal of the drug; taste disturbances, and hyperkalemia. The latter is usually not significant unless there is renal insufficiency or the patient is receiving a potassium-sparing diuretic. Allergic rashes of the pruritic maculopapular variety are seen, but more serious conditions like Stevens-Johnson syndrome are rare. Reports of angioneurotic edema and bone marrow depression are also rare. In the presence of bilateral renal artery stenosis or stenosis of the renal artery with a solitary kidney, ACE inhibition may cause severe renal insufficiency. This is of considerable importance following renal transplantation. Withdrawal of the drug usually restores the renal function.[160] Of special significance is fetal wastage and newborn anomalies reported with use during pregnancy, resulting in a recommendation that these drugs not be used during pregnancy.[149]

Captopril (Capoten®), the first marketed ACE inhibitor, is characterized biochemically by the presence of a sulfhydryl group which acts as a zinc ligand for enzyme binding-inactivation. Its action onset is a relatively rapid 20 to 30 minutes with a duration of about 12 hours.[161] Only oral dose forms are available.

Recommended dose for children is to begin with a 0.5 mg/kg dose adjusting by twofold increments to a maximum of 6 mg/kg per day or 75 mg/day in two or three doses (Table 7).[127] For adolescents, therapy is begun with 25 mg every 8 hours and increased at weekly intervals to a maximum of 150 mg/dose in monodrug treatment. When two drugs are used the dose can be kept small and side effects minimized. Concomitant use of a nonsteroidal anti-inflammatory drug will reduce the efficacy. Captopril is readily absorbed from the mouth or gastrointestinal tract and excreted in the urine. Doses in the presence of renal insufficiency are kept lower and less frequent.

The second generation ACE inhibitor, enalapril (Vasotec®) has a carboxyl group as the enzymatic zinc ligand, but similar effects and side effects in the treatment of hypertension as captopril.[162]

Enalapril actually is a prodrug. It is de-esterified in the liver to the active compound, enalapril. Thus, the drug has an action onset delay of about 2 hours with a peak at 4 to 12 hours and a duration of about 24 hours.[161] An analogue, lisinopril (Prinivil®, Zestril®) is said to be somewhat more effective.[163] Enalapril is available both in oral and I.V. forms (Table 7). For infants and children, dosage is begun with 0.1 mg/kg per day and adjusted to a maximum of 0.5 mg/kg per day over 2 weeks while for I.V. use 5 to 10 mug/kg per dose are given every 8 to 12 hours.[127] Adolescents are begun on 2.5 to 5 mg/day in one or two oral doses with increments to 10 to 40 mg/day.

Vasodilators

The drugs in this group of medications have a long history of use, some being used in the treatment of hypertension prior to diuretics. Included in this group are hydralazine, minoxidil, diazoxide, and sodium nitroprusside. The latter two drugs have been used frequently in hypertensive emergencies (Table 4). While formerly a mainstay in the treatment of hypertensive emergencies, difficulties in titration and side effects of diazoxide (Hyperstat®) have reduced its usage.[110] Sodium nitroprusside (Nipride®, Nitropres®) relaxes the vascular smooth muscle of both veins and arteries. The effect is both cardiac pre- and afterload reduction. Nitroprusside acts within minutes and loses its action soon after discontinuation. Both cyanide and thiocyanate toxicity are concerns with high doses over periods of 4 days or more. With monitoring for acidosis due to cyanide and maintenance of cyanide level below 20 µg/dL, as well as thiocyanate level below 10 mg/dL, toxicity is seldom seen.[164]

The sodium retention and tachycardia side effects of hydralazine (Apresoline®) formerly precluded its use. However, concomitant use of a β-blocker and diuretic obviates these effects. As a result, oral hydralazine is currently employed when triple therapy of moderate to severe hypertension is needed. An uncommon side effect is the development of a lupuslike syndrome which resolves when treatment is stopped.[165] The syndrome notwithstanding, hydralazine can be used in treatment of hypertension from nondrug-related systemic lupus erythematosus. The drug binds to smooth muscle and its effect may last as long as 12 hours although it is generally given every 6 hours. The initial oral dose is 0.75 mg/day divided every 6 to 12 hours and titrated to a maximum of 7.5 mg/day (Table 7).[127] For temporary I.V. use, as perioperatively, the dose varies from an initial 0.1 mg/kg per dose to a maximum 3.75 mg/kg per day in 4- to 6-hour divided doses. The adolescent oral dose is 10 to 100 mg every 6 to 12 hours with a maximum of 300 mg.

Minoxidil (Loniten®) is a rapidly acting vasodilator effective in acute hypertension.[166] Unfortunately, it has side effects of hypertrichosis, sympathetic overactivity with tachycardia, elevation of plasma-renin activity with salt and water retention, and, rarely, pericardial effusion among others. These side effects have curtailed its usage to the point of its being employed for serious refractory hypertension only and then with a β-blocker and diuretic.[167]

Follow-Up and Step-Down Program

When a hypertensive treatment program is begun, rather frequent follow-up visits are in order. At those assessments, blood pressure home measurements can be reviewed and compared with office evaluations. Drug doses can be checked and, if necessary, pill counts made. Since nonpharmacologic treatment should be part of every treatment program (if not the sole program), diet and weight control should be evaluated. Dietary consultation should be available. Maintenance of diet is the most difficult part of the program and much encouragement and support needs to be given. Exercise capability may also be evaluated by exercise testing and improvement noted.

These visits should occur at weekly intervals until blood pressure is approaching preset goals (< 95th percentile). Then they can be widened to biweekly, monthly, and even quarterly intervals.

If blood pressure medications are in use and adequate control has been achieved for about 2 years, an attempt at medication withdrawal can be made. If that is the case, closer follow-up is again in order. The patient must know that medication may have to be resumed.

Summary

Therapy directed at the prevention of target-organ damage in those afflicted with severe secondary hypertension is deemed important if not essential. Likewise, efforts directed at the prevention of hypertension offer enormous potential benefit to those at risk for the disorder. Unfortunately, those at such risk are hard to find although some clues are presented in Table 1. Additionally, the value of treatment of mild to moderate hypertension, especially of the primary variety, is yet to be proven. There appears to be some consensus for instituting nonpharmacologic therapy for most young people with moderate or severe hypertension as the sole treatment where possible and, when drugs are needed, as a means of reducing dosage.

Prior to the institution of any therapeutic program, it is necessary to characterize the level of blood pressure elevation and decide on a workup plan. The United States Task Force scheme (Fig. 1) is helpful for this purpose. If at all possible, treatment should be directed at an underlying condition. When indicated, surgical relief of conditions causing hypertension should be carried out, even in infants. Those with severe hypertension (blood pressure above the 99th percentile) will probably need drug therapy. They, like others with lesser blood pressure elevations, are likely to benefit from nonpharmacologic therapy. In all but urgent situations it is best to procrastinate with treatment while workup is in progress to allow for some "regression of the blood pressure toward the mean."

Among the nonpharmacologic measures, weight reduction, in those over the mean weight for age, is likely to be most beneficial and most difficult. Motivational problems, difficulty in maintenance of the loss, and avoidance of eating disorders plague such therapy. Use of a low fat, low sodium, and high fiber, high potassium diet with avoidance of calcium deficiency is reasonable despite the continued debate of these recommendations. It is generally agreed that certain subgroups will respond to some of these measures and that no harm will come from them. Endurance exercise also has been shown to be beneficial. All but those known to have extreme hypertension should be permitted to participate in all sports activities, with parental concurrence. Alcohol and smoking avoidance are recognized healthy habits which affect blood pressure favorably. Stress avoidance and relaxation while useful a priori, remain unproven as an adjunct to hypertension therapy.

About one in a thousand young persons will need drug treatment for hypertension. When very high blood pressure is found (30% to 50% over the 95th percentile), or in those with high blood pressure and overt signs of encephalopathy or cardiac failure signs, emergency drug therapy must be started at once. The latter will require I.V. nitroprusside and the former sublingual nifedipine (Table 4). Other measures such as diuretics and inotropic support may be needed as well.

Those with moderate to severe pressure elevation failing to respond to nonpharmacologic measures and for whom there is concern about target-organ damage, a pharmacologic program should be considered. At present, an individualized "stepped-care" approach is recommended. Selection of the initial drug for therapy can be from the traditional diuretic (hydrochlorothiazide–Table 5), β-blocker (atenolol–Table 6) groups, the more recently developed calcium entry blockers (nifedipine–Table 7), or angiotensin-converting enzyme inhibitors (enalapril–Table 7). The selected drug is begun in low doses along with continued nonpharmacologic treatment. The dosage can be titrated upward but generally, if the response is not optimal, it is best to substitute another drug or add a second drug. If a more complicated therapeutic program is needed, discretion calls for consultation with a specialist in pediatric hypertension.

A number of other drugs are available to treat hypertension. These include α-antagonists such as prazosin. It is of value, despite a first-dose postural hypotensive effect, in patients with bronchospasm, heart failure, and in diabetes mellitus and hypercholesterolemic states. The α-agonist, methyldopa, is useful in pregnancy. Of the vasodilators, hydralazine is now given as part of triple therapy. Low-dose reserpine, a peripheral α-antagonist, together with a diuretic, offers safe and inexpensive blood pressure reduction.

When considering the antihypertensive pharmacopeia, the practitioner is best advised to prescribe a few medications which he/she knows well. Regular follow-up evaluations for the treated patient are in order. After several years of successful treatment, a medication withdrawal program can be tried. By the outlined methodology, almost all hypertensive young people cannot only experience some relief of their disease process but also be guided into preparation for a healthy, productive adulthood.

References

1. Tobian L, Sugimoto T, Everson T. High K diets protect arteries, possibly by lowering renal papillary Na and thereby increasing interstitial cell secretion. *Hypertension* 20:403, 1992. Abstract 29.
2. Wu JN, Zhang L, King S, Edwards D, Berecek KH. Early treatment with captopril permanently alters hypertension in spontaneously hypertensive rats. *Hypertension* 20:401, 1992. Abstract 19.
3. National Heart, Lung, and Blood Institute's Task Force on Blood Pressure Control in Children. Report of the second task force on blood pressure control in children. *Pediatrics* 79:1-25, 1987.
4. Hohn AR, Riopel DA, Keil JE, Loadholt CB, Margolius HS, Halushka PV, Privitera PJ, Webb JG, Medley ES, Schuman SH, Rubin MI, Pantel RH, Braunstein ML. Childhood, familial, and racial differences

in physiologic and biochemical factors related to hypertension. *Hypertension* 5:56-70, 1983.

5. Kaas-Ibsen K. Normal and abnormal blood pressure in childhood. *Child Nephrol Urol* 12:90-95, 1992.

6. Stamler R, Stamler J, Gosch FC, Civinelli J, Fishman J, McKeever P, McDonald A, Dyer A. Primary prevention of hypertension by nutritional-hygienic means: final report of a randomized, controlled trial. *JAMA* 262:1801-1807, 1989.

7. Normal High Blood Pressure Education Program Working Group. Report on primary prevention of hypertension. *Arch Intern Med* 153:186-208, 1993.

8. Sinaiko AR, Wells TG. Childhood hypertension. In: Laragh JH, Brenner BM, eds. *Hypertension: Pathophysiology, Diagnosis, and Management.* New York: Raven Press; 1853-1868:1990.

9. Londe S, Bourgoignie JJ, Robson AM, Goldring D. Hypertension in apparently normal children. *J Pediatr* 78:569-577, 1971.

10. Staessen J, Fagard R, Lijnen P, Amery A. Body weight, sodium intake and blood pressure. *J Hypertens* 7(suppl I):S19-S23, 1989.

11. Schotte E, Stunkard AJ. The effects of weight reduction on blood pressure in 301 obese patients. *Arch Intern Med* 150:1701-1704, 1990.

12. Krieger DR, Landsberg L. Neuroendocrine mechanisms in obesity-related hypertension: the role of insulin and catecholamines. In: Laragh JH, Brenner BJM, Kaplan NM, eds. *Perspectives in Hypertension 2.* New York: Raven Press; 105- 128:1989.

13. Weinsier RL, James LD, Darnell BE, Dustan HP, Birch R, Hunter GR. Obesity-related hypertension: evaluation of the separate effects of energy restriction and weight reduction on hemodynamic and neuroendocrine status. *Am J Med* 90:460-468, 1991.

14. Fagerberg B, Anderson OK, Persson B, Hedner T. Reactivity to norepinephrine and effect of sodium on blood pressure during weight loss. *Hypertension* 7:586-592, 1985.

15. Rocchini AP, Katch V, Schork A, Kelch RP. Insulin and blood pressure during weight loss in obese adolescents. *Hypertension* 10:267-273, 1987.

16. Scherrer U, Nussberger J, Torriani S, Waeber B, Darioli R, Hofstter JR, Brunner HR. Effect of weight reduction in moderately overweight patients on recorded ambulatory blood pressure and free cytosolic platelet calcium. *Circulation* 83:552-558, 1991.

17. Clarke WR, Woolson RF, Lauer RM. Changes in ponderosity and blood pressure in childhood: the Muscatine Study. *Am J Epidemiol* 124:195-209, 1986.

18. Rocchini AP. Adolescent obesity and hypertension. *Pediatr Clin North Am* 40:81-92, 1993.

19. Sacks FM. Dietary fats and blood pressure: A critical review of the evidence. *Nutr Rev* 47:291-300, 1989.

20. Pacy PJ, Dodson PM, Kubicki AJ, Fletcher RF, Taylor KG. Comparison of the hypertensive and metabolic effects of bendrofluazide

therapy and a high fibre, low fat, low sodium diet in diabetic subjects with mild hypertension. *J Hypertens* 2:215-220, 1984.

21. Schlamowitz P, Halberg T, Warnoe O, Wilstrup F, Tyttig K. Treatment of mild to moderate hypertension with dietary fibre. *Lancet* 2:622-623, 1987.

22. Knapp HR, Fitzgerald GA. The antihypertensive effects of fish oil: a controlled study of polyunsaturated fatty acid supplements in essential hypertension. *N Engl J Med* 320:1037-1043, 1989.

23. Jenner DA, English DR, Vandongen R, Bjeilin LJ, Miller MR, Dunbar D. Diet and blood pressure in 9-year old Australian children. *Am J Clin Nutr* 47:1052-1059, 1988.

24. Rouse IL, Beilin LJ. Vegetarian and other complex diets, fiber intake, and blood pressure. In: Laragh JH, Brenner BM eds. *Hypertension: Pathophysiology, Diagnosis and Management.* New York: Raven Press; 241-255:1990.

25. Eliott P. Observational studies of salt and blood pressure. *Hypertension* 17(suppl I):I-3-I-8, 1991.

26. Pickering TG. Predicting the response to nonpharmacologic treatment in mild hypertension. *JAMA* 267:1256-1257, 1992. Editorial.

27. Final Report of the Subcommittee on Nonpharmacological Therapy of the 1984 Joint National Committee on Detection, Evacuation and Treatment of High Blood Pressure. Nonpharmacological approaches to the control of high blood pressure. *Hypertension* 8:444-467, 1986.

28. Swales JD. Non-drug therapy: salt, weight, alcohol, exercise and tobacco. In: Buhler FR, Laragh JH, eds. *Handbook of Hypertension 13: The Management of Hypertension.* New York: Elsevier; 334-350:1990.

29. Simpson FO. Blood pressure and sodium intake. In: Laragh JH, Brenner BM, eds. *Hypertension: Pathophysiology, Diagnosis and Management.* New York: Raven Press; 205-215:1990.

30. Hegsted DM. A perspective on reducing salt intake. *Hypertension* 17(suppl I):I-201-204, 1991.

31. MacGregor GA, Markandu ND, Sagnella GA, Singer DRJ, Cappucio FP. Double-blind study of three sodium intakes and long-term effects of sodium restriction in essential hypertension. *Lancet* 2:1244-1247, 1989.

32. The Trials of Hypertension Prevention Collaborative Research Group. The effects of nonpharmacologic interventions on blood pressure of persons with high normal levels: Results of the trials of hypertension prevention, phase 1. *JAMA* 267:1213-1220, 1992.

33. Omvik P, Lund-Johansen P. Comparison of long-term hemodynamic effects at rest and during exercise of lisinopril plus sodium restriction versus hydrochlorothiazide in essential hypertension. *Am J Cardiol* 65:331-338, 1990.

34. Rauh W, Levine LS. New MI. The role of dietary salt in juvenile hypertension. In: Giovanelli G, New MI, Gorini S, eds. *Hypertension in Children and Adolescents.* New York: Raven Press; 34-44:1981.

35. Tochikubo O, Sasaki O, Umemura S, Kaneko Y. Management of hypertension in high school students by using new salt titrator tape. *Hypertension* 8:1164-1171, 1986.
36. Ellison RC, Capper AL, Stephenson WP, Goldberg RJ, Hosmer DW Jr, Humphry KF, Ockene JK, Gamble WJ, Witschi JC, Stare FJ. Effects on blood pressure of a decrease in sodium use in institutional food preparation: the Exeter-Andover project. *J Clin Epidemiol* 42:201-208, 1989.
37. Lieberman E. Hypertension in childhood and adolescence. In: Kaplan NM, ed. *Clinical Hypertension, 5th ed.* Baltimore: Williams and Wilkins; 407-433, 1990.
38. Sinaiko AR. General considerations and clinical approach to the management of hypertension. In: Loggie JMH, ed. *Pediatric and Adolescent Hypertension.* Boston: Blackwell Scientific Pub; 119-126:1992.
39. Houtman PN, Dillon MJ. Medical management of hypertension in childhood. *Child Nephrol Urol* 12:154-161, 1992.
40. Meneely G, Battarbee HD. High sodium-low potassium environment and hypertension. *Am J Cardiol* 38:768-785, 1976.
41. Langford HG. Potassium in hypertension. *Postgrad Med* 73:227-233, 1983.
42. Tannen RL. Effects of potassium on blood pressure control. *Ann Intern Med* 98:773-780, 1983.
43. McCarron DA. Is calcium more important than sodium in the pathogenesis of essential hypertension? *Hypertension* 7:607-623, 1985.
44. Intersalt Research Group. Intersalt: an international cooperative study on electrolytes and blood pressure. *Br Med J* 297:319-328, 1988.
45. Criqui MH, Langer RD, Reed DM. Dietary alcohol, calcium, and potassium: independent and combined effects on blood pressure. *Circulation* 80:609-614, 1989.
46. Battarbee HD, Funch DP, Daily JW. The effect of dietary sodium and potassium upon blood pressure and catecholamine excretion in the rat. *Proc Soc Exp Biol Med* 161:32-37, 1979.
47. Young DB, Tipayamontri. Effects of high potassium intake on experimental angiotensin II hypertension. *Physiologist* 24:6, 1981.
48. Mark AL, Gordon FJ, Becker PA. Mechanisms of the antihypertensive action of high dietary potassium. *Clin Res* 29:525A, 1981. Abstract.
49. Overlack A, Muller H-M, Kolloch R, Ollig A, Moch B, Kleinmann R, Kruck F, Stumpe KO. Long-term antihypertensive effect of oral potassium in essential hypertension. *J Hypertens* 1(suppl 2):165-167, 1983.
50. Miller JZ, Weinberger MH, Christian JC. Blood pressure response to potassium supplementation in normotensive adults and children. *Hypertension* 10:437-442, 1987.
51. Beilin LJ. State of the Art Lecture. Diet and hypertension: critical concepts and controversies. *J Hypertens* 5(suppl 5):S447-S457, 1987.
52. Matlou SM, Isles CG, Higgs A , Milne GH, Murray GD, Schultz E, Starke IF. Potassium supplementation in blacks with mild to moderate essential hypertension. *J Hypertens* 4:61-64, 1986.
53. Kaplan NM, Carnegie A, Raskin P, Heller JA, Simmons M. Potassium

supplementation in hypertensive patients with diuretic- induced hypokalemia. *N Engl J Med* 312:746-749, 1985.

54. Kurtz TW, Morris RC Jr. Dietary chloride as a determinant of "sodium-dependent" hypertension. *Science* 22:1139-1141, 1983.

55. Svetkey LP, Klotman PE. Blood pressure and potassium intake. In: Laragh JH, Brenner BM, eds. *Hypertension: Pathophysiology, Diagnosis, and Management.* New York: Raven Press; 217-227:1990.

56. Khaw KT, Barrett-Connor E. Dietary potassium and stroke-associated mortality: a 12-year prospective population study. *N Engl J Med* 316:235-240, 1987.

57. Reed D, McGee D, Yano K. Biological and social correlates of blood pressure among Japanese men in Hawaii. *Hypertension* 4:406-414, 1982.

58. Ackly S, Barrett-Connor E, Suarez L. Dairy products, calcium, and blood pressure. *Am J Clin Nutr* 38:457-461, 1983.

59. Harlan WR, Hull AL, Schmouder RL, Landis JR, Thompson FE, Larkin FA. Blood pressure and nutrition in adults: the National Health and Nutrition Examination Survey. *Am J Epidemiol* 120:17-18, 1984.

60. Garcia-Palmieri MR, Costos R Jr, Cruz-Videl M, Sorlie PD, Tillotson J, Havlik RJ. Milk consumption, calcium intake, and decreased hypertension in Puerto Rico. *Hypertension* 6:322- 328, 1984.

61. Belizan JM, Villar J, Pineda O, Gonzalez AE, Sainz E, Garrera G, Sibrian R. Reduction of blood pressure with calcium supplementation in young adults. *JAMA* 249:1161-1165, 1983.

62. McCarron DA, Morris CD. Blood pressure response to oral calcium in persons with mild to moderate hypertension. *Ann Intern Med* 103:825-831, 1985.

63. Grobbee DE, Hofman A. Effect of calcium supplementation on diastolic blood pressure in young people with mild hypertension. *Lancet* 2:703-707, 1986.

64. Meese RB, Gonzales DG, Casparian JM, Ram CVS, Pak CM, Kaplan NM. The inconsistent effects of calcium supplements upon blood pressure in primary hypertension. *Am J Med Sci* 294:219-224, 1987.

65. Zoccali C, Mallamaci F, Delfin D, Ciccarelli M, Parlongo S, Iellamo D, Moscato D, Maggiore Q. Double-blind randomized, crossover trial of calcium supplementation in essential hypertension. *J Hypertension* 6:451-455, 1988.

66. Cappuccio FP, Siani A, Strazzullo P. Oral calcium supplementation and blood pressure: an overview of randomized controlled trials. *J Hypertens* 7:941-946, 1989.

67. Johnson NE, Smith EL, Freudenheim JL. Effects on blood pressure of calcium supplementation of women. *Am J Clin Nutr* 42:12-17, 1985.

68. Taufield PA, Ales KL, Resnick LM, Gertner JM, Laragh JH. Hypocalcemia in preeclampsia. *N Engl J Med* 316:715-718, 1987.

69. Dwyer JH, Dwyer KM, Scribner R, Hohn A. Effect of calcium supplementation on blood pressure in African American youth. *33rd Annual Conference on Cardiovascular Disease Epidemiology.* Santa Fe NM, 1993. Abstract.

70. Resnick LM. Uniformity and diversity of calcium metabolism in hypertension: a conceptual framework. *Am J Med* 82(suppl 1B):16-20, 1987.
71. Kaplan NM. Calcium and potassium in the treatment of essential hypertension. *Sem Nephrol* 8:176-184, 1988.
72. Garcia Zozaya JL, Padilla Viloria M, Vanezuela V, Castro A. Normotension with decreased plasma renin activity and low serum ionic calcium levels: a prehypertensive state? *South Med J* 82:686-691, 1989.
73. Hofman A, Walter HJ, Connelly PA, Vaughan RD. Blood pressure and physical fitness in children. *Hypertension* 9:188-191, 1987.
74. Fripp RR, Hodgson JL, Werner JC, Schuler HG, Whitman V. Aerobic capacity, obesity, and atherosclerotic risk factors in male adolescents. *Pediatrics* 75:813-818, 1985.
75. Fagard R, Bielen E, Hespel P, Lijnen P, Staessen J, Vanhees L, Van Hoof R, Amery A. Physical exercise in hypertension. In: Laragh JH, Brenner BM, eds. *Hypertension: Pathophysiology, Diagnosis and Management.* New York: Raven Press; 1985-1998, 1990.
76. Bonanno JA, Lies JE. Effects of physical training on coronary risk factors. *Am J Cardiol* 33:760-764, 1974.
77. Roman O, Camuzzi AL, Villalon E, Klenner C. Physical training program in arterial hypertension: a long-term prospective follow-up. *Cardiology* 67:230-243, 1981.
78. Kukkonen K, Rauramaa R, Voutilainen E, Lansimies E. Physical training of middle-aged men with borderline hypertension. *Ann Clin Res* 14(suppl 34):139-145, 1982.
79. Hagberg JM, Goldring D, Ehsani AA, Heath GW, Hernandez A, Schechtman K, Holloszy JO. Effect of exercise training on the blood pressure and hemodynamic features of hypertensive adolescents. *Am J Cardiol* 52:263-268, 1983.
80. Somers VK, Conway J, Sleight P. Physical training and ambulatory and sleep blood pressures in borderline hypertensive patients. *The 12th Scientific Meeting of the International Society of Hypertension.* 1183:1988. Programs and Abstract.
81. Fripp RR, Hodgson JL. Effect of resistive training on plasma lipid and lipoprotein levels in male adolescents. *J Pediatr* 111:926-931, 1987.
82. Hagberg JM, Ehsani AA, Goldring D, Hernandez A, Sinacore DR, Holloszy JO. Effect of weight training on blood pressure and hemodynamics in hypertensive adolescents. *J Pediatr* 104:147-151, 1984.
83. Maron BL, Roberts WC, McAllister HA, Rosing DR, Epstein SE. Sudden death in young athletes. *Circulation* 62:218-229, 1980.
84. Strong WB. Hypertension and sports. *Pediatrics* 64:693-695, 1979.
85. Nielsen B, Kubica R, Bonnesen A, Rasmussen IB, Stoklosa J, Wilk B. Physical work capacity after dehydration and hyperthermia. *Scan J Sports Sci* 3:2-10, 1981.
86. Ades PA, Gunther PGS, Meacham CP, Handy MA, LeWinter MM. Hypertension, exercise, and β-adrenergic blockade. *Ann Intern Med* 109:629-634, 1988.
87. Fagard R, Lijnen P, Vanhees L, Smery A. Hemodynamic response to

converting enzyme inhibition at rest and exercise in humans. *J Appl Physiol* 53:576-581, 1982.

88. Duffey DJ, Horwitz LD, Brammell HL. Nifedipine and the conditioning response. *Am J Cardiol* 53:908-911, 1984.

89. Paffenbarger RS, Hyde RT, Wing AL, Hsieh CC. Physical activity, all-cause mortality, and longevity of college alumni. *N Engl J Med* 314:605-613, 1986.

90. Blair SN, Goodyear NN, Gibbons LW, Cooper KH. Physical fitness and incidence of hypertension in healthy normotensive men and women. *JAMA* 252:487-490, 1984.

91. Strazzullo P, Cappuccio FP, Trevisan M, De Leo A, Krogh V, Giorgione N, Mancini M. Leisure time physical activity and blood pressure in schoolchildren. *Am J Epidemiol* 127:726-733, 1988.

92. Wilson JF, Straus R. Behavioral considerations in high blood pressure in the young. In: Kotchen TA, Kotchen JM, eds. Clinical Approaches to High Blood Pressure in the Young. Boston: John Wright; 277-299:1983.

93. Schnall PL, Pieper C, Schwartz JE, Karasek RA, Schlussel Y, Devereux RB, Ganau A, Alderman M, Warren K, Pickering TG. The relationship between "job strain," workplace diastolic blood pressure, and left ventricular mass index: results of a case- control study. *JAMA* 263:1929-1935, 1990.

94. Pickering TG, Harshfield GA, Klinert HD, Blank S, Laragh JH. Blood pressure during daily activities, sleep and exercise. JAMA 247:992-996, 1982.

95. Patel C, Marmot MG, Terry DJ, Carruthers M, Hunt B, Patel M. Trial of relaxation in reducing coronary risk: four year follow-up. *Br Med J* 290:1103-1106, 1985.

96. Goldstein IG, Shapiro D, Thananopavaran C. Home relaxation techniques for essential hypertension. *Psychosom Med* 46:398-414, 1984.

97. Cottier C, Shapiro K, Julius S. Treatment of hypertension with progressive muscular relaxation. *Arch Intern Med* 144:1954-1958, 1984.

98. Beutler JJ. Attevelt JTM, Schouten SA, Faber JAJ, Mees EJD, Geijskes GG. Paranormal healing and hypertension. *Br Med J* 296:1491-1494, 1988.

99. Julius S, Petrin J. Autonomic nervous and behavioral factors in hypertension: a rationale for treatment. In: Laragh JH, Brenner BM, eds. *Hypertension: Pathophysiology, Diagnosis and Management.* New York: Raven Press; 1985-1998:1990.

100. Benson H, Kotch JB, Crassweller KD, Greenwood MM. Historical and clinical considerations of the relaxation response. *Am Sci* 65:441-445, 1977.

101. Klatsky AL. Blood pressure and alcohol intake. In: Laragh JH, Brenner BM, eds. *Hypertension: Pathophysiology, Diagnosis and Management.* New York: Raven Press; 1985-1998:1990.

102. Sjtrogatz DS, James SA, Haines PS, Elmer PJ, Gerber AM, Browning SR, Amerman AS, Keenan NL. Alcohol consumption and blood pressure in black adults: the Pitt County Study. *Am J Epidemiol* 133:442-450, 1991.

103. Kaplan NM. Bashing booze: the danger of losing the benefits of moderate alcohol consumption. *Am Heart J* 121:1854-1856, 1991.
104. Criqui MH, Wallace RB, Mishkel M, Barrett-Conner E, Heiss G. Alcohol consumption and blood pressure: the Lipid Research Clinics Prevalence Study. *Hypertension* 3:557-565, 1981.
105. Friedman GD, Klatsky AL, Siegelaub AB. Alcohol, tobacco and hypertension. *Hypertension* 2(suppl III):143-150, 1982.
106. Ilses C, Brown JJ, Cumming AMM, Lever AF, McAreavey D, Robertson JIS, Hawthorne VM, Stewart GM, Robertson JWK, Wapshaw J. Excess smoking in malignant-phase hypertension. *Br Med J* 1:579-581, 1979.
107. Seltzer CC. Effect of smoking on blood pressure. Am Heart J 87:558-564, 1974.
108. Hohn AR. The Pasadena Study: Unpublished data, 1987.
109. Dwyer JH, Lippert P, Rieger-Ndakorerwa GE, Semmer NK. Some chronic disease risk factors and cigarette smoking in adolescents: the Berlin-Bremen Study. *MMWR* 36 (Suppl 4):S36-S40, 1988.
110. Houtman PN, Dillon MJ. Medical management of hypertension in childhood. *Child Nephrol Urol* 12:154-161, 1992.
111. Kotchen JM, Holley J, Kotchen TA. Treatment of high blood pressure in the young. *Semin Nephrol* 9:296-303, 1989.
112. Gruskin AB, Lerner GR, Fleischmann FE. Diuretic usage in hypertensive children. In: Loggie JMH, ed. *Pediatric and Adolescent Hypertension*. Boston: Blackwell Scientific Pub; 127-137:1992.
113. Grimm RH. Thiazide diuretics and selective α-blockers: comparison of use in antihypertensive therapy, including possible differences in coronary heart disease risk reduction. *Am J Med* 1A:26-30,1987.
114. Krakoff LR, Eison H, Phillips RH, Leiman SJ, Lev S. Effect of ambulatory blood pressure monitoring on the diagnosis and cost of treatment for mild hypertension. *Am Heart J* 116:1152-1154, 1988.
115. The International Committee of the Second International Symposium on Hypertension in Children and Adolescents. Recommendations for management of hypertension in children and adolescents. *Pediatr Nephrol* 1:56-58, 1987.
116. 1988 Joint National Committee (National High Blood Pressure Education Program). The 1988 report of the Joint National Committee on detection, evaluation and treatment of high blood pressure. *Arch Intern Med* 148:1023-1038, 1988.
117. Joint National Committee. The Fifth report of the Joint National Committee report on detection, evaluation and treatment of high blood pressure. *Arch Intern Med* 153:154-184, 1993.
118. McVeigh G, Galloway D, Johnston D. The case for low dose diuretics in hypertension: comparison of low and conventional doses of cyclopenthiazide. *Br Med J* 297:95-98, 1988.
119. Hawkins DW, Dieckmann MR, Horner RD. Diuretics and hypertension in black adults. *Arch Intern Med* 148:803-805, 1988.
120. Dillon MJ. Investigation and management of hypertension in children. *Pediatr Nephrol* 1:59-68, 1987.

121. Pollare T, Lithell H, Berne C. A comparison of the effects of hydrochlorothiazide and captopril on glucose and lipid metabolism in patients with hypertension. *N Engl J Med* 321:868-873, 1989.

122. Pollare T, Lithell H, Morlin C, Prantare H, Hvarfner A, Ljunghall S. Metabolic effects of diltiazem and atenolol: results from a randomized, double-blind study with parallel groups. *J Hypertens* 7:551-559, 1989.

123. Evans CE, Haynes RB, Goldsmith CH, Hewson SA. Home blood pressure-measuring devices: a comparative study of accuracy. *J Hypertens* 7:133-142, 1989.

124. Zachariah PK, Sheps SG, Ilstrup DM, Long CR, Bailey KR, Wiltgen CM, Carlson CA. Blood pressure load: a better determinant of hypertension. *Mayo Clin Proc* 63:1085-1091, 1988.

125. Houston MC. Abrupt cessation of treatment in hypertension: consideration of clinical features, mechanisms, presentation, and management of a discontinuation syndrome. Am Heart J 102:415-430, 1981.

126. Abrams JH, Schulman P, White WB. Successful treatment of a monoamine oxidase inhibitor-tyramine hypertensive emergency with intravenous labetalol. *N Engl J Med* 313:52, 1985.

127. Taketomo C. *Pediatric Dosing Handbook and Formulary. 7th ed.* Hudson Lexi-Comp; 1992.

128. Angeli P, Chiesa M, Caregaro L, Merkel C, Sacerdote D, Rondana M, Gatta A. Comparison of sublingual captopril and nifedipine in immediate treatment of hypertensive emergencies: a randomized, single-blind clinical trial. *Arch Intern Med* 151:678-682. 1991.

129. Cockcroft JR, Dollery CT. The diuretic dilemma. In: Buhler FR, Laragh JH, eds. *Handbook of Hypertension 13: The Management of Hypertension.* New York: Elsevier; 202-216:1990.

130. Wells TG. The pharmacology and therapeutics of diuretics in the pediatric patient. *Pediatr Clin North Am* 37:463-504, 1990.

131. Warram JH, Laffel LMB, Valsania P, Christlieb AR, Krolewski AS. Excess mortality associated with diuretic therapy in diabetes mellitus. *Arch Intern Med* 151:1350-1356, 1991.

132. Dorup I, Skajaa K, Clausen T, Kjeldsen K. Reduced concentrations of potassium, magnesium, and sodium-potassium pumps in human skeletal muscle during treatment with diuretics. Br Med J 296:455-458, 1988.

133. Ruilope LM, Alcazar JM, Hernandez E, Moreno F, Martinez MA, Rodicio JL. Does an adequate control of blood pressure protect the kidney in essential hypertension? *J Hypertens* 8:525-531, 1990.

134. McVeigh G, Galloway D, Johnston D. The case for low dose diuretics in hypertension: comparison of low and conventional doses of cyclopenthiazide. *Br Med J* 297:95-98, 1988.

135. Carlsen JE, Kober L, Torp-Pedersen C, Johansen P. Relation between dose of bendrofluazide, antihypertensive effect, and adverse biochemical effects. *Br Med J* 300:975-978, 1990.

136. Clementy J, Schwebig A, Mazaud C, Bricaud H. Comparative study of the efficacy and tolerance of capozide and monodiuretic adminis-

tered in a single daily dose for the treatment of chronic moderate arterial hypertension. *Postgrad Med J* 62(suppl 1):132-134, 1986.

137. Prebis J, Gruskin A, Baluarte J, Polinsky M, Katz S. Dual response to furosemide (F) in hypertensive children and its relationship to hyperuricemia. *Circulation* 60(suppl 2):II-207, 1979. Abstract.

138. Weinberger MH. Diuretics and their side effects. Dilemma in the treatment of hypertension. *Hypertension* 11(suppl II):II 16-II 20, 1988.

139. Ponce FE, Williams LC, Webb HM, Riopel DA, Hohn AR. Propranolol palliation of Tetralogy of Fallot: experience with long-term drug treatment in pediatric patients. *Pediatrics* 52:100-108, 1973.

140. Frishman WH. Beta-adrenergic receptor blockers: Adverse effects and drug interactions. *Hypertension* 11(suppl II):II 21-II 29, 1988.

141. Frohlich ED, Dunn FG, Messerli FH. Pharmacologic and physiologic considerations of adrenoceptor blockade. *Am J Med* 17:9-14, 1983.

142. Bolli P, Fernandez PG, Buhler FR. β-blockers in the treatment of hypertension. In: Laragh JH, Brenner BM eds. Hypertension: Pathophysiology, Diagnosis and Management. New York: Raven Press; 1985-1998:1990.

143. Saunders E, Weir MR, Kong BW, Hollifield J, Gray J, Vertes V, Sowers JR, Zemel MB, Curry C, Schoenberger J, Wright JT, Kirkendall W, Conradi EC, Jenkins P, McLean B, Massie B, Berenson G, Flamenbaum W. A comparison of the efficacy and safety of a β-blocker, a calcium channel blocker, and a converting enzyme inhibitor in hypertensive blacks. *Arch Intern Med* 150:1707-1713, 1990.

144. Velasco M, Hurt E, Silva H, et al. Effects of prazosin and propranolol on blood lipids and lipoproteins in hypertensive patients. *Am J Med* 80: 109-113, 1986.

145. Maruyama H, Saruta T, Koyama K, Kido K, Itoh K, Takei I, Kataoka K. Effect of α-adrenergic blockade on blood pressure, glucose, and lipid metabolism in hypertensive patients with non- insulin-dependent diabetes mellitus. *Am Heart J* 121:1302-1306, 1991.

146. Feher MD. Doxazosin therapy in the treatment of diabetic hypertension. *Am Heart J* 121:1294-1301, 1991.

147. Kaplan NM. *Clinical Hypertension, 5th ed.* Baltimore: Williams & Wilkins; 204-206:1990.

148. Participating Veterans Administration Medical Centers. Low doses vs standard dose of reserpine: A randomized, double-blind, multiclinic trial in patients taking chlorthalidone. *JAMA* 248:2471-2477, 1982.

149. Cunningham FG, Lindheimer MD. Hypertension in pregnancy. *N Engl J Med* 326:927-932, 1992.

150. Bartsch P, Maggiorini M, Ritter M, Noti C, Vock P, Oelz O. Prevention of high-altitude pulmonary edema by nifedipine. *N Engl J Med* 325:1284-1289, 1991.

151. Kaplan NM. Calcium entry blockers in the treatment of hypertension. *JAMA* 262:817-823, 1988.

152. Lerner GR, Gruskin AB. Calcium channel antagonists and ACE

inhibitors. In: Loggie JMH, ed. *Pediatric and Adolescent Hypertension.* Boston: Blackwell Scientific Pub; 159-177:1992.

153. Reams GP, Homory A, Lau A, Bauer JH. Effect of nifedipine on renal function in patients with essential hypertension. Hypertension 11:425-456, 1988.

154. Mimran A, Insua A, Ribstein J, Monnier L, Bringer J, Mirouze J. Contrasting effects of captopril and nifedipine in normotensive patients with incipient diabetic nephropathy. *J Hypertens* 6:919-923, 1989.

155. Williams GH. Converting enzyme inhibitors in the treatment of hypertension. *N Engl J Med* 319:1517-1525, 1988.

156. Dunn FG, Oigman W, Ventura HO, Messerli FH, Koterin I, Frohlich ED. Enalapril improves systemic and renal hemodynamics and allows regression of left ventricular mass in essential hypertension. *Am J Cardiol* 53:105-108, 1984.

157. Trachtman H, Gauthier B. Effect of angiotensin-converting enzyme inhibitor therapy of proteinuria in children with renal disease. *J Pediatr* 112:295-297, 1988.

158. Pollare T, Lithell H, Berne C. A comparison of the effects of hydrochlorothiazide and captopril in glucose and lipid metabolism in patients with hypertension. *N Engl J Med* 321:868-873, 1988.

159. Gavras H, Gavras I. Angiotensin converting enzyme inhibitors: properties and side effects. *Hypertension* 11(suppl II):II-37-II-41, 1988.

160. Collaste P, Haglund K, Lundgren G, Magnusson G, Ostman J. Reversible renal failure during treatment with captopril. *Br Med J* 2:612-613, 1979.

161. Kripalani KJ, McKinistry DN, Singhavi SM, Willard DA, Vukovich RA, Migdalof BM. Disposition of captopril in normal subjects. *Clin Pharmacol Ther* 27:636-641, 1980.

162. Vlasses PH, Conner DP, Rotmensch HH, Fruncillo RJ, Danzeisen Jr, Shepley KJ, Ferguson RK. Low doses vs. standard dose of reserpine: Double-blind comparison of captopril and enalapril in mild to moderate hypertension. *J Am Coll Cardiol* 7:651-660, 1986.

163. Conway J, Coats AJS, Bird R. Lisinopril and enalapril in hypertension: a comparative study using ambulatory monitoring. *J Hum Hyperten* 4:235-239, 1990.

164. Luderer JR, Hayer HH, Dubynsky O, Berlin CM. Long-term administration of sodium nitroprusside in childhood. *J Pediatr* 91:490-491, 1977.

165. Koch-Weser J. Hydralazine. *N Engl J Med* 295:736-742, 1976.

166. Strife CF, Quinlan M, Waldo FB, Fryer CJ, Jackson EC, Welch TR, McEnery PT, West CD. Minoxidil for control of acute blood pressure elevation in chronically hypertensive children. *Pediatrics* 78:861-865, 1986.

167. Sinaiko AR, O'Dea RF, Mirkin BL. Clinical response of hypertensive children to long-term minoxidil therapy. *J Cardiovasc Pharmacol* 2:S181-S188, 1980.

APPENDIX

The forgoing text was written to guide the provider of pediatric health care through the subject of hypertension in the young. While information concerning the great majority of disorders resulting in hypertension in this age group is contained in the presented material, a number of other conditions exist that are also associated with elevated blood pressure in the pediatric age group. Rather than expand the text-proper material, or omit those conditions, the author felt it best to offer the reader the opportunity to know of them from the list in Appendix A. The option exists to explore them by seeking additional information on a cause in question from the references provided in Appendix B or from a literature search.

A. Other Causes of Hypertension

1. Acromegaly
2. Burn injures.
3. Carcinoid
4. Cardiac surgery
5. Central nervous system disorders
    infections
    tumors
    dysautonomia (including Riley-Day syndrome)
    Guillain-Barre syndrome
6. Cold exposure
7. Elevated blood pressure in athletes.
8. Heavy metal poisoning (lead, mercury)
9. Hormonal replacement therapy
10. Hyperviscosity including polycythemia
11. Iatrogenic including volume overload
12. Orthopedic conditions including traction/immobilization
13. Pancreatitis
14. Porphyria
15. Psychogenic causes including hyperventilation syndromes
16. Sickle-cell crisis
17. Sleep apnea
18. Turner's syndrome (without aortic coarctation)

B. Other Texts on Hypertension

1. Berenson GS, McMahan CA, Voors AW, Webber LS, Srinivasan SR, Frank GC, Foster TA, Blonde CV, eds. *Cardiovascular Risk Factors in Children.* New York: Oxford University Press; 1980.

2. Buhler FR, Laragh JH, eds. *Handbook of Hypertension 13: The Management of Hypertension.* New York: Elsevier; 1990.

3. Genest J, Koiw E, Kuchel O, eds. *Hypertension Pathophysiology and Treatment.* New York: McGraw-Hill; 1977.

4. Giovanelli G, New MI, Gorini S, eds. *Hypertension in Children and Adolescents.* New York: Raven Press; 1981.

5. Ingelfinger JR. *Pediatric Hypertension.* Philadelphia: WB Saunders; 1982.

6. Kaplan NM. *Clinical Hypertension,* 5th ed. Baltimore: Williams & Wilkins; 1990.

7. Kotchen TA, Kotchen JM, eds. *Clinical Approaches to High Blood Pressure in the Young.* Boston: John Wright; 1983.

8. Laragh JH, Brenner BM, eds. *Hypertension: Pathophysiology, Diagnosis, and Management.* New York: Elsevier; 1990.

9. Loggie JMH, ed. *Pediatric and Adolescent Hypertension.* Boston: Blackwell Scientific; 1992.

10. Loggie JMH, Horan MH, Gruskin AB, Hohn AR, Dunbar JB, Havlick RJ, eds, NHLBI Workshop on Juvenile Hypertension. *Proceedings from a Symposium.* New York: Biomedical Information Corp, 1984.

11. Hypertension. *Pediatr Clin North Am 40,* 1993.

12. Soffer RL, ed. *Biochemical Regulation of Blood Pressure.* New York: John Wiley and Sons; 1989.

Index

Abdominal coarctation, 121
ACTH, 165
Adolescent
 primary hypertension, 211
 secondary hypertension, 213-214
Adrenal cortical hypertension, 159-161
Adrenal hyperplasia, congenital,
 hypertension, 170-171
Adrenal medulla, 172
Age, hypertension, 55
Alcohol
 childhood risk factors for hypertension, 89-91
 hypertension, 247-248
Aldosterone, 21
Aldosteronism, hypertension, 161-164
Algorithm, blood pressure, 48
Alpha-antagonist, agonists, 260-261
Ambulatory monitoring, blood pressure, 45-46
Analgesic-anti-inflammatory
 childhood risk factors for hypertension, 91
Anatomy, cardiac hypertension, 106-107
Angioplasty, 147,148
Angiotensin, 12-17
Angiotensin converting enzyme inhibitor,
 263-265
Antacid, hypertension, 91
Antiasthmatic, hypertension, 91
Antibiotic, hypertension, 91
Anticonvulsant, hypertension, 91
Antihistamine, 91
Antidiuretic hormone (vasopressin), 26
Anxiety, childhood risk factors for
 hypertension, 85-87
Aortoplasty, 118
Ask-Upmark kidney, 136
Atanolol, 258
Autoregulation, blood pressure, 19-20

Bainbridge reflex, 11
Balloon dilation aortoplasty, cardiac
 hypertension, 113-115
Baroreflexes, 7-9
Beta-adrenergic receptor stimulation blockers,
 258-260
Birth control, hypertension, 91
 algorithm, 48
Blood pressure risk factors, 74
 childhood risk factors for hypertension, 76-77
 control mechanisms, 6-27
 exercise pressure, 47
 hemodynamic principles, 2-4
 mercury manometer, 1
 neonate, influencing factors in, 187-188

neurotransmitters, 7
plasma-renin activity, influences on, 16
race, 17
renin-angiotensin system, 12-17, 20
resting pressure, 46-47
Blood pressure control mechanisms
 autoregulation, 19-20
 humoral factors, 11-17, 20-27
 kidney-blood volume, 17-19
 major factors affecting blood pressure,
  summary, 28
 nervous system, 6-11
Blood pressure measurement
 ambulatory monitoring, 45-46
 compression cuff, 38-39
 infant, 43-45
 instrumentation, 39-40
 "K" phase, 38
 newborn, 43-45, 185-187
 oscillometric devices, 40
 recording of, 40-43
  child, 40-43
 strain-gauge plethysmography, 40
 technique, 38-46
 ultrasound-Doppler systems, 40
Blood volume, 17
Bradykinin, 24
Bright, Richard, blood pressure, 1
Bright's disease, 1

Calcium, 26
 childhood risk factors for hypertension,
  84-85
 entry blocker, 261-263
 hypertension, 64-66
 supplementation, hypertension, 244-245
Captopril, cardiac hypertension, 113, 255
 contraindicated, 92
Cardiac hypertension, 105-125
Cardiac output measurement, 3
Catecholamines, 172
Cations, 84
Catheter-related hypertension, newborn, 197
Chemoreceptor, 9-11
Child. See also Infant, Newborn
 coarctation, cardiac hypertension, 110-111
 evaluation, 214-215
 history, 215-217, 223-230
 laboratory studies, 218-222
 physical evaluation, 217-218
 primary hypertension, 211
 secondary hypertension, 212-213
 treatment, 233-278

Childhood risk factors for hypertension, 76-77
  alcohol, 89-91
  analgesic, 91
  antacid, 91
  antiasthmatic, 91
  antibiotic, 91
  anticonvulsant, 91
  antihistamine, 91
  anxiety, 85-87
  blood pressure, 76-77
  calcium, 84-85
  decongestant, 91
  diabetes mellitus, 93
  diet, 82-85
  diuretic, 91
  drugs, 89-91
  exercise, 85-87
  heredity, 77-79
  left ventricular hypertrophy, 94
  magnesium, 85
  maternal factors, 91-93
  medications, 89-91
  obesity, 79-80
  potassium, 83-84
  race, 80-81
  smoking, 87-89
  sodium, 82-83
  stress, 85-87
  uric acid, 93
  vitamin supplement, 91
Clinical patterns, cardiac hypertension,
  109-111
Clonidine, 260
Coarctation
  abdominal coarctation, 121
  anatomy, 106-107
  balloon dilation aortoplasty, 113-115
  captopril, 113
  childhood coarctation, 110-111
  clinical patterns, 109-111
  coarctation, 106-107
  digoxin, 112
  embryology, 106-107
  hydralazine, 113
  infantile coarctation syndrome, 109-110
  mechanical factors, 107-108
  medication, 112-113
  neural mechanisms, 108-109
  nitroprusside, 113
  pathophysiology, 107-109
  postcoarctation repair syndromes, 116-119
  propranolol, 113
  prostaglandin, 113
  protocol for diagnosis, 111-112
  pseudocoarctation, 121-122
  recurrent coarctation, 120
  regional vascular factors, 109
  renal mechanisms, 108
  residual coarctation, 120
  surgical repair, 115-116
  treatment, 112-116
  recurrent, hypertension, cardiac, 120
  residual, hypertension, cardiac, 120
Cocaine, 91
Compression cuff, blood pressure
  measurement, 38-39
Conn's syndrome, 159
Contraceptives, 91
Control mechanisms, blood pressure, 6-27
Cortisol, 165
Cuff, blood pressure measurement, 38-39
Cushing's syndrome, hypertension, 165-170
Cyclosporin hypertension, 90
Cystic kidney disease, renal hypertension, 140

Decongestant
  childhood risk factor for hypertension, 91
  hypertension, 91
Diabetes mellitus
  childhood risk factor for hypertension, 93
  hypertension, 178
Diagnosis, hypertension, 236-237
Dialysis, 127
Diazoxide, 254
Diet
  childhood risk factors for hypertension,
    82-85
  influences, hypertension, 61-66
  low fat-high fiber, 240-241
Digoxin, cardiac hypertension, 112
Diuretic, 255-257
  hypertension, 91
Dopamine, 7, beta-hydroxylase, 7
Drugs
  childhood risk factor for hypertension,
    89-91
  for hypertension treatment, 247-248

Echocardiography, 129, 219
Eclampsia, 91
Ehlers-Danlos syndrome, renal hypertension,
  141
Embryology, cardiac hypertension, 106-107
Emergency, hypertension, 253-255
Enalapril, 264
Endocrinopathy, cause of hypertension,
  159-184
  adrenal cortical condition, 159-161

adrenal hyperplasia, congenital, 170-171
aldosteronism, 161-164
Cushing's syndrome, 165-170
diabetes mellitus, 178
glucocorticoid disorder, 165-170
hyperparathyroid condition, 177-178
hyperthyroid condition, 177-178
mineralocorticoid disorder, 161-165
pheochromocytoma, 171-177
Endothelin, 27
Endothelium-derived factor, 27
Ethacrynic acid, 257
Exercise
childhood risk factor for hypertension, 85-87
hypertension therapy, 245-246
Exercise blood pressure, 47, treatment 245

Familial influences, on hypertension, 57-58
Fibromuscular dysplasia, renal hypertension,
143-145
Fish oil, 241
Flush technique
infant blood pressure measurement, 44-45
newborn blood pressure measurement, 44-45
Follow-up program, 266
Furosamide, 257

Genetics, and hypertension, 57-58
Glomerular disease, renal hypertension,
137-142
Glomerulonephritis
acute, renal hypertension, 137
chronic, renal hypertension, 138-139
Glucocorticoid disorder, hypertension, 165-170
Goldenhar's syndrome, renal hypertension,
141
Guanethidine, 260
Gull, William, blood pressure, 1

Hales, Stephen, blood pressure measurement, 1
Harvey, William, blood pressure, 1
Hemodynamic principles, 2-4
Hemolytic uremic syndrome, renal
hypertension, 139-140
Heredity, childhood risk factors for
hypertension, 77-79
History, hypertension, sample form, 223-230
Humoral factors, blood pressure control
mechanisms, 11-17, 20-27
Hydralazine, cardiac hypertension, 113
Hydrochlorothiazide, 256
Hydronephrosis, renal hypertension, 136-137
Hyperparathyroid condition, hypertension,
177-178

Hypertension. *See also* Blood pressure
age, 55
alcohol, 247-248
alpha-antagonist, 260-261
analgesic-anti-inflammatory, 91
angiotensin converting enzyme inhibitor,
263-265
antacid, 91
antiasthmatic, 91
antibiotic, 91
anticonvulsant, 91
antihistamine, 91
beta-adrenergic receptor blockers,
258-260
birth control, 91
blood pressure regulation, 1-35
calcium, 64-66
entry blocker, 261-263
supplementation, 244-245
cardiac, 105-125
childhood risk factors, 76-77
decongestant, 91
defined, 194
diagnosis, 236-237
dietary influences, 61-66
diuretic, 91
diuretics, 255-257
emergency, 253-255
evaluation, 214-215
exercise, 245-246
familial influences, 57-58
first drug, 251-253
follow-up program, 266
genetics, 57-58
history, 215-217, 223-230
sample form, 223-230
laboratory studies, 218-222
low fat-high fiber diet, 240-241
medication, 247-248
natural history chart, 56
newborn, 185-207
normal blood pressure values, 189-193
treatment, 201-203
nonpharmacologic treatment, 239-249
obesity, 60-61
pharmacologic treatment, 249-250
primary
adolescent, 211
child, 211
infant, 211
newborn, 211
toddler, 211
young adult, 211
young persons, 210

Hypertension (*Continued*)
  race, 58-60
  relaxation, 246-247
  renal, 127-158
  risk factors in child, 75-104
  secondary
    adolescent, 213-214
    child, 212-213
    infant, 212
    newborn, 212
    toddler, 212-213
    young persons, 212-214
  smoking, 248-249
  sodium, 61-63
  sodium restriction, 241-242
  tracking, 55-57
  treatment, 233-278
  vasodilator, 265-266
  vitamin A, 66
  vitamin C, 66
  vitamin supplement, 91
  weight control, 240
  workup, 237-239
  young person, 209-231
Hypertrophy, ventricular, childhood risk
    factors for hypertension, 94

Infant. *See also* Child, Newborn
  blood pressure measurement, 43-45
    flush technique, 44-45
    oscillometric method, 45
    ultrasound-Doppler, 44
  primary hypertension, 211
  secondary hypertension, 212
Infantile coarctation syndrome, 109-110
Infantile polycystic disease of kidney, renal
    hypertension, 140-141
Instrumentation, blood pressure
    measurement, 39-40

Juxtaglomerular apparatus, 5

"K" phase blood pressure measurement, 38
Kallikrein-Kinin system, 23-25
Kidney-blood volume, blood pressure control
    mechanisms, 17-19

Labetalol, 254
Left ventricular hypertrophy, childhood risk
    factors for hypertension, 94
Lisinopril, 264
Loop diuretics, 257
Low fat-high fiber diet, 240-241

Magnesium, childhood risk factors for
    hypertension, 85

Major factors affecting blood pressure,
    summary, 28
Maternal factors, childhood risk factors for
    hypertension, 91-93
Medication
  cardiac hypertension, 112-113
  childhood risk factors for hypertension,
    89-91
  first, 251-253
  hypertension, 247-248
  renal hypertension, 134-135
  for treatment of hypertension, 249-250
Medullary cystic disease, renal hypertension, 141
MEN syndrome, 174
Mercury manometer, blood pressure
    measurement, 1
Methyldopa, 92, 254
Metolazone, 257
Metoprolol, 251
Mineralocorticoid disorder, hypertension,
    161-165
Minoxidil, 265

Natriuretic hormones, 26-27
Natural history of hypertension, 56
Nephrectomy, 128
Nephrotic syndrome, renal hypertension, 138
Nervous system, blood pressure control
    mechanisms, 6-11
Neural mechanisms, cardiac hypertension,
    108-109
Neurofibromatosis, renal hypertension, 145
Neurologic disorder, newborn hypertension,
    198-199
Neurotransmitters, blood pressure, 7
Newborn, 185-207. *See also* Infant, Child
  blood pressure measurement, 43-45, 185-187
    flush technique, 44-45
    oscillometric method, 45
    ultrasound-Doppler, 44
  catheter-related, 197
  causes of, 189, 194-199
  diagnosis of hypertension, 199-201
  incidence, 195
  influencing factors, blood pressure in
    neonate, 187-188
  neurologic disorder, 198-199
  "normal" blood pressure values, 189-193
  ophthalmoscopy, 194-195
  parenchymal disorder, 197-198
  primary hypertension, 211
  renal artery stenosis, 197
  renal artery thrombosis, 195-197
  risk factors for hypertension, 91-93
  secondary hypertension, 212
  treatment, 201-203

Nifedipine, 251
Nitric oxide, blood pressure, 27
Nitroprusside, cardiac hypertension, 113
Nonpharmacologic treatment, hypertension,
  239-249, 254
Norepinephrine, blood pressure, 7

Obesity
  childhood risk factor for hypertension, 79-80
  hypertension, 60-61
Obstructive uropathy, 130
Ophthalmoscopy, newborn, hypertension,
  194-195
Optic fundal abnormalities, 217
Oscillometric devices, blood pressure
  measurement, 40
Oscillometric method
  infant blood pressure measurement, 45
  newborn blood pressure measurement, 45

Paradoxical hypertension, 116-117
Paraplegia, postcoarctation repair
  syndromes, 119
Parenchymal disorder, newborn,
  hypertension, 197-198
Pathophysiology, cardiac hypertension,
  107-109
Pharmacology. See Medication
Pheochromocytoma, hypertension, 171-177
Plasma-renin activity
  influences on, 16
  and race, 17
Plasma renin activity, and renal
  hypertension, 130-132
Postcoarctectomy repair syndromes, cardiac
  hypertension, 116-119
  paradoxical hypertension, 116-117
  paraplegia, 119
  postcoarctectomy syndrome, 118-119
  postoperative hypertension, 117-118
  persistent, 119-121
Potassium
  childhood risk factor for hypertension, 83-84
  hypertension, 63-64
  increase, 242-244
Prazosin, 260
Preeclampsia, 91
Pregnancy, 91
Prevalence, of hypertension, 54-55
Prevention, hypertension, 234-236
Primary hypertension, young persons, 210
Propranolol, cardiac hypertension, 113
Prostaglandin, 22-23
  cardiac hypertension, 113
Pseudocoarctation, 121-122
Pyelonephritis, renal hypertension, 133, 136

Race
  childhood risk factors for hypertension, 80-81
  hypertension, 58-60
  and plasma-renin activity, 17
Radionuclide imaging, 130
Recording of blood pressure measurement, 40-43
  child, 40-43
Reflux uropathy, renal hypertension, 136
Regional vascular factors, cardiac
  hypertension, 109
Regulation, blood pressure, 1-35
Relaxation, treatment, 246-247
Renal architecture, 4-5
Renal artery stenosis
  newborn, 197
  reconstruction, 150-152
Renal artery thrombosis, 195-197
Renal causes, newborn, hypertension, 195
Renal corpuscle, 4-5
Renal disorders causing hypertension, 128
Renal hypertension, 127-158
  adult-type polycystic kidney disease, 141
  Ask-Upmark kidney. See Segmental
    hypoplasia
  clinical features, 145-146
  cystic kidney disease, 140
  diagnosis, 146-148
  fibromuscular dysplasia, 143-145
  glomerular disease, 137-142
  glomerulonephritis
    acute, 137
    chronic, 138-139
  hemolytic uremic syndrome, 139-140
  hydronephrosis, 136-137
  infantile polycystic disease of kidney, 140-141
  laboratory investigation for, 128-129
  medications, 134-135
  medullary cystic disease, 141
  nephrotic syndrome, 138
  neurofibromatosis, 145
  pathophysiology, 145
  plasma renin activity, 130-132
  pyelonephritis, 133, 136
  reflux uropathy, 136
  renal artery stenosis, reconstruction,
    150-152
  renal disorders causing, 128
  renal imaging, 130
  renal trauma, 142
  renal tumor, 142
  renovascular hypertension, 142-154
  scarring, renal, 132-133
  segmental hypoplasia, 136
  treatment, 148-154
  trisomy syndrome, 141
  tuberous sclerosis, 141

Renal imaging, for renal hypertension, 130
Renal mechanisms, cardiac hypertension, 108
Renal trauma, renal hypertension, 142
Renal tumor, renal hypertension, 142
Renin-angiotensin system, 12-17, 20
Renovascular hypertension, 142-154
Reserpine, 261
Resting blood pressure, 46-47
Risk factors for hypertension, newborn, 91-93

Salt sensitivity, 82
Scarring, renal, hypertension, 132-133
Segmental hypoplasia, renal hypertension, 136
Smoking
    childhood risk factors for hypertension, 87-89
    hypertension, 248-249
Sodium
    childhood risk factors for hypertension, 82-83
    hypertension, 61-63
    restriction, hypertension, 241-242
Sports participation, 246
Spironolactone, 257
Strain-gauge plethysmography, blood
        pressure measurement, 40
Stress, childhood risk factors for
        hypertension, 85-87
Sudden death, 246
Surgical repair, cardiac hypertension, 115-116
Sympathetic nervous system, 6

Thiocyanate toxicity, 265
Toddler
    primary hypertension, 211
    secondary hypertension, 212-213

Tracking hypertension, 55-57
Trisomy syndrome, renal hypertension, 141
Tuberous sclerosis, renal hypertension, 141
Turner's syndrome, 217

Ultrasound-Doppler, renal, 130
    blood pressure measurement, 40
    infant blood pressure measurement, 44
Uric acid, childhood risk factors for
        hypertension, 93
Urinary tubule, 4-5

Vasodilator, 265-266
Vasopressin, 26
Ventricular hypertrophy, childhood risk
        factors for hypertension, 94
Verapamil, 263
Vitamin A, hypertension, 66
Vitamin C, hypertension, 66
Vitamin supplement
    childhood risk factors for hypertension, 91
    hypertension, 91

Weight control, hypertension, 240
Workup, hypertension, 237-239

Young adult, primary hypertension, 211
Young person/child
    evaluation, 214-215
    history, 215-217, 223-230
    laboratory studies, 218-222
    physical evaluation, 217-218
    treatment, 233-278